COMPUTERS IN NURSING

Bridges to the Future

COMPUTERS IN NURSING

Bridges to the Future

Linda Q. Thede, PhD, RN,C

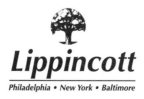

Lippincott

Philadelphia • New York • Baltimore

Acquisitions Editor: Lisa R. Marshall
Assistant Editor: Sandra Kasko
Project Editor: Gretchen Metzger
Senior Production Manager: Helen Ewan
Senior Production Coordinator: Nannette Winski

Assistant Art Director: Kathy Kelley-Luedtke
Indexer: Victoria Boyle
Compositor: Pine Tree Composition, Inc.
Printer: RR Donnelley Crawfordsville

9 8 7 6 5 4 3 2 1

Library of Congress Cataloging in Publications Data
Thede, Linda Q.
   Computers in nursing : bridges to the future / Linda Q. Thede.
      p.   cm.
   Includes bibliographical references and index.
   ISBN 0-7817-1557-1 (alk. paper)
   1. Nursing—Data processing.   I. Title.
   [DNLM: 1. Nursing.   2. Computers.   WY 26.5T375c 1999]
RT50.5.T48 1999
610.73′0285—dc21
DNLM/DLC
for Library of Congress   98-25817
                                                        CIP

Preface

Computers are changing all aspects of nursing. Today, computers are used in administration, research, education, and in clinical settings. For example, to access the latest in health care information, nurses are increasingly required to have the ability to search electronic databases, use the Internet, and to manage knowledge using a variety of software programs. Nurses must also become involved in the development of computerized health care information systems and classifications. These systems can then better fit their needs, and allow nurses a forum in which to clearly document what they add to health care. It is important that nurses embrace and use computers to the fullest, as this is the direction that health care, and indeed the world, has taken.

The focus on Unit One is to help nurses understand the basic characteristics of computers: hardware, software, and human input, which help nurses and other health care professionals manage information. Unit Two focuses on how computers enhance nurses' productivity. Word processing programs, spreadsheets, statistical packages, and presentation software are explored. Databases and special software are also examined as important aids to research and nursing education. Unit Three explores how the Internet greatly impacts the ability of nurses to retrieve and exchange information. The Internet provides ready access to the most recent research and information, and nurses must be familiar with these sources of information. Finally, Unit Four looks at computers as patient care tools and at how nurses must become involved in the development of information systems. The emerging field that combines nursing and computers is also explored.

Computers have many applications in health care, and as fifth generation computer systems are developed, they will assist nurses and others in ways yet to be known. Still, computers will continue to remain only a tool. Without human intervention, computers are ineffective. Computers are used in their highest capacity when individuals are able to understand and accept their possibilites as well as their limitations.

Computer usage ultlimately enhances patient care by allowing access to the latest research, quick communication between professionals, and the organization and presentation of this information. The ability to use computers is necessary in raising the professional image of nurses and for personal advancement in the field. When nurses gain confidence in the tools computers make available, they will begin to discover the infinite number of ways in which computers can be used to improve patient care and further the nurse's career. It is these discoveries that are the focus of this book.

Linda Q. Thede, PhD, RN,C

Acknowledgments

With the abundance of knowledge in today's society, one always needs experts to give the final word. This is especially true in writing a book. There are many people who patiently answered my many questions and encouraged me in this process. It would be impossible to mention everyone, but a few (given alphabetically) are in order. **Peg Allen**, who patiently waited for me to finish the database chapter so that she could build on it when writing the chapter about bibliographic resources, deserves my thanks. My neighbor, **Annie Clement**, an experienced author herself, gave me special encouragement and insights as to how to proceed. A close colleague, **Peggy Doheny**, worked with me to develop the database in Chapter 9 and to edit my information about NIC & NOC. **Vicky Elfrink** provided information about the Nightingale Tracker and patiently assisted me in writing about the Omaha system. **William Goossen** reviewed the information about the efforts being expended by the International Council of Nurses in creating the International Classification for Nursing Practice and filled in the missing pieces. **Mimi Hassett**, besides contributing a chapter, graciously reviewed the chapter about nursing informatics. **Judi Hornback** willingly and at short notice wrote the insert about a day in the life of a nursing informatics specialist. **Marion Johnson** reviewed and filled in pieces about NOC, and it is only appropriate to mention here **Joanne McCloskey** who did the same for NIC. **Karen Martin** willingly reviewed the section on the Omaha System. **Julie McAfooes** answered my questions about software directories. **Kathy Milholland** reviewed and offered corrections to the information about the Unified Nursing Language, and along with **Roy Simpson** assisted in developing the figure for Chapter 16. **Judy Ozbolt** was very helpful in my writing about the Patient Care Data Set and reviewed several versions.

The Quiggle family were my ultimate resource on many technical matters. **Adam Quiggle** reviewed and edited much of the information in chapter 12, always making certain that the information was technically correct as well as understandable. **Jim Quiggle** patiently answered questions as well as provided editing assistance on Java and other matters. **Susy Quiggle** waded through my first version of the chapter on hardware and made many helpful suggestions as to both content and wording. **Jeri Shaffer**, a colleague and neighbor, reviewed the very first draft of chapter one and made me very aware of "multiple guess pronouns," where you the reader are left to guess what they refer to. (I only hope that I learned that lesson.) **Jack Yensen** also lent encouragement and support including putting together a special web page, on how to discover your current IP address (http://www.langara.bc.ca/vnc/ipaddress.htm).

Credit also must be given to originators and maintainers of the PCWebopaedia website (http://www.pcwebopaedia.com/). I first found this site when working on information about hardware. I soon found that anytime I had a question remotely related to hardware or software, this site, not a search engine, was the first place to look. **Philip Margolis** of the Sandy Bay Software Company, which originated the site, was also responsive to my needs. The site is now owned by Mecklermedia.

Working with the Lippincott Williams & Wilkins staff has been a very positive experience. **Mary Ann Rizzolo**, who helped with the outline, has also encouraged me throughout this process. There would be no book without editor **Lisa Marshall**, who read my work and was gracious and encouraged my efforts; and who, along with **Sandy Kasko**, promptly answered the many questions I had as the work progressed. The efforts of **Julie Marusza** to tighten up the prose are also appreciated. I also want to voice my appreciation of my husband, **Dexter**, who never complained when I was preoccupied or when I constantly talked about how to approach various topics in the book.

To all those individuals and to others too numerous to mention, I can only say a heartfelt "Thank You!"

Contents

UNIT ONE

....

About Computers

IN the past few decades computers have become as much a part of modern life as the air we breathe. We use them in such things as cars, microwave ovens, and telephones without even being aware of it. When we use computers consciously however, as in health care, it is necessary to understand some of their basic characteristics for them to be effective. A computer system consists of hardware, software, and human input. In Chapter 1, the emphasis is on the need for computers in managing information. Some common misconceptions about computers are addressed. The focus of Chapter 2 is on the hardware that makes a computer. In Chapter 3, the various types of software are briefly introduced. With hardware, software, and human intelligence, computers help health care professionals and others manage information.

Computers: The Need to Manage Information

Objectives:

After studying this chapter you should be able to:

1 Describe the computer as an information tool

2 Gain an understanding of the history of computers

3 State some ways a computer helps manage information

4 Relate the development of the computer and hospital information systems to society's needs

5 Discuss some computer characteristics

6 Refute some common computer myths and anxieties

*L*ong ago, information that individuals needed was easily derived, understood, and passed on to successive generations through written and spoken word. The invention of the printing press in the 1450s started a slow transformation in the production of knowledge. Instead of one copy of a book on a subject, multiple copies could be produced in less time than it had taken to make one. Today, the printing press has given way to desktop publishing and Internet publications. The result is an explosion of information, the volume of which the world has never seen.

As the amount of information grew, the task of managing it manually became overwhelming. Although we tend to think of computers as a 20th century invention, they have a long history. In the 19th century, Charles Babbage designed a working computer that later served as the prototype for the first electronic computer. At the time however, society's perception was that the information available could be managed manually, and his computer was never built.

With the burst of information seen in the last quarter of the 20th century, the situation has changed. Managing the quantity of information in a useful way requires a tool: the computer. The computer is a device that assists people in finding and managing information and creating knowledge. But without human direction, interpretation, and manipulation, a computer is useless.

Learning the physical tasks associated with using a computer for managing information is only part of using a computer. Individuals need to become comfortable with the idea that although knowledge production is never ending, humans can organize information in ways that are more useful than ever before. Making this information available for health care practitioners and when caring for patients is one of today's challenges. In order to justify to a cost-conscious society that nursing is a highly professional skill and is crucial to quality health care, nurses need to be able to identify, define, and retrieve information about their practice from patient care settings. The ability to use a computer to attain these ends is a necessity.

▼ Computers in Health Care

The value of computers first became evident after World War II. In peacetime it did not take long for businesses to see the time savings and accuracy that resulted from using computers. The earliest computer health care applications were developed in the late 1950s and early 1960s. The focus of these programs was finance management but later moved into patient care (Saba, Johnson, & Simpson, 1994). By the late 1960s, some hospital information systems were starting to include patient diagnoses, other patient information, and care plans based on physician and nursing orders.

It was the amendment of the Social Security Act to include Medicare and Medicaid in 1965 that started the accelerated use of computers in health care. This legislation proved to be a boon to nursing information systems, because nurses were required to provide data to document the care that was delivered (U.S. Department of Health and Human Services, 1983). The push by the federal government for information continues to hasten the growth of computers in health care.

One of the interesting early uses of computers in patient care was the problem-oriented medical information system (PROMIS), begun in 1968 by Lawrence Weed at the University Medical Center in Burlington, Vermont (McNeill, 1979). This system was important because it was the first attempt to provide a total, integrated system. Based on Weed's problem oriented medical record (PROM), the system was implemented in 1971 on a gynecology unit at the University of Vermont hospital, then re-developed for use on a medical unit.

PROMIS provided a wide array of information to all professionals involved in health care, including the cost of procedures and laboratory tests. Documentation was focused on the problem list, in which individuals in all disciplines recorded their observations and plans, thus breaking down barriers between disciplines. The PROMIS system also made it possible to see the relationship between conditions, treatments, costs, and outcomes. This system did not have wide acceptance. To embrace it meant a change in the structure of health care, something that did not begin to happen until the advent of managed care in all its variations in the 1990s, which has reinvigorated a push toward patient-centered information systems.

Today, to meet many demands, the computer is continuing to gain importance in patient care. Just as institutions cannot survive without computerizing, no one who intends to progress in a career can succeed without integrating computers into practice.

▼Managing Information

Computers assist in many tasks involving information management. They help find information and move, rearrange, and store data; also, with appropriate instructions, they can create knowledge.

FIND INFORMATION

Computers allow people to find all kinds of information easily. When information is online, or in a computer, a simple search can provide what is needed in a fraction of the time it would take to do a manual search. Computers locate information by comparing user requests with available knowledge at high rates of speed. Computers have the ability to compare millions of pieces of information, often in seconds.

MOVE AND TRANSFORM INFORMATION

Computers can move information from one computerized source to another. They can also take information from external sources, such as a printed document, and place it in a word processing file or other application program through the use of an optical character reader (OCR), or scanner, as they are commonly known.

Computers also have the capability to use one piece of information in many different ways. For example, a name and address entered into a computer can be used for a mailing label or in the salutation of a letter. If there are many addresses in this data bank, the computer can be told to count all the people who live in a given city.

Looking at data in this manner is called "analyzing data in the aggregate." It is done by drawing comparisons among small pieces of information from many records. For instance, when all the people who live in a particular city are counted, the information that x number of people reside in that city is produced. Using data in the aggregate, patterns can be seen that are not visible when records are looked at individually.

COMPUTE INFORMATION

Computers are excellent at performing mathematical functions. To do this, they follow simple algebraic rules of formula calculation. For calculations that would take humans hours even with a calculator, a computer takes seconds. Spreadsheets, or the computer equivalent of accounting papers, now allow budgeting to be less of a mathematical chore and more of an analytical and conceptual function. Health care professionals and other individuals who prepare budgets or financial forecasts can try various combinations of items before determining the final document. Computers have also made statistical analysis substantially easier. By using computers, professors can now teach statistics classes that focus more on when to use each statistical test, instead of focusing on how to perform the calculations. Computers are excellent at performing any task that involves repeated actions that can be precisely stated.

How Do Computers Help Nurses?

Computers serve nurses in tasks such as word processing, locating resources, and creating budgets. They are also useful for more complex operations. Computers are needed to organize and generate information systems that aid in the collection, storage, process, retrieval, display, and communication of information. A well-designed computer-based information system provides the nurse with knowledge to enhance patient care. Planning, designing, and implementing systems to serve health care professionals requires input from those who use them.

 Some Computer Characteristics

Computers are not infallible. Being electronic, they are subject to electrical problems. Humans build computers, program them, and enter data into them. For these reasons, many situations can cause error and frustration. Two of the most common challenges with computers are "glitches" and the "garbage in, garbage out" principle (GIGO).

COMPUTER GLITCHES

Everyone has heard of a computer that "went down." Unless the user was purposefully engaged in a destructive act, the user did not create the problem. A flaw inadvertently created by the programmer was just found in the system.[1] There are times when glitches occur for seemingly no reason.

GIGO

One infallible principle to which computers adhere is the garbage in, garbage out (GIGO) principle. If inaccurate data are entered, the output will be erroneous. The output of a computer is neither better nor worse than the quality of information on which the output was computed. For instance, if a mistake was made in entering names and addresses into a computer, this error will show up whenever the data are used.

 Computer Myths

Some of the difficulties that many people face when they are starting to use computers are due to computer myths that have been created. A few of the most common

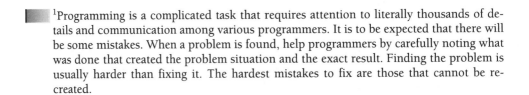

[1]Programming is a complicated task that requires attention to literally thousands of details and communication among various programmers. It is to be expected that there will be some mistakes. When a problem is found, help programmers by carefully noting what was done that created the problem situation and the exact result. Finding the problem is usually harder than fixing it. The hardest mistakes to fix are those that cannot be recreated.

misperceptions that have developed about computers include the following:

- ▼ Computers can think
- ▼ Only mathematical geniuses can use computers
- ▼ Computers make mistakes

Computers cannot think, and they are not smart. Incidents such as Deep Blue (the nickname given to an IBM computer specially designed to play chess) winning a game of chess against world chess champion Garry Kasparov lead to such misperceptions. Consider the game of chess. There are a given set of moves, rules, and goals that make it a perfect forum for displaying the potential of computers. Deep Blue is a very powerful computer, capable of analyzing hundreds of millions of possible moves each second. It made use of these qualities to beat Kasparov. It did not use thinking in the human sense.

The myth that only mathematical geniuses can use computers, although just as false, continues to flourish. This belief is linked to the development of the first computers as a means to merely "crunch numbers," or process mathematical equations. Hence, in colleges and universities, many computer departments are still housed in, or closely related to, math departments. It did not take experts long to translate the mathematical concepts into everyday language, an accomplishment that made the computer available to everyone, regardless of their proficiency in math. The last myth, that computers make mistakes, makes a wonderful excuse for human error. Computers do not make mistakes; they only do what they are told. A computer requires complete, definitive directions.

Tasks that have simple, clear-cut rules and goals provide the perfect conditions for computers to shine (Horgan, 1997). Computers do very poorly under circumstances that necessitate complicated or ambiguous data, rules, and goals. No computer has ever written a novel, and computers cannot even begin to replicate the human ability to process language or solve problems (Cohen, 1997). But when properly instructed, computers can and do manage prodigious amounts of information. It is unlikely that anything resembling human intelligence will be seen in computers in the next 50 years. This does not mean that computers cannot be very useful in decision making. It means that human beings will need to continue to mediate and analyze all computer input and output.

▼ Overcoming Computer Anxiety

The attitudes people have toward computers range from dislike and frustration to curiosity and excitement. Although media and acquaintances convey both aspects, people seem to remember the negative. As with all new experiences, becoming comfortable with a computer or a new application can produce anxiety (Display 1-1). The breadth of this problem in nursing can be seen by the variety of studies that explore computer anxiety and attitudes in nurses (Focus, 1995; McBride & Nagle, 1996; Jayasuriya & Caputi, 1996; Simpson & Kenrick, 1997).

▲●▼●▲●▼●▲●▼●▲●▼●▲●▼●▲●▼●▲●▼●▲●▼●▲●▼●▲●▼●▲●▼●▲●▼●▲●▼

Display 1-1 • OVERCOMING COMPUTER ANXIETY

"My great-great grandfather rode a horse, but was afraid of a train. My great-grandfather rode the train, but was afraid to drive a car. My grandfather drove a car, but was afraid to fly. My father flew in an airplane, but is afraid of computers. I use a computer, but am afraid to ride a horse. . . ."

What we fear is often what we are unfamiliar with, or something with which we have had a bad experience. It is not unusual to be unfamiliar with computers, and it is quite possible that some of us have had a less than pleasant encounter with a computer. Unpleasant experiences with computers are often related to a lack of meaningful help when trying to figure out how to accomplish a task. Not too long ago, documentation for software told the user about a function but neglected to say how to perform it. Fortunately, today's online documentation has progressed to a point where it is much more helpful.

Another thought that can impede a person in using a computer fully is a fear that one will break the computer. In truth it is very difficult to break a computer. Unless of course you dump a cup of coffee or other liquid on it, throw it out the window, or hit it with a baseball bat.[1] At times everyone has been tempted to do at least one of these things: Computers can be frustrating! Breaking the computer or erasing an entire system by means that do not involve physically attacking it, such as by pressing a key, is not something users can do accidentally in a well-designed system. In the rare instance that this should happen, it is NOT the user who has created the problem, it is the software (or hardware) producers who have failed to produce a robust system. Creating good software involves trying to anticipate all the various ways that a user could act when he or she misunderstands what is required, and providing "error traps" to assist the user in these instances. An error trap is a programming sequence that responds to erroneous keystrokes or actions with feedback about the difficulty and how to correct it.

Not knowing what to do when using a computer is where we all begin. This also occurs when we learn a new program or when we need to learn a new version of an existing program. We all stumble and make false starts as we learn new things. We were not born knowing how to walk, read, or write. Yet, today we can do all these things because we learned how. In the same way, anyone who wants to can learn to use a computer. Just as many false starts were made when learning to do any of the aforementioned tasks, when learning to use a computer, we will not always accomplish our objectives on the first or even the third try.

One source of frustration in using computers is their lack of ability to discriminate shades of gray. With a computer, an action performed either produces the desired result or it does not. This behavior, however, is no different from that of the other technologies with which you are familiar. If you are in an elevator and push the number five, the elevator will stop at the fifth floor whether you really wanted it to go to the fifth floor or not—even when you realize you have made a mistake and push six for the sixth floor. This exactness, however, produces a machine of great predictability, which is what makes the computer functional. A given command produces a given function.

When you think of learning to use a computer, think of trial and error. It is this process that produces the knowledge and competency that you are seeking. If you perform an action and what you expected to have happened does not, observe what *has* happened. Then try again. It may be necessary to use any of the help systems available to you before you gain your goal. Try to look at your situation as though you have made a discovery, not a mistake. This of course is not the model of learning with which most of us are familiar (Simpson, 1960). Prior experience has led us to fear "mistakes," and to regard them as a sign of failure.

Educational experience has often conditioned us to expect a teacher to impart the knowledge we need to function. In learning to use a computer, didactic information can give only a small part of the picture. As thinking human beings, we need to apply this infor-

(continued)

---

[1]There was one frustrated owner who, forgetting that the computer was inhuman, or maybe because of that, shot his computer "dead." He put four bullets into the hard drive and one into the monitor, whereupon he was taken to a mental hospital for observation. (Computer shot dead by frustrated owner [1997, July 12]. *Cleveland Plain Dealer*, 8A.)

●▼●▲●▼●▲●▼●▲●▼●▲●▼●▲●▼●▲●▼●▲●▼●▲●▼●▲●▼●▲●▼

Display 1-1 • OVERCOMING COMPUTER ANXIETY (Continued)

mation by actively experimenting, observing the results of our experimentation, and reflecting on this information.

Also, try to remember that as humans we cannot open our heads and have information or skills poured in. We have to work at learning. Senge (1994) tells us that real learning occurs only when we struggle with feeling incompetent and ignorant. We need to accept the fact that we will make many "discoveries" before we

feel comfortable. And we will feel frustrated at times. A good rule of thumb is to take a break when frustration threatens to disable you. Many problems are solved when an individual takes a break and lets the subconscious work. When your frustration level gets high, take a break and remember that you have learned to ride a bike and drive a car, both potentially far more dangerous to your health than usuing a computer. You can also learn to "drive" a computer.

▼Summary

Not only are we in the Information Age but we are also in the Computer Age. Just as the past 5 years have found nurses engaged in discussions about hospital finances, operating budgets, profitability, and accounting issues, it has also become imperative for nurses to be computer literate.

The computer is not smart or infallible, nor does it require that a user to be a mathematical genius. The sheer volume of information that has been and continues to be developed has created a society in which computers are vital to the management of knowledge. This factor has created a solid place for the computer in society, and is contributing to the acceleration of its development.

EXERCISES

1. When Jacquard invented the weaving machine in the 19th century, the workers, fearful of losing their jobs, rioted and broke the machine. How does this relate to today's climate?

2. Weed's PROMIS system was a radical departure from organizational thinking in health care. The current health care environment, however, is undergoing radical changes. Why, or why not, do you think the PROMIS system would be accepted today?

3. What evidence would you give that we are in the Computer Age?

4. What are some ways computers are being used to manage information by health care professionals in:
   a. Clinical practice?
   b. Administration?
   c. Education?
   d. Research?
   e. Entrepreneurial work?

REFERENCES

Brechner, I. (1983). *Getting into computers: A career guide to today's hottest new field.* New York: Ballantine Books.

Cohen, S. L. (1997, December 22) Man vs. machine. *Cleveland Plain Dealer,* p. B9.

Focus. (1995). The impact of computer anxiety and computer resistance on the use of computer technology by nurses. *Journal of Nursing Staff Development, 11*(3), 172–175.

Horgan, J. (1997, May 7, 1997) Future of mastering mastermind. *Cleveland Plain Dealer,* p. B13.

Jayasuriya, R., & Caputi, P. (1996). Computer attitude and computer anxiety in nursing: Validation of an instrument using an Australian sample—Nurses Computer Attitudes Inventory (NCATT) Computer Attitude Scale (CATT). *Computers in Nursing, 14*(6), 340–345.

McBride, S. H., & Nagle, L. M. (1996). Attitudes toward computers: A test of construct validity—Stronge and Brodt's Nurses' Attitudes Toward Computerization (NATC) questionnaire. *Computers in Nursing, 14*(3), 164–170.

McNeill, D. G. (1979). Developing the complete computer-based information system. *Journal of Nursing Administration 9*(11), 34–46.

Moye, W. T. (January, 1996). *ENIAC: The army-sponsored revolution.* Available: http://ftp.arl.mil/~mike/comphist/.

Saba, V. K., Johnson, J. E., & Simpson, R. L. (1994). *Computers in nursing management.* Washington, D.C.: ANA.

Senge, P. (1994). *The fifth discipline: The art and practice of the learning organization.* New York: Currency Doubleday.

Simpson, G., & Kenrick, M. (1997). Nurses' attitudes toward computerization in clinical practice in a British general hospital. *Computers in Nursing, 15*(1), 37–42.

Simpson, R. (1996). Creating a true learning organization. *Nursing Management, 27*(4), 19, 20.

U.S. Department of Health and Human Services. (1983). *1st national conference: Computer and technology and nursing.* (NIH Publication No. 83-2412) Washington, D.C.: U.S. Government Printing Office.

CHAPTER 2

Hardware:
The Machine Computer

Objectives:

After studying this chapter you should be able to:

1 Differentiate among uses for various types of computers

2 Explain different types of memory and storage in computers

3 Identify input and output devices for a computer

4 Define terms associated with a computer

A complete computer system is the integration of human input and information resources using hardware and software. It is easiest to discuss each of these aspects separately. In computer terms, hardware refers to objects such as disks, disk drives, monitors, keyboards, speakers, printers, mice, boards, chips, and the computer itself.

 Types of Computers

Computers come in many different sizes and shapes— from a simple microprocessor (chip that controls the device) to a supercomputer. Various types of computers have different characteristics. In some cases, the lines between different types of computers are getting murkier as technology progresses.

SUPERCOMPUTERS

Technically, supercomputers are the most powerful type of computer, if power is judged by numerical calculations. Supercomputers can follow hundreds of millions of instructions per second. They are used in applications that require extensive mathematical calculations, such as weather forecasting, fluid dynamic calculations, petroleum exploration, and nuclear energy research. Supercomputers are designed to execute only one task at a time; hence, they devote of all their resources to this one situation. This gives them the speed they need for their tasks.

MAINFRAMES AND MINICOMPUTERS

Mainframes are designed to serve many users concurrently and are also able to run a number of programs at the same time. These computers form the backbone of many hospital information systems. A few years ago, the "computers" found on clinical units were not really computers but video-text terminals. A video-text terminal consists of a display screen, keyboard, and modem, or a device that connects it to the mainframe. Information is entered on the keyboard and transmitted to the mainframe, which is located somewhere else, often in the basement in a secure, temperature-controlled room. Any processing done to the information is done by the mainframe, which returns the results to the screen of the video-text terminal.

Minicomputers were a phenomena of the 1960s, 1970s, and early 1980s. They were used like a mainframe in that they were multi-user machines which served video-text terminals, but they were smaller and less costly. Unlike the large mainframe, they did not require a special temperature controlled room, and were useful in situations with fewer users. Minicomputers were displaced by smaller and less costly mainframes and personal computers (PCs).

PERSONAL COMPUTERS

PCs are designed for the individual user and are relatively inexpensive. Unless the individual is part of an information processing department, this is the type of computer that the consumer is most likely to purchase. PCs are based on microprocessor technology, which enables manufacturers to put an entire processing unit on one chip, thus permitting the small size. These computers have many uses, including word processing, accounting, desktop publishing, graphics design, database management, and communicating on the Internet. When PCs were adopted, they freed users from the resource limitations of the mainframe computer and allowed data processing staff to concentrate on tasks that needed a large system. In businesses, personal computers are often connected (networked) to other personal computers or to larger machines. They still process information, but when they are put on a network, data can be shared between computers.

There are essentially two different types of personal computers: descendants of the IBM PC, now often known as "Windows™ computers"; and descendants of the Macintosh™. Although Windows computers are used in most business applications, the Macintosh computer continues to be the computer of choice for those who produce artwork or multimedia. Multimedia is an integration of text, graphics, video, animation, and sound in one program.

TRANSPORTABLE, LAPTOP, AND NOTEBOOK COMPUTERS

Once individuals became accustomed to the savings in time and effort that computers produced, they wanted machines that were more mobile. The first such type of machine was a transportable PC. These computers were subsequently replaced by the much smaller and more portable laptop, so called because it can fit on a lap. Notebook computers are even more compact. These machines are small enough to fit inside a briefcase and typically weigh less than 6 pounds.

Notebooks essentially have the same microprocessor, memory capacity, and disk drives as a desktop computer, giving them nearly the same amount of computing power. Putting all this in a small package is expensive. A notebook, therefore, usually costs more than a comparable PC. Like laptops, notebook computers have batteries that allow users to work for several hours without an outside power source. The life span of these batteries continues to increase with advances in technology.

The performance level of notebook computers is also improving and varies between vendors and models. The quality of the display screen is an important consideration if the computer is used for long periods of time. Keyboards also vary. Most laptop keyboards are compressed and do not have the numerical entry keyboard found on desktop machines. To overcome these drawbacks, yet still retain portability, some individuals purchase a monitor and keyboard to use with their notebook while at their more permanent location. When they are at home base, they use the external monitor and full-size keyboard, thereby giving them a system similar to a regular PC. When these users want to take the computer with them, they detach the keyboard and monitor, and use the display screen and keyboard that are part of the notebook.

Personal Digital Assistants

Personal digital assistants (PDAs) are small computers. They range in size from "palmtops," or those small enough to fit easily into one hand; to "handhelds," which are a little larger than a checkbook; to those the size of a small book. Although there are specialized uses for these devices (point-of-care documentation is one), they are most often employed as personal information managers (PIM). In this use, PDAs function as a kind of automated notebook. They enable users to enter, organize, and easily access various types of information, such as reminders, lists of names, addresses, and dates. They may also include scheduling and calculator programs.

Given the small size of PDAs, they usually do not contain disk drives, although some have attachments that allow the transfer of information with a full-size computer. PDAs may not have a keyboard. If there is no keyboard, data entry is done by selecting from a menu. In addition to basic database functions, some PDAs have cellular telephone/fax capabilities and networking features. There are even PDAs capable of voice recognition. These computers are often powered by regular batteries.

▼ Personal Computer Systems

Desktop, laptop, and notebook computers consist of three units. These parts include system components, a keyboard for entering data, and a display screen. These units make up a complete computer system, and they can be classified as system, input, and output devices. In a desktop computer, these three units are usually separate, whereas in a laptop and notebook, they are all one piece.

SYSTEM DEVICES

The system box houses components such as the central processing unit (CPU), disk drives, hard drives, connectors, and slots for special purpose cards. These devices are all mounted on a motherboard. A motherboard is the physical component in a computer through which all other devices communicate. It is a flat, rectangular board with slots for the cards that provide the connectivity for the system components. Another term for the motherboard is system board.

Central Processing Units

The CPU is the hardware heart or brains of the computer. The CPU controls the interpretation and execution of commands. It is sometimes referred to as the "processor" or "central processor." Without a CPU, a computer cannot function. Computers such as supercomputers or mainframes may have many CPUs. Personal computers, however, have a single CPU, which consists of a microprocessor. These chips, which are smaller and thinner than a baby's fingernail, may be referred to by manufacturer and number or manufacturer and name, for example, the Intel™ 486 or the Intel Pentium II. Differences in microprocessors may include power management modifications for battery-run computers, or the speed at which the chip accomplishes its tasks.

An additional capability, called MMX, has been added to many computers that have at least a Pentium Pro chip. MMX is a set of instructions built into the Pentium Pro processor that enables the computer to run multimedia programs without a separate sound and video card. To be compatible with the MMX chip, software must be specifically written to use these instructions. Each increase in the number of the chip from a manufacturer denotes a rise in computing power. The chips are generally "backwardly," but not "forwardly," compatible. That is, a computer with an Intel Pentium chip can run software designed for an Intel 386, but a 386 cannot run software designed for the Pentium. Higher chip numbers and more computing power will continue to be seen. Even before a chip is released, the next generation is on the drawing board.

The CPU consists of an arithmetic logic unit (ALU), a control unit, and some memory registers. The ALU performs all arithmetic and logical operations. The control unit directs the flow of information in the computer. It can be thought of as a combination between a switchboard and traffic officer, in that it gets instructions from memory, interprets them, sends them to the appropriate location, and makes certain that they are properly executed. The control unit performs these operations in nanoseconds (one billionth of a second); so, to a user, the results appear instantaneous.

The speed with which the computer processes instructions is determined not only by the number of the chip but also by the clock speed of the computer. The name for the measure of clock speed is megahertz (MHz). The clock speed determines how often a pulse of electricity "cycles" or circulates through the circuits, and thus, how fast information is processed. The more cycles per given time period, the greater the processing speed. Because the processing speed is also determined by the chip technology, a Pentium Pro chip that operates at 66 MHz will complete tasks much faster than a 486 chip that operates at 66 MHz. Processing speed is very important to those who calculate spreadsheets, do statistical calculations, work with complex graphics, or desire a fast response time for all activities.

The speed of processing is also affected by what is called "word size." This is not related to a word as known in reading but to the number of bits a computer processes at one time. When a CPU processes 16 bits of information at one time, it is said to be a 16-bit computer. Its word size is 16 bits. However, a computer that processes 32 bits of information at one time is a 32-bit computer and has a word size of 32 bits. The 32-bit computer is faster than the 16-bit machine.

▼ How a CPU Works With Data

A computer does all its work based on whether electronic circuits are on or off. In giving information to the computer, these conditions are represented by a one (1) if the circuit is on, and a zero (0) if it is off. Because only 1s and 0s are used, the data are said to be binary data. The familiar decimal system is a base 10 number system, whereas a binary system is a base 2 number system. Two other numbering systems in computers include octal, or base 8, and hexadecimal, which is base 16.

BITS AND BYTES

The amount of data that can be represented by one circuit is formally called a binary digit and is usually referred to as a bit. Bits hold only one of two values: 0 or 1. They are the smallest unit of information that a machine can hold. When eight of these bits are combined, there is enough memory, or on-off switches, to represent a letter, number, or other character. This amount of memory is called a byte.

ASCII

To make it possible for data to be exchanged between computers, standards were set for how the on and off switches in a byte would be used for each character. The standard for personal computers is the American Standard Code for Information Exchange (ASCII). Under this system, each character on the keyboard is represented by a number. The decimal equivalent of a capital "A" is 65. In the binary system, it would be represented by 01000001, or a byte in which the first bit is off, the second on, the third through seventh off, and the last switch on. Capital "B" is 66, whereas a lower case "b" is 98, each of which can be represented in binary data. All characters, including the space bar, arrow keys, and the return have a numerical value in ASCII. Large IBM mainframes use a somewhat similar code, called the Extended Binary Coded Decimal Interchange Code (EBDIC).

▼ Memory

The memory required to store even one document would be a large number if it was measured in bytes. To overcome this problem, memory is talked about by using prefixes in front of the word byte which denote increments of approximately 1000. A

TABLE 2-1 ● The Bytes	
Name	**Number of bytes**
Kilobyte	1024 bytes
Megabyte	1,048,576 bytes
Gigabyte	1,073,741,824 bytes
Terabyte	1,099,511,627,776 bytes
Petabyte	1,125,899,906,842,624 bytes
Exabyte	1,152,921,504,606,846,976 bytes
Zettabyte	1,000,000,000,000,000,000,000 bytes (approx.)
Yottabyte	1,000,000,000,000,000,000,000,000 bytes (approx.)

kilobyte is 1024 bytes, a megabyte is a little more than one million bytes, and a giga-byte approximately one billion bytes (Table 2-1). A kilobyte is abbreviated as "K" and a megabyte as "MB"—though it is often referred to as "meg."

If a computer is to process information, it needs to be able to store the data. To provide these services, there are several different types of memory. To prevent confusion, the term memory is used to denote operational memory, and the term storage is used when talking about the amount of data a given storage device will hold.

RANDOM ACCESS MEMORY

Random access memory (RAM) is the primary working memory of the computer. RAM is temporary memory. Once a program is opened, such as a word processor, the user is actually working from a copy of the program in RAM. Any documents created with the application are also stored in RAM. When after saving the information, the document is closed, it is erased from this memory. Information contained in RAM is also erased when power to the computer is lost, either when the computer is turned off or from a power outage. Anything not saved to a more permanent form of storage is lost.

RAM comes in many varieties—dynamic RAM, known as DRAM (pronounced D Ram), and SRAM, or static RAM (pronounced S Ram). Although SRAM is much faster, it is also more expensive and larger in size. To meet the need for speed without the overhead required by SRAM, newer forms of DRAM have been developed. The current form of DRAM in use is SDRAM (Synchronous DRAM). It too, however, will be replaced, probably by either RDRAM or SLDRAM. Anything contained in any form of RAM is lost when the computer is turned off. However, work is underway to develop a form of RAM supported by a battery that will not lose its contents when the computer is turned off.

The measurement unit used to describe RAM is megabytes but expect to see it ex-pressed in gigabytes in the not too distant future. As the functions that software per-forms increase in number and quality, the amount of RAM needed keeps creeping upward. In 1997, 16 megabytes of RAM was believed to be adequate, but computers with 32, 64, and even 128 megabytes are becoming the new standards. The more RAM a computer has, the more functionality, and often speed, it will have. Lack of RAM is one of the causes of computer "crashes."

Another condition that increases the amount of RAM needed is that users are no longer satisfied to have just one application open at a time. Users may want to move data from their spreadsheet to their word processor or database, or capture information from the Internet and use it in a presentation. Additionally, those working with graphics files or multimedia need a large amount of RAM because such files are very large.

Generally, the amount of RAM a computer requires depends on the use to which it will be put. For many people, once they purchase a computer, they discover more uses for it than they had originally considered. Although RAM can be added at a later date, the entire memory may have to be replaced to upgrade the system.[1]

READ ONLY MEMORY—BASIC INPUT OUTPUT SYSTEM

Read only memory (ROM) is a permanent form of storage and is used to store the programs needed when the computer is started. ROM is where all those words on the screen originate when the computer is first turned on. The computer can read information saved in ROM but cannot write to it or add anything. Personal computers have only a few thousand bytes of ROM. This form of memory is contained on a chip and is programmed by the computer manufacturer. ROM is also used in calculators and laser printers.

The BIOS, which is an acronym for Basic Input Output System, is usually placed on the ROM chip. The BIOS is built-in software that determines what the computer can do without accessing any additional software. The last instruction the BIOS executes is to look for an operating system and install it. On personal computers, the BIOS contains all the programming necessary to control the keyboard, display screen, disk drives, serial communications, and a number of miscellaneous functions.

CACHE

In reading a computer advertisement, the word cache (pronounced "cash") may be seen with the amount given in kilobytes (K). Cache is a special memory mechanism that allows the CPU very rapid access to information. There are two types of memory "caching": RAM or disk.

RAM cache is a portion of memory that stores data or instructions the computer has determined that the user will use repeatedly. The term disk caching is misleading, because data is not stored on a disk as we think of one but in a place in RAM known as a "disk cache" that has been set aside for this purpose.

Getting information from RAM is thousands of times faster than accessing information from a disk. Cache, therefore, serves the purpose of decreasing response time to provide a better response. Some microprocessors have a built in memory cache.

---

[1]For example, if you order a computer with 32 megabytes of RAM that is upgradable to 128 megabytes (meaning that there are eight memory chip slots available, each capable of holding a 16-megabyte chip), the manufacturer may insert eight 4-megabyte chips instead of two 16-megabyte chips. Thus, some of the original memory chips, which are still perfectly good, may be discarded to make room for the upgrade.

This type of cache is called L1, or level one, cache. When additional cache memory is added, it is called L2, or level two, cache.

MASS STORAGE DEVICES

Owing to the volatile nature of RAM and the inability of users to add anything to ROM, permanent forms of data storage are needed. The main types of mass storage are magnetic and optical disks, although tape drives are still used in some instances. Optical disks often only allow a user to retrieve or read data, although read and write optical disks are becoming more widely available. Magnetic disks offer the user the ability to save and retrieve data. The types of disks used with a desktop computer are diskettes, Zip™ or Jaz™ diskettes, and hard or fixed disks. The amount of storage they provide varies.

Magnetic Disks

Lower storage capacity magnetic diskettes are made of a sheet of plastic, whereas larger capacity disks often have a glass or aluminum core. No matter what core is used, the base is covered with a thin coating of a magnetizable substance. A device called a "read/write" head, which is part of the disk drive, transfers information to the disk by magnetizing or not magnetizing a *bit* (a very small section) on the disk. When information is retrieved, or "read," the read/write head transforms these magnetized bits into the information that was originally saved. Because magnetizable material is used, the disk can be remagnetized (rewritten) to store different information (Fig. 2-1).

Before being used, a magnetic disk needs to be formatted. Formatting puts the magnetic covering of the disk into a pattern so the type of operating system with which it will be used can send or retrieve information from it. Formatting also tests the disk to be sure that all areas on it are in working order. If it finds any areas that

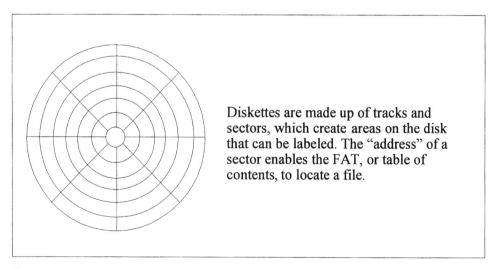

Diskettes are made up of tracks and sectors, which create areas on the disk that can be labeled. The "address" of a sector enables the FAT, or table of contents, to locate a file.

Figure 2-1 • A diskette.

Display 2-1 • CARING FOR A DISKETTE

To preserve data on diskettes, keep them 12 to 18 inches from

1. Magnets (the storage is based on whether a spot is magnetized or not, consequently any magnet can destroy the
   memory).
2. Electric motors, including a ringing telephone; they have a
   magnetic field.
3. Televisions; they too give off magnetism.

Care for diskettes by

1. Keeping them dry.
2. Refraining from sliding the protective metal piece covering the
   read-write surface back and forth. The surface underneath can
   be scratched.

---

are unreliable, it makes them inaccessible. This process then creates what is called a FAT, or file allocation table. The FAT is the portion of the disk that contains the table of contents or the area used to record where on the disk the beginning of a file is stored. Diskettes are one form of "permanent" storage. But this storage is not always permanent, because a user can chose to delete information from a diskette.

The 3.5-inch (or 5.25-inch) slot on the front or side of a computer is called a disk drive. A disk drive is the slot into which a diskette is inserted. The computer can then be directed to save or retrieve information from the diskette. (See Display 2-1 for information on caring for diskettes.)

Diskettes are a portable form of storage in that they can be used in more than one computer. The computers, however, must be of the same type. If the disk was written to by a Macintosh, it cannot be read by a PC.[2]

The most common diskette in desktop personal computers is the 3.5-inch type. Diskettes in use today will store about 1.4 megabytes of data. In practical terms, one such diskette will store around 300 pages of single spaced text. Adding tables or graphics reduces this number. If the text is broken up into several files, this number is also reduced because each file requires a given amount of disk space.

Many people who work with graphics files have found that the files they create have become too big to transport using a 3.5-inch diskette. To meet this need, drives that read and write larger diskettes have been developed. One, the SuperDisk™, can store 120 megabytes. The advantage to this disk is that the drives that support it are also capable of reading and writing to regular 3.5 diskettes. The drives that support the other two types, Zip and Jaz diskettes, however, can only read and write to their respective disks. A Zip disk will store 100 megabytes of data. The new Jaz drive, which is capable of writing to a disk that will store two gigabytes of data, will read and write to the original Jaz diskettes, which only stored one gigabyte.

---

[2]Some Macintoshes are capable of reading information from PC disk.

Hard Disks

A hard, or fixed, disk found inside the computer, is the main form of storage for users. A hard disk consists of several nonflexible disks that are housed along with the read/write head in a hermetically sealed device. Hard disks come in varying memory sizes, sizes that are today measured in gigabytes. Besides the large storage capacity of a hard disk, retrieving data is considerably faster than trying to get the same data from a 3½-inch diskette.

Optical Diskettes

Data is recorded on optical diskettes by using a laser to burn microscopic holes onto the surface. To read them, another laser beam is shone on the disk. The holes are then detected by changes in the reflection pattern. When a reflection is detected, the bit is on; when there is no reflection, the bit is off. Optical diskettes have a very large storage capacity, but the access time is generally longer than with a hard diskette. The ones most commonly available are read only type. Optical diskettes are not affected by magnets, but they can be damaged by scratches.

CD-ROM

There are several types of optical diskettes, but the ones in use most frequently with personal computers are CD-ROMs. Because most software sold today is on a CD-ROM, a CD-ROM drive is considered standard equipment. A single CD will store 630 megabytes of information, which is equivalent to about 700 1.4-megabyte, 3.5-inch diskettes. CD-ROM drives vary in how fast data can be accessed. The speed is expressed as a number followed by an "x." A single-speed CD drive takes 600 milliseconds (or 6 tenths of a second) to access 150K of memory, while a 16x speed drive will access 2.4 megabytes in one to two tenths of a second.

In computers, CD-ROM is being replaced by what is called DVD-ROM (digital versatile disk or digital video disk). Although it is presently a read only disk, it can store a minimum of 4.7 gigabytes of information, which is enough for a full-length movie. This new format also has the potential to hold 17 gigabytes, with access rates from 600 kilobits per second to 1.3 megabits per second. One of its best features is that CD-ROM disks can be used with a DVD-ROM drive.

A Bus

A computer bus is a mode of transportation for data. Physically, it is a collection of wires that transmit data from one part of a computer to another, such as from the CPU to the main memory. Buses are referred to by the number of bits of data that can be transferred at the same time, which is also called the width of the bus. For example, a 16-bit bus will move 16 bits (2 bytes) of data at one time, and a 32-bit bus will move 32 bits of data. In addition to this bus, many PCs include a local high-speed bus that is connected directly to the CPU for data that requires very fast transfer speeds, such as video data. Depending on the configuration of a computer, there may be more than one bus. The current standard for buses is the peripheral component interconnect (PCI).

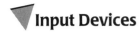Input Devices

There are many ways that data can be entered into a computer, and some may be more familiar to you than others.

KEYBOARD

Probably the most familiar data entry tool for a computer is the keyboard (see Appendix A). A computer keyboard has different keys depending on the type of machine used. Although they are similar to typewriter keyboards, computer keyboards have more keys.

The keys and layout on a keyboard vary with the type of computer being used. In specially designed applications, in which the keyboard serves only one purpose, the function keys (top row of keyboard, labeled with an F plus a number on PCs) have a label that designates exactly what they do. Keyboards for the PC vary, from the screen-based keyboard found on a handheld computer, to the 104-key keyboard (and there are some with even more keys) that was introduced with Windows 95. Keyboards shaped in a widespread V are also available for PCs. These keyboards were designed to be more ergonomically suited to the normal position of the hands.

Macintosh keyboards are called ADB keyboards, because they connect to the Apple Desktop Bus (ADB). There are two main types of Macintosh keyboards—the standard keyboard and the extended keyboard. The extended keyboard has 15 additional keys that correspond to the F keys on a PC keyboard.

MICE

A regular computer mouse is a device with a moveable ball in the bottom. As the user rolls the mouse over a flat surface, the ball rotates, moving the screen pointer in the direction the mouse is moved. The screen pointer can be positioned over a selection, at which time the user quickly depresses and releases the mouse button, a procedure called "clicking the mouse." When holding the mouse button down instead of releasing it, a selected object can be dragged to another location. Mice contain from one to three buttons, the number and type depending on the computer type and mouse manufacturer. Macintosh mice have only one button, whereas PC mice can have two or more buttons.

Instead of a separate mouse, some keyboards, particularly those on laptops, have built-in mice. These come in several varieties. One is a trackball, which is a ball moved with fingers that directs the screen pointer. Another alternative is a flat box built into the keyboard that is approximately 2 by 3 inches. To move the screen pointer, a finger is moved over the box. Laptop computers may also have what is called an "eraser" or "mouse button." This is a small projection in the keyboard that looks like the top of a pencil eraser. Like the external mouse, these devices all have buttons that are pushed to indicate a choice.

JOYSTICKS

Another input device is a joystick, but this device is used primarily for computer games. A joystick is composed of a stick (or lever) that protrudes vertically from a box. The stick is moved in the direction that the user wishes the screen pointer to move. Once the lever is in a given position, the screen pointer will continue moving in that direction until the lever is moved to the 90-degree vertical position. Joysticks may also contain buttons called "triggers."

SCREEN "TOUCH" METHODS

In an effort to make data entry easier, some systems are set up to allow the user to make selections from a menu through some method of touching the screen. The two most common are a touch screen and a light pen. A touch screen has a touch-sensitive transparent panel covering the screen. Instead of moving a mouse pointer to a selection and clicking the mouse, users touch the screen in the desired location.

The light pen is another device that allows the user to enter data by communicating with the screen. The user moves a pen with a light-sensitive detector to the desired choice and selects it by clicking the pen.

SCANNERS

A scanner is a device that translates information on paper into a computer image. The quality of the transformation is measured by resolution. Resolution refers to how many dots per inch (DPI), or in the case of a scanner, points of light per inch, are used to create an image. Scanners come in different sizes and shapes. The least expensive are handheld scanners, which are useful for small pictures or photos but are difficult to use with an entire page. Flatbed scanners consist of a large piece of glass on which the paper containing the image to be converted to a computer image is placed.

When they are scanned, all images are represented as one graphical object. For this reason, text that has been scanned cannot be edited directly. If a user wishes to edit the text, it is necessary to have a special program that will translate the image to text. Called optical character recognition (OCR) programs, today most scanners come with these packages. OCRs do very well with most machine-produced text, but the ability to decipher handwriting is still in the developmental stage.

Bar codes are another form of scanning. A bar code is a printed pattern of wide and narrow bars that represent numerical codes. The bars conform to the universal product code (UPC), which is the standard code for products. When a special type of scanner is passed over the bar code, it transforms into a number that is entered into the computer. The computer can then match the number with the appropriate item. For instance, if a nurse removes a catheter tray from a hospital supply cart and passes the bar code on it over a scanner, the results can be sent to the supply department, allowing that department to have a running total of how many catheter trays are left on the unit. The supply department can use this information to know when to restock the equipment cart. If the nurse also adds information about the patient for whom the catheter tray is intended, the appropriate amount can be charged to the patient's account.

DIGITAL CAMERAS

Digital cameras are devices that record images digitally on a disk instead of on film. The picture can then be transferred to a computer, where it may be placed in a file or a database for easy retrieval. It can also be viewed on a computer monitor or printed. The quality of the photo depends on the quality of the camera, monitor, and printer.

Digital cameras are finding a wide variety of uses in health care. One outpatient wound center uses them to photograph the wounds at each visit (Brooks & Bryant, 1998). The photos are filed in a computer database, then retrieved for comparison at each subsequent visit. This enables the patient and health care professionals to see the progress that has been made and to have evidence of the results from various types of treatment. The photos can also be transmitted to referring physicians as documentation of the patient's progress.

VOICE

Voice recognition is the ability of a computer to recognize spoken words. It does not mean that the computer understands what is said, only that it can translate the spoken word into a text word. There are two types of voice recognition: discrete and continuous speech processing (Voice recognition, 1997). The most common and least expensive form of voice recognition is discrete speech processing. When using a discrete speech processing system, the user utters one word at a time, pausing briefly after each word. In continuous speech processing, the user can speak at a normal rate. Continuous speech processing systems are less tolerant of background noise than discrete systems.

Many systems still require the speaker to train the computer to understand his or her language. The training consists of repeating the words the user wants the computer to understand until the word is recognized. Some systems today are capable of acknowledging many variations of a spoken word without this special training. The claim is made that for most people, they will be 95% accurate. Several companies have introduced systems that have a large built-in vocabulary focused on a specific field, such as radiology (Voice recognition, 1996). Voice recognition is finding many uses in the health care system, from recording medical histories to nursing documentation.

▼ Output Devices

In computers, output refers to anything that comes out of a computer. An output device is any machine capable of representing information derived from a computer. This includes plotters, monitors, and printers. A plotter is simply a mechanism that draws pictures on paper as directed by a computer. Plotters are used most often in computer-aided design (CAD).

MONITORS

A monitor is the box that contains the display screen for a computer. Monitors come in many varieties with different properties that reflect the quality of the display. Some of these characteristics are screen size, resolution, dot pitch, refresh rate, and whether the screen is interlaced. Of the other factors used in judging a monitor, screen size is the easiest to understand. Measured diagonally, many users prefer large screens with high resolution. Resolution refers to the number of pixels, or dots of light, that make up the basic picture element of any screen. Computer screens are made up of thousands (in very high resolution, millions) of dots arranged in a series of rows and columns. As the number of dots per line increases, so does the clarity of letters and other objects. Dot pitch refers to how much vertical distance there is between each pixel. The smaller the dot pitch, the sharper the image. If, however, the distance is too small, the screen brightness and contrast will be lessened.

The monitor interfaces with the computer through a video adapter, or a board that plugs into the motherboard inside the computer. The display capabilities of the computer depend not only on the monitor but also on this video adapter. The display on some monitors can be improved with a higher quality video card, but there is a limit to this. The ability of the monitor and the video board must be coordinated.

There are two types of monitors—a cathode ray tube (CRT) and liquid crystal display (LCD), each of which displays an image a little differently. Generally, CRTs are found with desktop computers, and LCDs with laptops and other smaller computers.

Images on CRT screens are produced by an electron beam that moves across each row of pixels. The beam begins at the upper left corner of the screen and moves over the first row of pixels, lighting only those pixels needed for the image. The beam then moves to the beginning of the next row, lighting those needed in the second row, and continues until the entire screen has been scanned, at which time the process is repeated. The number of times per second each row is scanned by the beam is known as the refresh rate. If this rate is too low, the screen will flicker. Although the refresh rate at which a screen appears to flicker is often an individual perception, generally if the refresh rate is below 70 to 75 hertz (Hz), most people will complain.

Another term usually heard when talking about monitors is "noninterlaced." Interlacing is a technique in which only half the horizontal lines are refreshed with each pass, thus enabling twice as many lines to be displayed per refresh cycle. Interlacing actually produces higher resolution, but it slows down the speed with which the computer shows images and, as a result, may produce screen flicker. Most monitors are noninterlaced.

On an LCD screen, instead of being constantly refreshed, all of the pixels are continuously lighted by backlighting, which produces a gray screen. An image is displayed on an LCD screen when the appropriate pixels are turned off, which is just the opposite of a CRT. Besides resolution, the terms encountered when buying a computer with an LCD screen are passive or active matrix display. In a passive matrix display, the light to the pixels is blocked to turn it on. In an active matrix display, a transistor controls each pixel, a technique that permits a higher quality image. A passive matrix display is less expensive.

PRINTERS

There are many different types of printers; the ones that are most commonly used today are dot matrix, ink-jet, and laser printers. Dot matrix printers produce characters by striking pins against an ink ribbon, which prints closely spaced dots in the appropriate form. Dot matrix printers are relatively fast and inexpensive to use, but their output is low quality. These printers are relatively noisy and can easily become jammed if the paper feed is not perfectly aligned with the tractor feed device.

Ink-jet printers work by spraying ionized ink on a sheet of paper in the desired shapes. An ink-jet printer produces a page almost equal to the quality of a laser printed-page. The initial cost of an ink-jet printer is considerably less than a laser printer, but they require a special type of ink that can smudge on inexpensive copier paper. Because of their small size, ink jets are popular as portable printers.

Laser printers use the same technology as a photocopy machine. A laser beam produces an image on the drum, which is rolled through a reservoir of toner. The toner is then transferred to the paper through a combination of heat and pressure. Laser printers produce the highest quality printing. Because of the way a page is prepared for printing, laser printers require RAM. They come with a certain amount, but if graphics are printed, additional RAM may be needed.

Color printers are generally either ink-jet or laser printers. Color printing is much slower than regular printing. Most color printers are based on what is called the CMYK model, that is, they print in four colors: cyan, magenta, yellow, and black. Different combinations of these are used to produce a specific color. A lower priced printer may print only cyan, magenta and yellow, but this printer cannot print true black, and the colors it prints tend to be somewhat faded.

▼ Input and Output Devices

Some devices, such as synthesizers, ports, and modems, defy categorization as either input or output devices because they are used both to enter and output information. Synthesizers allow both the input and output of sound to a computer. The most common usage of synthesizers is for music or voice data. A music synthesizer records music in a digitized format, whereas a voice synthesizer records voice.

A "port" is a socket to which can be attached specially designed plugs that connect a device to a computer. Ports can be serial, parallel, or the new universal serial bus (USB).

Serial ports are referred to as RS-232C ports. They transmit data one bit at a time, whereas a parallel port transmits 8 bits at a time. For this reason, parallel ports are faster. Printers can be connected to either port but are usually connected to a parallel port. Zip and Jaz drives are connected to a parallel port, whereas mice and modems (devices that allow computer data to be sent over a telephone line) are connected to a serial port.

A cable attached to the port is used to make the external connection. They are specific to the type of port, that is, serial or parallel. Most connectors used to attach these cables have been designed so they will fit only the port for which they are designed, thus leading to worry-free connections. The USB (universal serial bus) will eventually replace serial and parallel ports. Not only does it transmit data at very fast

●▼●▲●▼●▲●▼●▲●▼●▲●▼●▲●▼●▲●▼●▲●

Display 2-2 • ANALOG-DIGITAL

Analog and *digital* are terms that describe types of information. Analog information is continuous, whereas digital information is discrete numbers (see Fig. 2-2). A glass oral thermometer is analog; it registers anywhere on the thermometer that the mercury stops. However, an electronic thermometer is digital; it gives you readings in exact numbers. Anything in between is rounded either up or down.

speeds (12 million bits per second), but devices of all kinds can be connected to this port. It makes it possible to add and remove devices without the hassle of different types of cards—all while the computer is running (called hot plugging).

The word modem is actually a shortened version of the term modem-demodulator. A modem is a device that permits a computer to communicate with other computers via a telephone line. The modem converts the digital output of a computer to an analog signal that can be sent on telephone wire. For incoming data, the modem converts the analog signal to a digital signal that the computer understands (Display 2-2, Fig. 2-2). One of the most important quality indicators for modems is the speed of data transfer, which is measured in bits per second. Typical telephone modems operate at a speed of 28.8 or 33.3 kilobits per second, although 56.6 kilobits per second telephone modems are now available, as are other types of faster modems.

▼Computerese

There are many computer-related terms that are often used in discussion, instruction, and advertising. Although they are not strictly hardware terms, they can often be confusing.

If one watches a computer when it has just been turned on, one will see different types of information flashing across the screen. This information is produced by what

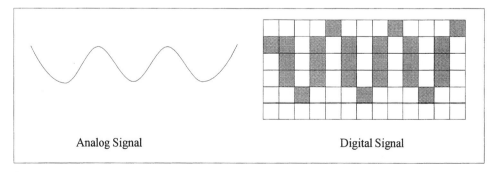

Analog Signal   Digital Signal

Figure 2-2 • Analog and digital signals.

is called the "booting" process. Booting refers to all of the self-tests that a computer performs and the process of retrieving from the disk the software necessary for work to begin.

The term reboot means to restart the computer.[3] Turning off the computer as a means to reboot should be avoided when possible. The jolt of electricity received each time a device is turned on may shorten its life span. Rebooting the computer without turning it off is known as a "warm boot." This procedure is often used to return the computer to its initial state, which erases information in RAM and eliminates memory conflicts that may be causing problems. These conflicts are often caused by different programs trying to store data in the same location. If a warm boot fails to notify the programs that it is time to stop fighting and give the user back the computer, the machine must be turned off for a "cold boot."

A "bug" is a defect in either the program or hardware that causes a malfunction. It may be as simple as presenting the user with a weight chart when blood pressure was requested, or something that causes the entire system to crash.

Compatibility refers to whether programs designed for one chip will work with an older or newer chip, or whether files created with one version of a program will work with another version of the same program. When discussing computer chips earlier, it was mentioned that most chips are backwardly compatible. Software, too, is usually backwardly compatible. This means the files created with older versions of a program can be edited with newer versions. Software producers generally try to keep their products backwardly compatible, so files created with an older version will not be lost when a user upgrades.

A "driver" is a software program that allows data to be transmitted between the computer and a device that is connected to the computer. Drivers are generally specific to the brand and model of the device, whether it be a printer, disk drive, mouse, or keyboard.

"Hacker" originally meant someone who was a very technically sophisticated computer enthusiast. Today, the term refers to an individual who illegally gains access to others' computer systems and steals data or creates problems by corrupting data. True hackers are individuals who are challenged by solving the problem of breaking into a system. When they succeed, rather than corrupt or steal data, they notify the system administrator and provide information needed to prevent further breeches of security. The correct term for those who maliciously hack is cracker.

The terms logical and physical often refer to where data in the computer are located. The physical structure is the actual location, whereas a logical structure is where users access the data and how it is presented to us. For example, when a user requests information about a laboratory test, he or she may see the indications for the test, the normal values, the cost of the test, and if asked, a patient's test results. Although this information may be presented as one screen, which would be its logical structure, different pieces have been retrieved from different files in different locations, which is the physical structure of the information.

---

[3]In some instances, it may mean to restart a program.

A "peripheral" is any external device attached to a computer. Printers, scanners, digital cameras, and Jaz drives are peripherals. Setting up peripherals can be a frustrating job. Not only must the correct driver be present, but often jumpers and switches need to be adjusted. To overcome these difficulties, efforts are now being made to make all peripherals "plug and play." Theoretically, a plug and play device will be operable once it is attached (plugged) to the computer.

▼ Summary

As technology increases, it is getting difficult to classify computers. Computer sizes vary from supercomputers, which are intended to process large amounts of data for one user at a time; to mainframes, which serve many users simultaneously; to PCs; laptops; and notebooks. Each of these types of computers have their niche in health care.

EXERCISES

1. Look at a manual for using a software product, and determine how you would perform any commands that use a combination of keys, such as Alt-Shift-F9. (Hint—when the Alt, Shift, or Control keys are used in combination, use them exactly as you would if they were alone, that is, hold down both of them and tap the last key.) See the Appendix.

2. Compare three or more computer advertisements and decide which offers the most value for the least money.

3. What are some ways the information in this chapter can be used by health care professionals in
   a. Clinical practice?
   b. Administration?
   c. Education?
   d. Research?
   e. Entrepreneurial work?

REFERENCES

Brooks, T., & Bryant, J. (1998). Personal communication.
Voice recognition takes off. (1996). *Health Care Informatics, 13*(11), 18.
Voice recognition. (1997). Automatic Identification Manufacturers International, Inc. Available: http://www.aimi.org/voice.htm.

CHAPTER 3

Software:
What Makes the Computer Work

A fter hardware, software is the second part of the computer connection, the third being human interaction. Computer software comes in many varieties, but all allow the use of a computer for a specific purpose. Without software, a computer is like a camera without film. When purchasing a computer, software is too often the forgotten item. It is not unusual for an individual to pay $2000 or more for the latest model computer but neglect to budget anything for software. Salespeople are very good at saying the computer comes with word processing, a spreadsheet, and a database. Most today do. The abilities of such software, however, is usually very limited.

 Types of Software

Although there are many kinds of software (also known as "applications"), there are two overall types—systems software and application programs (Fig. 3-1). Systems software includes those programs and utilities that reside in ROM that enable the computer and the operating system to start, and those that control the computer. Application software includes those programs used to do work, such as creating a document. There are many different types of application programs, but they generally can be classified into one of five groups: word processing, spreadsheets, database management, presentation software, and programs that enable computer-to-computer communication. Many of these categories can be subdivided further.

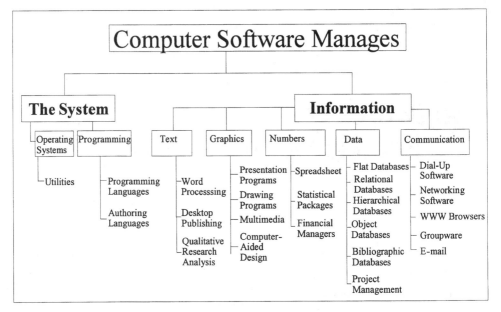

Figure 3-1 • Programming languages are not true system software, but are used to create applications.

There are various brands of each of the above-mentioned types of software, all of which will do the basic job for which they are intended. Some excel in one feature, others in another. There are differences in how a specific package organizes the various tasks within applications.

▼ Operating Systems

The most important program on the computer is the operating system. It is the operating system that coordinates input from the keyboard with output on the screen, responds to mouse clicks, heeds commands to save a file, and transmits commands to printers and other peripheral devices. The operating system is the platform on top of which other application programs run. Application programs are written to work with a specific operating system. Thus, the operating system a user selects determines which applications can be run. On PCs of recent vintage, a user is most apt to find a version of Windows, although computers from the 1980s may still use DOS. The Macintosh uses a different operating system, as do larger computers.

DOS

DOS is the acronym for disk operating system. Although it can refer to any operating system, it is generally associated with the type of personal computer introduced by IBM in the 1980s. Developed by Microsoft™ and originally termed just DOS, it is now referred to as MS-DOS (Microsoft Disk Operating System). Using DOS required users to remember a set of commands such as delete, run, copy, and rename. Unlike

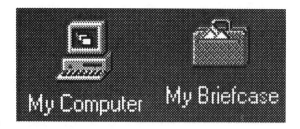

Figure 3-2 • Icons.

today's operating systems, DOS allowed only one program at a time to be operational. Moving information between programs was difficult and time consuming, as was using anything that was not text.

GRAPHICAL USER INTERFACES

Modern operating systems use what is called a graphical user interface, which is usually referred to as a GUI.[1] A GUI uses computer graphics to facilitate using the computer. Whereas DOS users had to memorize commands, a GUI user can often just "point and click." Pointing and clicking refers to moving the mouse so the pointer on the screen is on the desired object and quickly tapping the left mouse button. Graphical user interfaces include the various versions of Microsoft Windows, the Apple Macintosh™ system, and OS/2™.

No matter which brand of GUI one uses, they have much in common. They all have pointers, icons (small pictures), a working area called a desktop, menus, and boxes called windows, that can be active or inactive.

A pointer is a symbol, usually an arrow, whose movements correspond to a pointing device, usually a mouse. Icons are small pictures that represent such things as application programs, files, windows, or commands (Fig. 3-2). When the mouse pointer is over them, clicking the mouse causes an action to occur. On PCs, the action is dependent on whether the left or right mouse button is clicked and if the user clicks once or twice.

Because of the ease of use of GUIs, many health care information systems are moving to a GUI environment, usually a version of Microsoft Windows. For this reason, as well as the computer literacy demanded of today's health care professional, it is appropriate to review some of the basics of using Windows.

Opening and Exiting Windows

On most computers, when the computer is booted, Windows starts automatically. Exiting Windows, however is another matter. In the DOS days when one was through using the computer, it could simply be turned off. But Windows objects to this type of treatment. Although it is invisible to users, Windows actually works

---

[1]Interface is how one device communicates with another, or with a human. A human computer interface is the actions a user employs to make the computer do his or her bidding.

● ▼ ● ▲ ● ▼ ● ▲ ● ▼ ● ▲ ● ▼ ● ▲ ● ▼ ● ▲ ● ▼ ● ▲ ●

Display 3-1 • EXITING WINDOWS

To close Windows properly, close the application programs you are using, then access the Start (ridiculous, isn't it?) menu by clicking on start. The bottom-most entry on the menu will be "Shut down." When you click on it, a dialog box appears (see Fig. 3-3). If you are on a single-user computer, or shutting down a network computer for the day, click on the circle followed by "Shut down the computer." If you are on a network and others will be using the computer, click on the circle followed by "Close all programs and log on as a different user." If you are using an information system computer, instead of shutting down, you will probably log out. Be sure you understand how to do this correctly. Failing to log out can leave your account open for anyone to use, including those bent on mischief.

very hard behind the scenes to provide its many functions, as do many of the application programs. To do this, these programs have to remember a great number of things. Often this is accomplished by creating what are called files, that is, the programs place information they need to remember on the hard disk. These files are temporary and unknown to the users. They are created, changed, and deleted as users change what they are doing. Before quitting Windows, the application programs need to be able to shut these files down. If users do not exit all programs and close Windows properly, these temporary files are left on the disk (Display 3-1, Fig. 3-3).

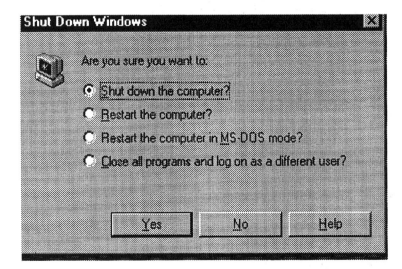

Figure 3-3 • Shut Down dialog box in Windows.

Starting a Program

As with all things in Windows, there are at least two different ways to open a program—from an icon or from the start menu. If the screen display is the desktop and the program the user wishes to start is represented by an icon, place the mouse pointer over the icon and click with the left mouse button. Or, if another program is open, click on start, then on programs. This last click causes a list of the programs to appear. Click on the name of the program to be started. Some of the programs, particularly those that are together in a suite (such as Corel™ Office, Lotus Smart Suite™, or Microsoft Office™) may be on a secondary menu under the name of the suite.[2] Names that lead to other menus are indicated on the programs menu by a black triangular mark pointing to the right.

When many of the combination suites are installed, a group of icons appear in a corner of the screen. Any program in that suite can be started by clicking on the appropriate icon. Like many icons, if the mouse pointer is left over one of these icons for a few seconds, the name of the program they launch will appear.

Windows and More Windows

If using a PC, the term Windows may refer to the operating system or to the various content boxes that appear on the screen. Each program that is open creates its own window. If a word processor and spreadsheet program are open simultaneously, two program windows are open. In a word processor, a user also may have more than one document open (Fig. 3-4).[3] These document windows are windows within the word processor program. If desired, the user may choose to see more than one document window at the same time (Fig. 3-5). Additionally, the user may add a window from another program to the screen display so that he or she can see parts of all the windows on which they are working. One of the hardest things for those just starting to use GUIs to grasp is that it is not only possible to have many different windows open at one time but that using this option is an aid to productivity.

To close a window, click on the appropriate icon. There are closing icons for the whole program and for all documents within the program window. If a user wishes to close a document within a program but leave the program open, he or she would click on the closing icon for the document. The shape and position of the icon to close a window depends on the GUI used.

Sometimes when a program is open, the window for that application does not fill the entire screen. If a user wants the window to fill the entire screen, he or she must click on the "maximize" icon. Like the closing icon, the location and shape of this icon varies with the operating system. Clicking again on the icon in the same position also reduces it to the size it originally was. If clicking on the minimize or maximize button does not produce a window of the desired size, a user can further resize it by passing the mouse pointer over the borders of the window until it becomes a double

---

[2]A suite is the name used to refer to a group of products designed to work together. Suites generally consist of a word processor, a spreadsheet, a database, a presentation program, a scheduler, and other utilities.

[3]Note, most word processors can have many more than two documents open at one time.

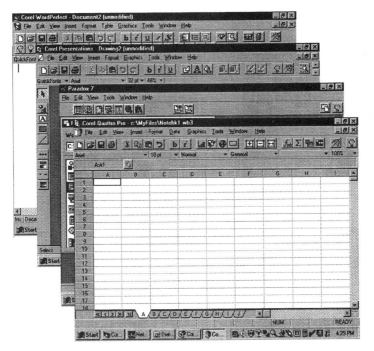

Windows stacked on the desktop. "Clicking" on any part of any window will bring it to the front and make it the active window.

Figure 3-4 • Stacked windows.

edged arrow. Then depress the left mouse button and drag the window border in either direction until it is the desired size. Windows can also be moved anywhere on the screen. To move a window, place the mouse pointer over the title bar, which is the top line of the window, then depress the left mouse button, and drag the window to the chosen location.

It is also possible to switch easily between windows within a program. Although how this is accomplished varies with the version of the program, this can always be done by clicking on the word "window" on the menu line and selecting from a list of the documents that are open. Some versions provide icons that represent the various windows open within an application program from which a selection can be made.

Switching between application programs is also fairly straightforward. In some GUIs, an icon representing all open windows is on the bottom of the screen. To move to another application, click on the appropriate icon. In other GUIs, there are key presses that can be used. In Windows 3.11, for example, tapping Alt-Tab rotates through all the open windows with each tap of the tab key. When the name of the desired program is on the screen, release the Alt key.

To reduce a window to an icon or just a name on the task bar, minimize it. Again, the GUIs vary in how this is accomplished, but all provide an icon for this purpose. When a window is minimized, it is easily reactivated. It is not necessary to minimize

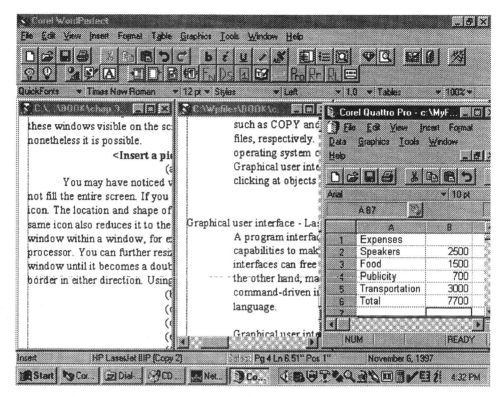

The window with the darker title bar is the active window. "Clicking" on any other window will make it the active window.

Figure 3-5 • View of some open windows.

a window before moving to another. Once a new window is selected, the GUI automatically minimizes the window in which the user is working.

Most documents, whether text in a word processor, or data in a spreadsheet or a database, are too large to be seen in their entirety on the display screen. To allow the user to scroll to other parts of a document, Windows provides "scroll boxes." A vertical scroll bar is on the right side of the screen, and a horizontal scroll bar is at the bottom. To use the scroll bar, place the mouse pointer on the box within the bar, depress the left mouse button, and drag it in the desired direction. It is also possible to scroll in more controlled increments by clicking on the arrowhead at either end of the scroll bars. The vertical scroll box serves another function. It allows the user to judge how far down a document they are by its placement on the scroll bar. If it is halfway down the bar, the user is at the middle portion of the document.

In many cases, the keyboard can also be used to scroll. The up and down arrow keys move one line up or down, and the left and right arrow keys move one character to the left or right in a text program, or one column in a spreadsheet or database.

Dialog Boxes

Windows application products and Windows itself make use of what are called dialog boxes. A dialog box is a window that pops up when the program wants more information. Dialog boxes appear in response to a request made when the user clicks on a menu item that has three dots after it. To respond, type in the requested information and either tap the enter key or click on the appropriate box. Error messages appear in boxes that pop up, which are called message boxes. After reading the message, the user may need to click "ok" before they can be closed.

Other Windows Conventions

"Pop up" or "drop down" menus are also a staple of Windows. Words on the menu line, or the second line on the screen, all produce a menu when they are clicked. When an entry is followed by a gray square with a black triangle in it, clicking on that square will produce another drop down menu (Fig. 3-6).

These conventions are often used in health care information systems that are GUI based to save the user from typing data. For instance, in an ICU, when a nurse clicks on the black triangle under "tubes," a drop down list may appear of all possible tubes that might be used. Similarly, clicking on another black triangle for drainage may produce a list of possible entries. What is on these lists is determined by nurses who work in these areas. Good information systems result from a partnership between the nurses who work in an area and those who are involved with designing and implementing the system.

ACCESSORIES

Operating systems usually come with some built-in software, some of which may be useful for small tasks. Paint™, a simple drawing program that creates a type of graphic file called a bitmap, is one of these types of software. A user can create drawings or various shapes, such as a circle, square, or triangle in any of the available col-

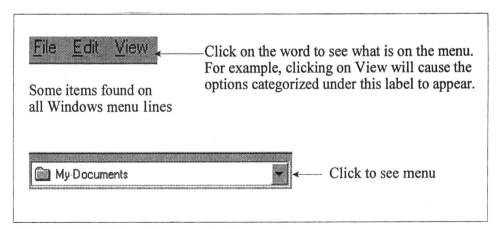

Figure 3-6 • Drop down menus.

ors. Notepad™ is a product that is useful in creating files in a format that can be read by most programs, and WordPad™ is a program designed for memos.

▼ Application Programs

Besides programming languages, there are five overall types of application programs. With the exception of communication packages, several vendors offer versions of each of these as one package. These suites may or may not include a database manager, depending on the version of the suite purchased. Buying the application programs as one package is not only less expensive but ensures that the products will work well together. In suites, the lines between programs are often blurred. A table in a word processor, for example, can easily become part of any of the other programs, and vice versa. Graphs or charts can be created with many of the different application programs, and visuals can be inserted into all of them. All are tools for information management. It is not unusual to use bits and pieces of several different programs to complete a project.

WORD PROCESSORS AND DESKTOP PUBLISHERS

A computer word processing program is a quantum step up from electric typewriters. Word processors simplify creating, editing, and formatting documents. They also are capable of many functions that allow the user to construct attractive and effective documents. One of the advantages of word processing is that when a mistake is made or editing is necessary, changes can be made without retyping the entire document.

Although some would say that desktop publishing software is a separate category of software, it is closely related to word processing. Desktop publishing software simplifies all the tasks involved in designing professional-looking pages for printing. Before GUIs, only desktop publishing programs offered the ability to insert pictures into a page of text and see the results. For high-quality page designing, desktop publishing still offers more control over the appearance of a page than a word processing package. They are, however, losing popularity as word processors become more powerful and flexible.

SPREADSHEETS

Perhaps the next most popular type of program is a spreadsheet. A spreadsheet is a program that facilitates manipulating numbers. The screen in a spreadsheet resembles a ledger with rows and columns, creating a series of boxes or "cells." The user enters values in a cell as in a paper ledger. The user creates relationships between the cells by writing formulas that specify what should be done with the contents of each cell, such as adding one cell to another. As with word processing, the user can change anything in the spreadsheet. If the contents of the changed cell are mentioned in a formula, the formula recalculates, putting a new result based on the current values in the cell. Spreadsheets are also very good at creating graphical displays of values.

PRESENTATION PROGRAMS

A presentation program is software designed to allow users to create visuals, such as a "drawing" or a graph, for use when giving a presentation. Presentation programs facilitate designing a series of visuals. They provide templates, or layouts, for different types of visuals, such as a title page, bulleted points, and even an organizational chart. Using these programs, one can create transparencies, printed material, or 35-mm slides.

DATABASE MANAGERS

Database application programs are designed to facilitate the management of information. Databases permit manipulations that are so large, they could never be done manually. An example of a simple database is a telephone book. With a database application, items in a telephone book could be sorted by phone number or address. Some types of information, because of their unique requirements, need specialized database management systems. Project management is one of these systems. Software designed to monitor ongoing projects is called project management software.

COMPUTER-TO-COMPUTER COMMUNICATION PROGRAMS

As soon as computers could store information in memory, the desire to share this information between computers arose. It was, however, the development of a standard method of computer communication and inexpensive modems that made this interaction available to the general public.

Email
Email, or electronic mail, was one of the first ways that computers communicated. Email can consist of data of all sorts, such as letters, numbers, or even pictures. When an individual sends email to someone, unlike regular mail, a copy of the message is sent, and the sending computer retains the original. The data that are sent can be entered from the keyboard, from information stored in memory, or from a storage device.

Networking
The PC was originally intended as a stand-alone computer. As more and more tasks fell to computers, the need to share data more easily than by diskettes became obvious. To meet this need, multiple computers in one location were linked together. This required a physical wire connection, or wireless transmission, and software to manage the linking. In a network, a user on Computer A can access the same files as an individual using Computer B. There are several different ways of networking and several vendors who supply the software.

Groupware
Groupware is software that permits a group discussion. This category was introduced in 1989 when Lotus introduced Lotus Notes™, an outgrowth of an earlier product used on the mainframe (Woolley, 1996). The current term refers to software that

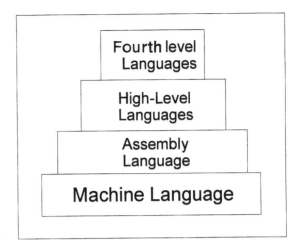

Figure 3-7 • Language levels.

promotes not only group discussion but an array of activities such as scheduling and document sharing. There is a wide variety in the features that vendors provide in groupware. Some are suites of ready-made applications, whereas others are toolboxes for creating collaborative applications with customizable templates included. These products have found use in business and education.

Programming Languages

There are different computer languages and levels of languages (Fig. 3-7). Levels represent the degree to which the language approaches natural language. The higher the level, the closer to regular language. Machine language is the lowest level of language. Machine language is a translation of higher levels of code to the zeros and ones required by the computer. Table 3-1 shows some decimal, binary, and hexadecimal representations of numbers. There would be great difficulty in programming if each letter in each statement had to be represented by a binary number. To avoid this problem, higher level languages and programs to convert them to machine language were created.

The next level of programming is called assembly language. In assembly language, the programmer uses cryptic names instead of numbers. In the example in Table 3-2, the programmer's aim is to move the contents of one storage box to another area.

TABLE 3-1 ● *Binary Hex Table*		
Decimal	**Binary**	**Hexadecimal**
Base 10	Base 2	Base 16
1	1	01
2	10	02
3	11	03
4	100	04

TABLE 3-2 ● *Assembly Language*
MOV AX,0006h
MOV BX,AX
MOV AX,4C00h
INT 21H

MOV translates to Move. The other code designates the location to which the box should be moved. Programs written in assembly language run fast. The code is compact, and it is easier to write than machine language.

Both machine and assembly language programs must be written for a specific type of computer. To ease the chore of programming and to make it possible for programmers to write programs that were somewhat independent of a particular computer, higher, or third-level languages were developed.

The further from machine language, the closer the programming language is to natural language. The trade-off is that higher level languages are very specialized and not multipurpose. An example of a next-generation, or fourth-generation, language is the Structured Query Language (SQL). SQL was designed to be a standard interface for querying relational databases and was intended to make designing queries as close as possible to natural language (Collen, 1994).

There are two terms often mentioned when programming is discussed: algorithm and infinite loops. An algorithm is a specific set of steps, or rules, that if followed, will yield a specific result. The flow chart in Figure 3-8 is an algorithm. To be useful, the steps must be very detailed and inclusive.

Looping is a programming procedure in which the computer repeats a given set of instructions until a stated condition has been met. The computer, for instance, may be instructed to keep asking the user to enter names until the user types in the word quit. If the programmer forgets to set a condition in which the program will stop looping, the computer goes into an infinite loop. It will never stop asking the user to enter names. The only recourse is to use an emergency exit to stop the program, or to turn off the computer.

PROGRAMMING

All application programs are created by a process known as programming. Programming is the providing of step-by-step instructions that tell the computer what to do. More specifically, programming means defining the problem, developing a flow chart of instructions to create the desired functionality, writing the code, and testing and debugging the code (the process of finding errors and correcting them).

As a health care professional, a nurse may be called on to assist in defining a problem or testing an end result. Defining a problem with enough accuracy and detail so the computer can be used to solve it is a difficult task. Perhaps a nurse wants a computer to flag any vital signs that require nursing attention. Before this task can be done, the nurse needs to determine what are normal limits. This may sound easy until the nurse remembers that in some cases, an elevated temperature of 2° F may

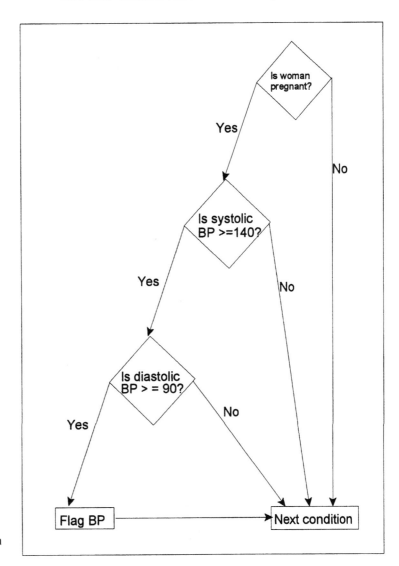

Figure 3-8 • An algorithm in a flow chart.

not be of any concern. In the same vein, the nurse must also define what are normal pulse and respiration rates and blood pressures. To do this, the nurse has to come up with a set of rules stating what readings need flagging under which conditions, using "If/Then/Else" statements.

An If/Then/Else statement is one that tells the computer what to do if a certain condition exists. With this information, the programmer can create a set of conditions that determine when to flag a given reading. In the scenario given in the previous paragraph, one rule the nurse might have written is that when the blood pressure is taken from a pregnant woman, if the systolic pressure is greater than 140 and the

```
REM IF BP = 1 then do not flag the blood pressure
REM IF BP = 2 then flag the blood pressure


BP = 1
IF A$ = "pregnant" THEN
     IF SysBP > = 140 THEN
          IF DiastBP >=90 THEN
               BP = 2
          ENDIF
     ENDIF
ENDIF
```

Figure 3-9 • Some programming statements.

diastolic pressure is greater than 90, the reading should be flagged. A flow chart showing the decisions the program will need to make is seen in Figure 3-8.

When code is written, the computer follows it linearly, unless directed otherwise. The computer completes the actions prescribed in line 1, then proceeds to line 2, and so on. An example of one way to write an if/then code is seen in Figure 3-9.[4] The programmer used A$[5] to represent the client, and decided that if the blood pressure needed to be flagged, a variable named BP would have a value of 2, otherwise it would have a value of 1. In the first statement, the program uses information it received earlier about whether the client is pregnant. If the client is not pregnant, the program skips the rest of the steps, gives the variable BP a value of 1, and goes to the next evaluation condition. If the client is pregnant, the computer first evaluates the systolic blood pressure (SysBP) to determine whether it exceeds or is equal to 140. If neither of these conditions are met, the variable BP keeps the value of 1, and the program goes to the next condition. If the systolic blood pressure is greater than or equal to 140, the program then evaluates the diastolic blood pressure (DiastBP). If this is below 90, the variable BP keeps the value of 1, and the program goes to the next condition. But, if the diastolic blood pressure is 90 or more, both conditions have been met, and the variable BP is given a value of 2 before the program moves onto the next condition. The computer will store a value for BP in its memory. When the program reaches the lines of code that tell the computer whether it should flag the blood pressure, if it finds that the variable BP = 1, it will not flag the blood pressure. If the variable BP = 2, it will flag the blood pressure, probably by giving it a different color.

[4]These code lines are written in a version of the Basic language. Other languages would have different words, but the concepts would be the same. That is, if the correct combination of conditions were met, the variable would be given a value of 2, and the blood pressure would be flagged.

[5]When variables represent anything but numbers, they are often designated with the use of a $ and referred to as strings.

When evaluating the output of a computer, it is important to understand that this output is dependent on both the lines of code and the values given. In the preceding example, the user would want to know the computer flags the blood pressure for a pregnant woman only when the systolic is above 140 and the diastolic is above 90. When the user knows what the rules are that the computer follows, it is easier to evaluate the output. Because it is highly unlikely that every condition can be programmed, it is imperative that computer users do not rely solely on computer output for determining anomalies. There is no substitute for critical thinking by a perceptive health care professional.

What sounds like a simple assignment, therefore, is in reality a very involved task. Because it is extremely easy to omit an important detail, extensive testing of any code is necessary. When code for an information system is tested, those involved create a "play hospital," in which they create many different patient scenarios to determine how the system will handle them. Not only do the testers, some of whom are nurses, invent "regular" patients, they also create patients whose conditions create unusual situations. It is inevitable that testers will find problem areas, or bugs. Even after the system is installed, problems may be found. A health care information system is a living phenomenon that needs continual maintenance.

USER GROUPS

When learning to use a program, sources of help can be extremely useful. Whether seeking help from a book, a teacher, or an acquaintance, there are times when everyone needs a question answered. One excellent source of help is a user group. A user group is a gathering of people who meet regularly for the purpose of sharing information. There are user groups for application programs and information systems. User group members range from novices to those who make a living as a consultant for the program. The degree of formal organization varies with the size and purpose of the group. Most user group meetings have an agenda in which a member or invited guest discusses some topic of interest, followed by a question-and-answer session.

There are few areas today in the United States that do not have a computer user group of some type for application programs. In large cities, there may be one umbrella group with smaller significant interest groups (SIGs) that meet independently to learn more about a specific program. For more information about user groups and how to find a group, see the web site for the Association of Personal Computer User Groups at http://www.apcug.org/, or call a local computer store. Computer stores usually have information on the groups in the area. In fact, they may even be the site for meetings.

Like commercial application programs, there are user groups for health information systems. There are two types of information system user groups—internal and external (Simpson, 1990). An internal group consists of users of a system within a given institution, whereas an external group has members from health care institutions all over the country (or even the world). Like other software user groups, they share experiences both positive and negative. If a nurse is not a member of a user group for the information system in his or her institution, the nurse is overlooking an opportunity to be a powerful advocate for nursing.

▼ Copyright of Programs

When buying software, many vendors believe that the user is not buying it but that they are rather buying a license to use it. In this thinking, breaking the shrinkwrap means the user agrees to the conditions of the license. These licenses generally state that the software cannot be sold or given away without the permission of the vendor. Depending on the vendor, a user may be told they can install the software on only one computer, or in some cases, on more than one computer if only one copy will be used at a time.

Given the ease of installing software, many people are not aware that not following the license agreement is called software piracy. A decade or more ago, most software was "copy protected." Under this scheme, the vendors placed algorithms on the disk that made it difficult to reproduce the program. With the advent of hard disks on which users installed programs, this approach became impractical. Some people mistakenly believe when the copy protection is removed from programs, so is the copyright. Today vendors rely somewhat on users' honesty to preserve their right to be reimbursed for their efforts.

The Business Software Alliance estimates that the software industry loses billions of dollars each year due to software piracy (Business Software, Undated). According to the alliance, piracy is defined as the illegal distribution or copying of software for personal or organizational use. This group makes a concerted worldwide effort to find and prosecute those involved in this act. Since their founding in 1988, the Business Software Alliance has filed more than 600 lawsuits against suspected software copyright infringers.

The Software Copyright Protection Bill, which Congress passed in 1992, raised software piracy from a misdemeanor to a felony (Nicoll, 1994). Penalties of up to $100,000 for statutory damages and fines of up to $250,000 can be levied for this crime, plus those responsible can be sentenced to a jail term of up to 5 years. Software vendors are very serious about copyright violations. Like all organizations, health care and educational organizations are not immune from prosecution. One western university paid $130,000 to the Software Publishers Association when it was found to have illegal software in a lab. A hospital in Illinois was fined about $161,000 when they were found engaging in unauthorized software duplication (Chicago Hospital, 1997). Organizations without an enforced software oversight policy are possible candidates for investigation.

Some software is distributed as shareware. Software of this type is often found on the Internet. The publishers of shareware encourage users to give copies to friends and colleagues to try out. They request that anyone who uses the program after a trial period pay them a fee. Registration information is included in the program. Continuing to use shareware without paying the registration fee is considered software piracy.

Freeware is an application the programmer has decided to make freely available to anyone who wishes to use it. Although it may be used without paying a fee, the author usually maintains the copyright, which means a user cannot do anything with it other than what the author intended. There are some freeware programs available on the Internet. When a user accepts software through any channel but a reputable reseller, they should be certain they know whether the software is proprietary, shareware, or freeware. Software that is in the public domain can be used any way the user desires; changes may be made to it.

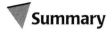

Summary

There are many different types of software that are useful in managing information. Yet, it can be said that there are two overall types of software: systems and application programs. Systems software consists of utilities and operating systems. Application software can be roughly classified as word processors, spreadsheets, database managers, presentation packages, and computer-to-computer communication. There are different vendors for application programs, each of which approaches the task of implementing functions a little differently. Several vendors offer office suites, which consist of a word processor, spreadsheet, presentation package and databases—all designed to work well together.

Programming languages can be classified as machine language, assembly, high-level, or fourth-generation languages. Machine language consists solely of zeros and ones, whereas assembly language, which is one level higher, uses some wordlike characters in its code. Fourth-generation languages come the closest to natural language. Ultimately, no matter which level language or which language a program is written in, it must be translated to machine language in a process called compiling.

Most of the software used is proprietary and is copyrighted. Using a copy of a proprietary program for which a user does not hold a license is software piracy. Shareware is software that can be tried for free, but a registration fee should be paid if it is regularly used. Only freeware can be used without cost.

EXERCISES

1. If you have access to a computer with a GUI, experiment with the various options, such as opening more than one window, resizing, moving, tiling, cascading, and closing windows.

2. Write down as many rules as you can think of that define when deviations either above or below the normal temperature of 98.6° F (37° C) are a cause for action by a nurse.

3. Create an algorithm by writing a series of steps for making muffins. Include mundane but necessary steps, such as lining the baking cups, finding the recipe or mix, preheating the oven, breaking an egg, disposing of the shell, and so on. Use a flow chart.

4. A friend gives you a CD-ROM with a program on it and tells you to install the program on your computer. What things should you consider before doing so?

5. You wish to install a program that you have at home on your computer at work. What things need to be considered?

REFERENCES

Business Software Alliance (Undated). *Anti-Piracy Information.* Available: http://www.bsa.org/ piracy/piracy.html.
Chicago Hospital Caught Pirating. (1997, January). *Healthcare Informatics,* 20.

Collen, M. (1994). The origins of informatics. *Journal of the American Medical Informatics Association, 1*(2), 91–107.

Nicoll, L. H. (1994). Modern day pirates: Software users and abusers. *Journal of Nursing Administration, 24*(1), 18–20.

Simpson, R. (1990). What are user groups and how can they help you wield more power? *Nursing Management, 21*(10), 24, 28.

Woolley, D. R. (1996). *Choosing Web Conferencing Software.* Available: http://freenet.msp.mn.us/people/drwool/wcchoice.html. Retrieved March 12, 1998.

UNIT TWO

Computers as Productivity Tools

COMPUTERS can greatly increase the productivity of nurses. Because communication is such a vital part of health care, knowing how to work effectively among word processing programs, spreadsheets, statistical packages, and presentation software is a necessity in advancing in nursing. These topics are explored in Chapters 4, 5, 6, 7, and 8. Chapter 9 explores databases, which are the basis for all hospital information systems. The focus in Chapter 10 is on how nurses can quickly access the latest information and apply it to practice by learning to search electronic databases and manage knowledge. In Chapter 11, specialty software is examined as an important aid to research and nursing education.

Word Processors

Software programs that are designed to help a user manipulate written text, edit, rearrange, and retype documents on a personal computer are called word processors. The popularity of word processing attests to the fact that written communication is still the primary means of spreading information and knowledge. Because communication is such a vital part of health care, using a word processor effectively has become a necessity to advance in nursing.

Word processing software packages vary in the features they offer. All packages, however, even the text editing software that comes with an operating system, offer the ability to insert, delete, cut, and paste text; search and replace words; store and retrieve documents; and word wrap (the automatic insertion of line breaks when text exceeds the width of the page). Full-featured word processors such as Corel's WordPerfect™, Lotus' Word Pro™, and Microsoft's Word™ offer the writer many more features.

 Characters and Fonts

A character is any symbol that can be entered from the keyboard, including a space. Besides entering and deleting printable characters, in word processing programs, attributes can be applied to them. An attribute is a characteristic that changes the appearance of a printable symbol. Attributes that can be applied to characters in most word processors include boldfacing, italicizing, and underlining. Attributes can be turned on before or

Different Fonts and Sizes		
8 point	12 point	20 point
Arial	Arial	Arial
Courier	Courier	Courier
Times New Roman	Times New Roman	Times New Roman
Ribbon	Ribbon	Ribbon
Swiss	Swiss	Swiss
Century Schoolbook	Century Schoolbook	Century Schoolbook

Figure 4-1 • Fonts and point sizes.

after characters are typed by choosing from the tool bar. To remove an attribute, select the text and unselect the attribute from the tool bar.

A font is the typeface that is used for the characters (Fig. 4-1). The font and the size of the print can be changed for the entire document, or for just a small section. Changes can be made before or after text is entered. A drop down box for both fonts and size is generally on the top of the screen. Some word processors use the term "point" to refer to the size of the print. The fonts and sizes available are a function of the printer in use as much as the application program. Laser jet and bubble jet printers have more fonts than dot matrix printers.

▼Entering Text

There are two modes for entering text in a word processing program. The mode the word processor naturally uses is the insert setting. In this mode, when the user enters new text in a line, the original text automatically makes room for it. In typeover (may be called overtype) mode, any new characters will replace those already in the document. Sometimes, as a result of an accidental tapping of the insert key, a user may be in overtype mode when this is not desired. To remedy this, tap the insert key. If in doubt about which mode a user currently is in, the status line usually provides this information.[1]

[1]The status line in on the bottom of the screen. It provides information such as what page you are on, how far from the left margin your insertion point is, whether you have the CAPS lock on, and so on.

TABLE 4-1 ● *Editing Text*	
Using the delete key	**Using the backspace key**
Remove the character that is to the *right* of the insertion point.	Removes the character that is to the *left* of the insertion point.

▼ Editing Text

Basic editing involves "navigating" around a document and using the editing keys. Navigation entails using the arrow keys or the mouse to move the insertion point (Table 4-1).[2] These actions allow the user to move the insertion point without disturbing any text. To insert new text, the user places the insertion point where he or she wishes the new words to be and then starts typing. Characters can be erased with either the "delete" or the "backspace" key.

DELETING TEXT

Deleting a block of text involves placing the mouse pointer at the beginning or end of the unwanted text, holding down the left mouse button, and dragging the pointer to the other end. The text will change color to show it has been "selected." Release the mouse button when the text is highlighted. With the text selected, tap the delete key or depress the right mouse button and choose "delete" from the pop-up menu.[3]

CUTTING OR MOVING TEXT

With word processing, the user has the ability to move sentences, paragraphs, and entire pages. Cutting can be achieved in several ways. Windows word processors have a pair of scissors on the tool bar that cut selected text. Or after selecting text, click "edit" on the menu line, and choose "cut" from the drop down menu. Ctrl-X also cuts text from a document. Cutting text removes the selected text from its original location and places it on the clipboard. The clipboard is a portion of the computer's memory that holds any items that are being moved or copied.

COPYING TEXT

There are also two ways to copy text. After selecting text for copying, click on the copy icon, or select "copy" from the edit menu. Either of these actions leaves the original text in place but places a copy of it on the clipboard.

[2]The insertion point is the place where the next character to be typed will be placed. Before Windows™, this was called a cursor.

[3]Actually, once text is selected, if the user types in any letter, number, or symbol, it will replace the text. This principle holds true in any program.

PASTING TEXT

Once an item is on the clipboard, move the insertion point to the location in the document where the text is to be copied, and paste it there by clicking on the paste icon or by selecting "paste" from the edit menu. Items remain on the clipboard even after they are pasted until they are displaced by another item. Once an item has been placed on the clipboard, it can be pasted many times or until another item is placed on the clipboard by cutting or copying.

▼Word Wrap

Instead of asking the user to determine the end of a line, word processors and many other computer applications use "word wrap." Word wrap is the automatic insertion by the computer of a line break at the point where the computer finds that the word added to the line will cause it to exceed the line length for that font and margin. This line break is called a "soft return" and is not permanent. When the user edits the document by either adding or deleting text, the line break changes its position to accommodate. Line breaks can also change if the user switches the margins, font, font size, or font attributes.

Tapping the enter key is called entering a "hard return." When a user enters a hard return, the computer skips down to the next line and begins a new paragraph. In word processing, use the enter key to start a new paragraph or insert a blank line. In other instances, let the computer word wrap.

▼Page Breaks

To force a new page, called a "hard page" by some word processors, hold down Ctrl and tap the Enter key. Do not force a new page to keep text together. Instead, select the text and then access the format menu. In some word processors, the command to keep text on one page will be found under "paragraph," and in others, it is found under "page." The online "help" can be used to discover how a word processor activates this function.

MARGINS

The original term for alignment of text along a margin is "justification." Word processors vary in which term they use to designate this function. There are four main ways that text can be aligned. When text is "left aligned" or left justified, the left margin is flush. When the text is right justified, the right margin is flush. In center alignment, each line of text is centered. "Justification" or "full justification" are terms that mean both the left and right margins are flush. Justification can be changed for one line, any part of a document, or the whole document (Fig. 4-2).

The most important justification for readability is left justification. When the left margin is not flush, the reader has to work harder to comprehend the text. Full justification can result in lines with unequal spacing between the words, like that occasionally seen in newspaper columns (Table 4-2). This problem occurs most frequently when the printer cannot accommodate what are called "proportional fonts."

> **Left Justification (Alignment)**
> There are four main ways that text can be justified. When text is left justified, the left margin is flush; when it is right justified, the margin is flush with the right margin. In center justification each line of text is centered, while in full justification both the left and right margins are flush.
>
> **Right Justification (Alignment)**
> There are four main ways that text can be justified. When text is left justified, the left margin is flush; when it is right justified, the margin is flush with the right margin. In center justification each line of text is centered, while in full justification both the left and right margins are flush.
>
> **Center Justification (Alignment)**
> There are four main ways that text can be justified. When text is left justified, the left margin is flush; when it is right justified, the margin is flush with the right margin. In center justification each line of text is centered, while in full justification both the left and right margins are flush.
>
> **Full Justification (Justified)**
> There are four main ways that text can be justified. When text is left justified, the left margin is flush; when it is right justified, the margin is flush with the right margin. In center justification each line of text is centered, while in full justification both the left and right margins are flush.

Figure 4-2 • Justification styles.

In a proportional font, each character only uses the space required for that character. In "monospaced fonts," or "nonproportional fonts," each character takes a given amount of space, regardless of the size of each character.

Default margins, or those that the word processor automatically uses, vary from word processor to word processor. Access the margin dialog box, and enter the appropriate number for any or all of the four margins. Use the help function if the margin dialog box cannot be found.

HEADERS, FOOTERS, AND PAGE NUMBERS

Headers and footers are text that are printed on the top or bottom of every page. Some formal documents require headers on all of the pages. On others, the user may want to use a header as clarification for the reader. Manually entering headers and footers results in them moving to a location other than the top of a page with any editing of the document that either adds or deletes a line. For this reason, headers and footers should be inserted using the word processor "header" function. Headers and footers can have any attributes that can be applied to text, and can be left, center, or right jus-

TABLE 4-2 ● *Comparison of Proportional and Monospaced Fonts in Full Justification*		
Type of font	**Font**	**Results of full justification**
Proportional	Times New Roman	The most important justification for readability is left justification. When the left margin is not flush, the reader has to work harder to comprehend the text.
Monospaced	Courier	The most important justification for readability is left justification. When the left margin is not flush, the reader has to work harder to comprehend the text.

tified. Some word processors print a header above the margin, thus creating a smaller top margin. This can be reset. A header or footer can include page numbers, or page numbers may be inserted without using headers or footers. If both a header and a page number are needed, include the page number as part of the header. The page number will then not try to print in the same location as the header (Fig. 4-3). Check the help function for header, footer, or page numbers to learn to use these functions.

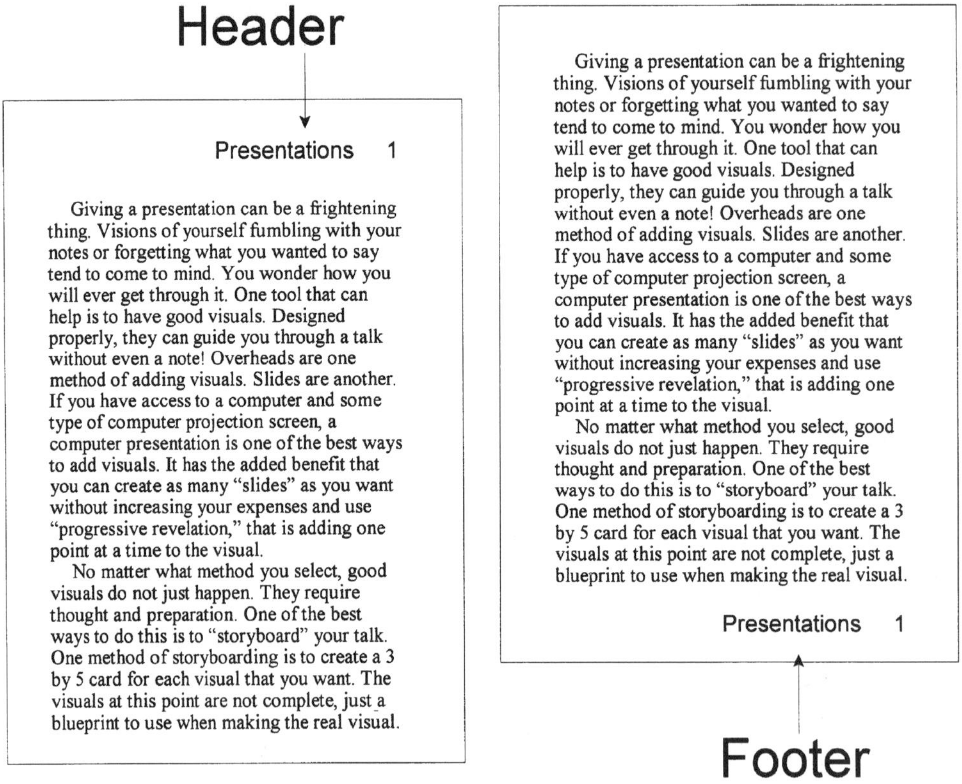

Figure 4-3 ● Headers and footers.

▼Some Common Word Processor Features

When communication involves a written document, it is important that the document appears professional. Word processors provide many features that help accomplish this task.

SPELL CHECK

There are many misconceptions about how spell check works. A computer does not think, it only makes comparisons (Fig. 4-4). When spell check is used, the computer compares each set of characters with the "words" that are in its dictionary. If it finds a set of matching letters, it assumes that the word is spelled correctly. If it does not find them, it presents the user with a list. If one of those words is the correct one, the user selects and inserts it. Users can add words to the dictionary.

The newer versions of word processors use a red line to underline any words that are considered misspelled at the point of data entry. To find out how the word processor thinks the word should be spelled, place the mouse pointer over the word and click the right button. A list of suggestions will appear. It is also possible to add another dictionary, such as a medical dictionary, to the spell check function.

One function that is related to the speller is the ability of word processors to change automatically what is seen as a misspelled—or more usually, mistyped—word, to what is considered the correct format. This function is often referred to as auto correct or quick correct. To provide for this function, the word processor stores a list of common misspellings together, with the correctly spelled word. If a word is typed in a way that matches the misspelling, the correct word is automatically substituted for the misspelled one. New words can also be added at this function, and words that may not be a misspelling in a certain context can be deleted.

THESAURUS

The thesaurus operates just as effectively as a printed one, and is much quicker to use. Like the spell check, the thesaurus is located under "tools" on the menu, or it may also be represented on the tool bar. To use the thesaurus, place the insertion

> I have a spelling checker
> I disk covered four my PC.
> It plane lee marks four my revue
> Miss steaks aye can knot see.
>
> Eye ran this poem threw it.
> Your sure real glad two no.
> Its very polished in its weigh,
> My checker tolled me sew.

Figure 4-4 • Speller peccadilloes.

point on the word for which the user wishes to find a substitute, and access the thesaurus. A window pops up that lists some possible synonyms. Some word processors also provide antonyms. Select the proper word, and click on the box that tells the computer to replace.

GRAMMAR CHECKERS

Perfect functionality has not yet been reached with grammar checkers. Still, using one does not hurt. They are excellent at picking up syntax errors such as subject-verb disagreement and run-on sentences. Grammar checkers may be found under "tools."

FIND AND REPLACE

Find and replace is also a very useful tool. Perhaps in writing, a user typed the word "nurse" when he or she really wanted to write "registered nurse." By accessing find and/or replace on the "tool" menu, the word processor finds every instance of "nurse" and replaces it with "registered nurse." The user has a choice in making the replacement. The user can allow the computer to replace in every instance automatically, or the user can decide on alternative replacements.

FOOTNOTES AND ENDNOTES

Footnotes and endnotes are different features, but each is accessed and entered the same way. A footnote is a piece of text printed at the bottom of a page. It is usually additional information that may add to a reader's knowledge. An endnote is a piece of text that is printed at the end of a document, for instance, a list of references. Word processors automatically place these notes in the proper position and number them accordingly. The drop down box for this feature is found on the "insert" menu.

TABLES

Tables can be created by accessing "table" on the menu line, or placing the pointer on the appropriate icon on the tool bar and dragging to create the number of rows and columns wanted. Extra columns can be added or deleted at any time. If the default column size does not match a need, columns can be resized by placing the mouse pointer on the grid line between columns, depressing the left mouse button, and dragging the line. To enter text into a table, simply type. The rectangle, or cell, will enlarge as needed. There are many options for formatting a table (Fig. 4-5). Whereas some word processors have detailed features, all of them provide the following functions:

- ▼ Adding a row to the bottom of the table by placing the insertion point in the cell in the bottom row that is farthest to the right, and tapping the tab key.
- ▼ Navigating the table, by tapping the tab key to go to the cell on the right, shift-tab to go the cell on the left, or using the arrow keys to move the insertion point up or down a row.
- ▼ Changing the appearance or style of a table. Accessing this function depends on the word processor.

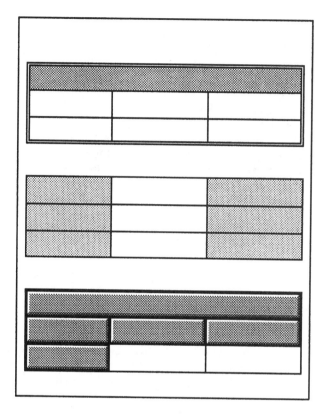

Figure 4-5 • Some table styles.

COLUMNS

See Figure 4-6.

GRAPHICS

The term "graphic" in the computer world applies to any item that is not text or a table. Usually this item is a picture (Fig. 4-7), but text can also be placed in a frame and then treated as a graphic. Additionally, there are options to draw a picture, either within the word processor itself or using the presentation package that is a part of the suite. Most suites also come with "clip art," or small pictures or symbols that can be used in a document.

SORTING

When typing a list of names, it is not always convenient to enter them in alphabetical order, yet with the "sort" function, they can automatically be alphabetized. The sorting function is also useful in listing references for a paper. Use the "help" function to learn how to sort.

Newspaper Columns

This text is in a format called a newspaper column. These are easily created in a word processor. When newspaper columns are used, the text automatically moves to the top of the next column when it has exceeded the page length, or you enter a forced page break.

You can create a column for an entire document, or just a selected portion of it. Word processors differ on how this feature is invoked; use the help function and search on columns to find out how to do this. In all word processors, columns can be formatted either before or after you enter text.

Figure 4-6 ● Newspaper columns.

MAIL MERGE

Mail merge takes a set of data and places the different pieces into a desired form. In using names and addresses to write a form letter, the user creates a set of data that includes "fields" such as title, first name, middle name, last name, address, and so forth. A letter, or form, is then planned in which these items are placed appropriately (Fig. 4-8).

OUTLINE

The outline function is useful for creating an outline for text, a multiple choice test, or any list that requires numbers to be ordered or reordered. The outline option is selected from the "tool" menu. When the outline function is on, tap the enter key and the next number at that level appears automatically. To move to a level below, tap the tab key, and the symbol reverts to the next lower level. To change to a level above, tap shift-tab. Check help to learn how to use this feature (Fig. 4-9).

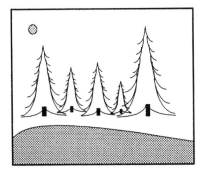

Figure 4-7 ● A graphic.

```
(Title)Ms.
(First Name)Lucy
(Middle Name)X.
(Last Name)Caro
(Address)25 East Southwick Drive
(City)Anywhere
(State)Any State
(Zip)42424-1001
```

Sample of one record in a data set

```
(Title) (First Name) (Middle Name) (Last Name)
(Address)
(City), (State) (Zip)

Dear (Title) (Last Name):

        You have been selected from many people to
enjoy a special vacation at our new resort at the beautiful
sea shore. (First Name), we know that you will not object
to paying a small fee of $2000 for this privilege. You
need to contact us by Friday at the latest to take part in
this great opportunity. Call us anytime at 1-800-
BELIEVE.

Sincerely,


Joe Barnum
A sucker is born every minute
```

Sample of a form letter

```
Ms. Lucy X. Caro
25 East Southwick Drive
Anywhere, Any State 42424-1001

Dear Ms. Caro:

        You have been selected from many people to enjoy a special vacation at our new
resort at the beautiful sea shore. Lucy, we know that you will not object to paying a small
fee of $2000 for this privilege. You need to contact us by Friday at the latest to take part
in this great opportunity. Call us anytime at 1-800-BELIEVE.

Sincerely,


Joe Barnum
A sucker is born every minute
```

Form letter after it has been merged

Figure 4-8 • Data set, form letter, and result of merge.

1. This is level one of an outline
   a. This is level two
   b. And so is this
2. Shift-tab moved back to the first level.
   a. Level two again
      i. Level three
         (1) Level four
            (a) Level five
3. Now we are back at level one again.

Typical outline with various levels

I. This is level one of an outline
   A. This is level two
   B. And so is this
II. Here shift-tab was pressed to move back to the first level.
   A. Level two again
      1. Level three
         a. Level four
            (1) Level five
III. Now we are back at level one again.

Same outline converted to regular outline markings

This is level one of an outline
This is level two
And so is this
Shift-tab moved back to the first level.
Level two again
Level three
   Level four
   Level five
Now we are back at level one again.

Outline converted to headings (Of course there would be text under each of these headings!)

Figure 4-9 • Some outline styles.

TEMPLATE

In creating documents with the same styling, a user may wish to create a template. A template is a document that has all the formatting and headings in place. A template, for example, can be constructed for a newsletter. The template option is listed under the "tool" menu.

MACRO

A macro is a small program that automates a function. If the same functions are continually accessed, such as creating a superscript, a macro can be created that will automatically perform this function. Although complex macros are programmed, it is also possible to create a macro by recording keystrokes as a function is performed. After creating a macro, it can be placed on the tool bar or assigned to a key. To place an item on the tool bar, place the mouse pointer on the tool bar and click with the right mouse button, then follow the directions. To record keystrokes, click on "tools/macro/record."

Printing

Any document created with a word processor can be printed. In Windows compliant programs, tapping Ctrl-P will automatically print the document or start the printing process. The "file" menu also contains a print function. A block of text, one page, a range of pages, or the entire document can be selected for printing.

Saving Files

Many Windows programs, not just word processors, are designed so documents can be saved by tapping Ctrl-S. Files can also be saved by selecting "save" from the file menu or by clicking on the appropriate icon on the tool bar. The first time a document is saved, it must be named.

It is always safe to use letters and numbers in a file name. When the save command is issued, what is stored is the document as it is at the moment of the save. If changes are made, the file needs to be saved again. Computer users should save their work frequently (Fig. 4-10). Many word processors have a provision for an automatic backup. That is, after a given number of minutes, the computer will automatically save.

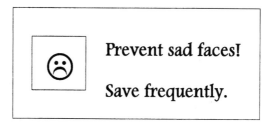

Figure 4-10 • SAVE!

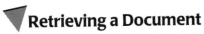

Retrieving a Document

To retrieve a document, the user needs to know the location and name of the file. If a file is saved to a diskette with "a:\" preceding it, it can be retrieved by tapping Ctrl-O and entering the file name (including the a:\) and tapping enter (Table 4-3). For ex-

---

TABLE 4-3 ● *Universal Commands in Word Processors*

Want to?	Use
Navigate a document	
Move the insertion point without changing any of the text?	Arrow keys or the mouse
Move from beginning of a word to beginning of the next?	Ctrl-right or left arrow key
Move from paragraph to paragraph?	Ctrl-up or down arrow key
Delete and insert characters	
Delete a character that is to the left of your insertion point?	Backspace
Delete a character that is to the right of your insertion point?	Delete key
Select some text?	Place mouse pointer at beginning or end of the text, depress and hold left mouse button, and drag to the opposite end of the text. Release mouse button.
Select the entire document?	Ctrl-A
Type over the existing text?	Insert key (use this key to toggle back to the regular insert mode too).
Force line and page breaks	
Force a new line?	Enter key
Force a new page?	Ctrl-Enter
Format a paragraph	
Indent the first line of a paragraph?	Tab key
Create a hanging paragraph?	Format/Paragraph
Miscellaneous	
Find a phrase in the document?	Ctrl-F
Print?	Ctrl-P
Save a document?	Ctrl-S
Record a macro?	Tools/Macro/Record
Cut, copy, and move text	
Copy a selected portion of text?	Ctrl-C
Cut out a selected portion of text?	Ctrl-X
Paste anything on the clipboard to a new location?	Ctrl-V
Work with tables	
Create a table?	Tables/Insert table or place pointer on icon and drag until correct number of rows and columns are selected
Move from cell to cell within a table?	Tab to go forward, shift-tab to go backwards
Add a row at the end of a table?	Place insertion point in last cell on the right and tap the tab key.

ample, if a file was named mypaper and saved to a diskette in the "a" drive, to open the file, enter a:\mypaper in the appropriate box. If the file is in the current working folder, or the user knows its location and how to change working folders, it can also be retrieved by using the "open file" option.

▼ Summary

Using a word processor makes editing easier. Taking the time to explore what a word processor can do will result in saved time and professional looking documents. Learning to use a word processor is not done overnight. The best approach is to learn features as needed. If a function works, it will work under many different scenarios. Following are some good rules to remember.

▼ Use the enter key to force a new line. This is done after a title, to start a new paragraph, to add a blank line, or any time the next section of text should be on the following line.

▼ Use a forced (hard) page break (Ctrl-Enter), not repeated hard returns, to create a permanent page break.

▼ Unless the page break will always be needed (such as when you are beginning a reference page), do not create hard page breaks until you are ready to print. Use the "keep text together" function instead.

▼ Use the tab key to indent the first line of a paragraph.

▼ Tell the word processor to insert headers, footers, and page numbering automatically instead of laboriously doing them manually.

EXERCISES

1. Experiment with
   a. Creating page breaks using both the enter key and Ctrl-Enter for a hard (forced) page, and editing a full page of text above it.
   b. Using the overtype (typeover) and insert mode of text entry.
   c. Using the outline mode of entry.
   d. Creating a macro by recording your keystrokes.
2. Use the help function to learn to justify a paragraph.
3. What are some ways word processing is being used by health care professionals in
   a. Clinical practice?
   b. Administration?
   c. Education?
   d. Research?
   e. Entrepreneurial work?

CHAPTER 5

Understanding Computer Concepts

Objectives:

After studying this chapter you should be able to:

1 Apply computer conventions when faced with new situations

2 Use the help option to learn to perform new functions

3 Use the right mouse button appropriately

4 Use "save" and "save as" appropriately

5 Employ the file organizational principles in copying files

Remember the first time you cared for a patient? Everything took a long time and required absolute concentration while you moved through each procedure step by step. By gaining experience, procedures were modified according to each patient's needs. Similarities in tasks became apparent, and these principles were then applied to all patients.

In taking blood pressure measurements, for example, wrapping the cuff, pumping up the manometer, properly placing the stethoscope, and slowly releasing the pressure require concentration for the beginner. After some experience, blood pressure is viewed as a part of the total assessment picture and is evaluated accordingly. When a nurse is able to judge when to take a blood pressure that is not ordered, the action is beyond required recording of the results. This knowledge is freedom from a dependence on procedures and allows nurses to practice professionally.

The same thing happens in working with computers. At first, a user may be very concerned about the keystrokes needed to perform each function. As more experience is gained, specific procedures (such as creating headers) become just another tool. In experimenting with different application programs, similarities and differences are recognized. Tasks that used to require full concentration become automatic.

Learning to Use a Computer

In learning to use computers, without realizing it, the user internalizes perceptions which often translates to the quicker understanding and mastery of other programs. With the hope of facilitating the process of seeing computer use as a whole instead of a series of functions, each requiring a different procedure, it is useful to explore concepts encountered in many different computer applications.

Learning a good word processing program is a useful tool, because many concepts are transferable to other software products. For example, the use of the delete and backspace keys to edit text or numbers applies, in some way, to all other computer programs, as does selecting attributes such as bold or italics, or changing fonts and point size. Word wrap is another concept encountered in countless other applications, as is selecting text and saving work.

DEFAULT

One universal concept a user may not be aware of is the "default" function. Defaults are properties or attributes that can be changed but that are employed by the program unless otherwise specified. When using a word processor, the "default" mode for entering text is the insert mode. That is, unless this is specifically changed by tapping the insert key, any text entered is inserted at the location of the insertion point. The new text does not overwrite any text that is already there, it just pushes the text already there ahead of it. Also found are default margins, usually 1 inch, and a default font, often Times Roman or Arial.

When a change is made, whatever characteristic is assigned becomes the new "default" for that document. The default margin, for instance, is 1 inch on all four sides. Perhaps when writing a paper, a user decides to change the margins to 1½ inches. One and one-half inches, therefore, becomes the default margin for that document. Most of the properties changed will only alter the default for that characteristic for the active document. Very few will affect the overall action of the program. If something different than the default is frequently used, most programs provide a way to change the default so it will affect all documents.

SCREEN APPEARANCE

Screen design is very similar in most programs. All programs have title bars, menu lines, and tool bars (Fig. 5-1). Many also have a status line on the bottom. Since Windows 95™, PCs also have a task bar at the bottom of the screen. In between the top

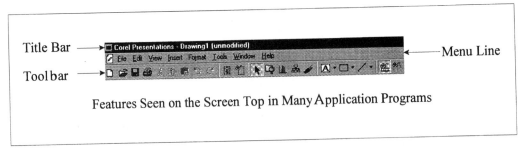

Features Seen on the Screen Top in Many Application Programs

Figure 5-1 ● Screen tops in many application programs. (Printed with permission of Corel.)

TABLE 5-1 ● *Focus of Menu Functions*					
	File	**Edit**	**View**	**Insert**	**Format**
Focus of functions found on the menu	Functions pertaining to a file	Functions that allow you to edit the text	Functions that affect the screen display	Functions that can be inserted into the file	Functions that affect how the printed file will appear
Some functions found on the menu	Open a file Save a file Print Exit	Cut Copy Paste Find	Zoom Bars that are visible	Graphics (pictures) Footnotes Endnotes	Page size Margins Paragraph styles

Although there are differences between vendors, these functions are generally found on the drop down menus from these menu items.

and bottom lines is the work space, or the place where the user can enter or edit the document. There are some variations between programs and operating systems, but generally these tools are available in all programs. Another similarity that programs share is that in most Windows programs, there are usually at least two ways to perform a function.

MENUS

Not only are the screen layouts very similar in most programs but the menu choices are, too (Table 5-1). Although what a user may find on the drop down menu varies among programs and vendors, there is much that is the same. On the menu line, most Windows programs place, in the following order, "files," "edit," "view," "insert," and "format." Understanding the focus of the functions on given menus makes it easier to find specific commands in a program.

TOOLBARS

As with menus, toolbars also have many similarities. The majority start with the same four icons, which include, "open a new document," "retrieve a file," "save a document," and "print."[1] These icons represent functions that can also be found on a file menu. Although their exact placement may differ, generally the next group of icons will enable cutting, copying and pasting, or items also found on an edit menu. These icons are followed by a symbol for undo and one for redo. Figure 5-2 shows these icons. Many programs also provide the ability to edit the toolbars by either removing objects that are not used or adding those that are used frequently.

[1]The exceptions to this rule are applications that only allow one open document at a time, such as some statistics programs. In those programs, the first icon, "open a new document," is missing. The next three, however, are there.

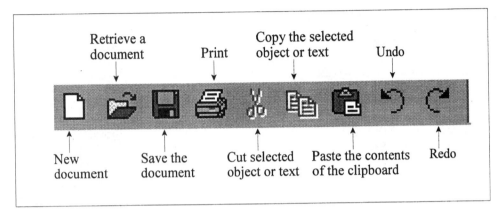

Figure 5-2 ● Some fairly universal icons.

STATUS BAR OR LINE

The line at the bottom of the screen is called the status bar or status line. The status line gives information that varies among programs and vendors. In many word processors, this line indicates the page of a document, the line of text on that page, or how far from the left margin the insertion point is located. The status line may also indicate whether the user is in insert or overtype mode or if the CAPS lock is on.

UNDO AND REDO

Two commands many applications have, especially word processors, spreadsheets, and graphics programs, are "undo" and "redo." By clicking on the undo icon, the last "edit" or change becomes undone. Clicking once again will undo prior changes in some programs. The number of changes that can be undone is program dependent. Redo also puts changes back in the order in which they were removed. The exact look of the icons for these functions differs from program to program. Commands to accomplish these functions are also found on the edit menu.

HELP

Feeling comfortable using a computer is often a matter of getting help when it is needed. Classes may provide some beginning skills, but when a user tries to employ the functions learned or experiment with new functions, problems may arise. Help, however, is often just a mouse click away. Most programs provide online help, or help that is available by clicking on a word on the menu line.

Help is an option on the title bar in earlier versions of Windows. For Windows 95, help is an option on the start menu. Both versions provide a short tutorial that is very useful, and both allow searching for topics in which help is needed. Among many applications today, manuals no longer come with the program, although one is sometimes available for a fee. Instead, users are expected to use the help feature.[2]

---

[2]Some products feature a choice called "help online," which can connect the user to the Internet and then to their home page. Some vendors have excellent help sites with frequently asked questions and other helpful information.

Help is usually available by clicking the right-most item on the menu line or tapping F1. The contents of the drop down menu vary among programs, but the menu almost always contains an item that starts with "about." Clicking on the "about" item presents information about the program. This information may contain the serial number of the program, the exact version of the program in use, and possibly how much RAM is available.

To find out how to perform a function, use the "find" or "index" features. With these options, a user can browse through an entire list or enter a request for clarification in the space provided. Whether index or find works best will probably depend on how a search is phrased.

To use help, on the appropriate screen, enter the word or words which describe the function. In learning to insert a header, enter the word "header" in the box provided (Fig. 5-3), and then either tap the enter key, or click on the option provided that will start the search. This could be "ok," "search," or "go." The program will respond with a list of choices. Click on the one that matches the information needed, and then click on display. The ability to print the help information will be found under options.

For some features, instead of receiving printed information, a "wizard" or "expert" will lead the user through each step of performing the function. This automatic help

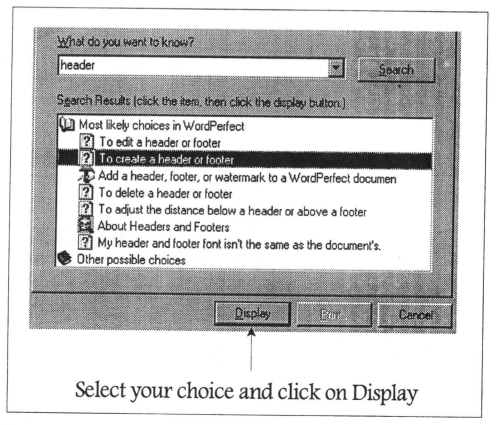

Figure 5-3 ● Results of a search.

is carried even further in some programs that lead the user through programmed steps. A presentation program, for example, may assume a user is going to make regular slides, and therefore, moves step-by-step toward accomplishing this goal without the user having to make many program-related decisions.

Books about the software in use are also helpful. Many texts about popular software products are available; however, there are so many that making a decision about which book to use can be complicated. Some are written for beginners, whereas others are complete references for a program. Keep in mind that the beginning books are very limited in their coverage of a program's functions. They are helpful when one is first starting to use a program, but it might be more cost effective to buy a more complete book.

The type of support available from a vendor varies. Some provide an 800 number that can be used for a given length of time after an initial call. Others use a toll number for the same purpose. All provide web sites, although the quality of help available at these web sites varies. User groups are also a great source of help.

If one is using an institutional copy of a program, the way it is licensed may stipulate that only specific people can call the vendor. In these cases, there will usually be a help desk for the program within the institution. It is important that the user locate the sources of help available and take advantage of them.

CUTTING, COPYING, AND PASTING

Cut, copy, and paste functions work in all Windows software products. It is even possible to use the copy function in a situation in which there are no icons or menu items from which to select copy or paste (Fig. 5-4). In these cases, to copy something after the text has been selected, tap Ctrl-C. This places it on the clipboard, from which it can be pasted where desired, including in another program, by tapping Ctrl-V or Shift-Insert. These keystrokes work in most Windows programs, whether the program is a word processor or a web browser (ie, program that makes it possible for the user to see documents on the World Wide Web [WWW]).

THE RIGHT MOUSE BUTTON

Mice on PCs have two buttons. The left mouse button is clicked to select items. The right button reveals a list of functions that can be activated for the "active object." For example, in placing the mouse pointer on the toolbar and right clicking, a list of options that can be applied to the toolbar is seen. If text is selected, a right click pro-

Function	Key Strokes
Copy	Ctrl-C
Paste	Ctrl V or Shift-Insert

Figure 5-4 • Universal copy and paste commands

duces another menu for functions such as cut, copy, paste, and delete. In word processors, a right click with the pointer over a misspelled word produces a list of possible spellings. In graphics programs, the right mouse button is sometimes the only way to access a command. In these applications, to find out what can be done with an object, select it and right click the mouse.

GRAPHICS

Graphics, or nontext items, can be encountered in word processing programs, spreadsheets and databases, as well as presentation or graphics programs. Like text, graphical objects share many similarities, no matter which application is in use. Once they are selected, when the right mouse button is clicked, a list of properties and functions for the selected object is displayed. The properties, however, will be different depending on the program and type of object.

When an object or objects are selected, they can be cut, copied, pasted, or dragged just like text. Once selected, some objects can be dragged anywhere with the mouse pointer inside of them; others do not allow this, unless the pointer is on the edge of the object, or the pointer changes its shape to a hand. Depending on the type of program, other functions can be performed with a selected object. In a drawing program, the user can usually rotate the object, change its color, or resize it. Resizing of an object is done in the same manner as resizing a window—by moving the mouse pointer until it is shaped like a double-edged arrow, then dragging the side. To resize a graphical object without distorting it, drag one of the corners. Dragging a side will lengthen or widen the object and leave it out of proportion.

If designing a form in a database or a chart in a spreadsheet, the user may encounter nested objects. A nested object is one contained inside another object. In order to differentiate between the overall object and its contents, one left click selects the overall object, and a second click selects whatever object the mouse pointer is on within the overall object.

SAVING

When a file is saved, a copy of the current document is put on a disk where it can be retrieved for future use. To make it easier to find the file the next time it is needed, the name chosen should reflect its contents. DOS and Windows 3.11 permit only eight characters, none of which can be a space, whereas Windows 95 allows the use of spaces and increases the number of characters a name can have to 256.

When a file is saved, there are two choices for saving: "save" and "save as." The first time a file is saved, it matters little which function is selected. After that, there is a great deal of difference. Save does what is called a repeat save, that is, it saves the document using the same name with any changes that may have been made. This action replaces what is on the diskette under that name with the current contents of that document.

Use "save as" when you wish to keep the version of the file that was originally saved, but have made modifications that you also wish to save. See Figure 5-5 for a decision tree to use when faced with the choice of using "save" or "save as."

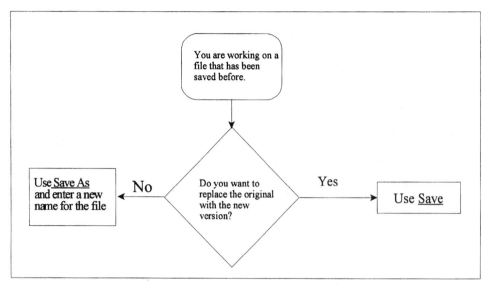

Figure 5-5 ● Decision tree for using *save* or *save as.*

Sometimes when a file is saved for the first time, the user will receive a message stating a file by that name already exists. The program also asks if the file should be replaced. Unless the user knows what is in the current file that has that name, and does not mind losing it, they should type "no," and select a new name.

FILE FORMATS

Applications from different vendors create files that are often incompatible with other programs, the same applications from other vendors, and even different versions of the same program.

Proprietary File Formats

When a document is saved in a word processor, a file is created that is specific to the brand of software and sometimes the version. In other words, the file is saved in a proprietary file format, or one the software vendor owns. If using Microsoft Word™, the file will have been assigned an extension of ".doc," which tells the world this is a Microsoft Word document. If a diskette with this file on it is taken to another computer and the user attempts to retrieve the file with a different word processor, there are often difficulties.

The first difficulty occurs when the user goes to the open file screen, and the word processor is set to show only files it created. This can be remedied by finding the box on the open files screen that has a label that uses the word "type," clicking on the down arrow at the right end of the box, and selecting "all files" from the menu. Generally, newer versions of applications read files created by older versions of the same program.

The results of attempting to open a file on another computer is more successful if the same brand and version of a word processor is used. Opening files created with different types of application programs, such as opening a word processing document in a spreadsheet, is even more dependent on circumstances. Generally, between the applications in an office suite from the same vendor, a spreadsheet can be opened in a word processor, but it will open as a table. Unless a file is a table or very small, a word processing file cannot be opened with a spreadsheet.

ASCII File Formats

The one format that is universally accepted by most programs is the ASCII format. ASCII contains only text, and each line is regarded as a separate paragraph, which means that editing will be difficult. But ASCII can be a very useful format for structured data (data organized by rows and columns), because it can be easily opened in a spreadsheet or a database. Rich text format, or RFT, is a type of ASCII file that does retain formatting information, such as fonts and margins.

PRINT

Printing is another function that is available in all computer programs. When printing things such as spreadsheets or databases, it is easy to forget that a piece of paper has a finite size. Although this is not usually a problem with word processors, because the formatting is tied to paper size, with both spreadsheets and databases, this can present difficulties. It is common with either program to design a document that is wider than any paper a printer can use. When an attempt is made to print the document, the part that is too wide to fit on one sheet may be completely omitted.

If the spreadsheet or database in question is not too large, there are two possible ways to solve this problem. One is to change the paper orientation from the default portrait to landscape. In landscape orientation, the longest side is horizontal instead of the shortest side. Although this approach can take care of some width problems, it still cannot accommodate all cases. More room can be created by making the fonts smaller, but this solution has its limitations in readability. The best solution is to remember paper size when designing any item for printing.

FILE ORGANIZATION

Managing files is not as complicated as it seems. There is an organizational scheme to where files are located on a disk. Imagine that inside each computer is a very large filing cabinet. This filing cabinets has drawers. Folders can be placed in the drawers and files in folders. If anyone is going to be able to find anything in this filing system, it is necessary to devise some way of naming the various items. Because there may be more than one filing cabinet, it is necessary to give each a name. One that happens to be a gray color might be called "GRAY." Then to avoid confusion about the drawers, they are also named. The top drawer in GRAY may be called "TOP," the next drawer "MIDDLE," and the bottom drawer "LOWEST." The folders that go into these drawers also need to have names. One of the folders that is placed in the MIDDLE drawer may be named "DIABETES." Inside that folder is a document that is ti-

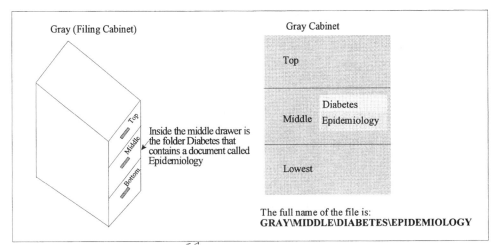

Figure 5-6 • Comparison of filing systems.

tled "EPIDEMIOLOGY." In describing how this document may be found, one could say to go to the GRAY filing cabinet, look in the drawer named "MIDDLE" for the folder named "DIABETES," and pull out the document titled "EPIDEMIOLOGY." Because the instructions are thorough, this document could be located. A shortened way of giving retrieval instructions using the same system would be "GRAY:\MIDDLE\DIABETES\EPIDEMIOLOGY."

Now imagine that although the filing cabinet has a finite size, the number or size of drawers and folders within drawers are not constrained by any physical size beyond the fact that together, they cannot exceed the overall size of the filing cabinet (Fig. 5-6). Instead, the number of drawers, folders, and files can be increased or decreased to meet current filing needs.

This is a perfect analogy of the way items are named and organized on a disk. Instead of the different divisions being called filing cabinets, drawers, folders, and documents, the big filing cabinet is called a disk, the drawers first-level folders, the folder a second-level folder, and the document a file (Table 5-2). Where disk storage varies greatly from a physical filing cabinet is that the folders can increase or decrease in size as needed. If you are using Windows 3.X or DOS, folders are referred to as directories.

TABLE 5-2 ● *File Type Comparison*	
Your filing cabinet system	**Your computer disk system**
Gray filing cabinet	A **disk** named with a letter; if the hard disk, usually a "C:" A smaller external diskette is usually called "A:"
Middle drawer	A **first level folder**
Diabetes folder	A **second level folder**
Epidemiology document	A **file**

This organizational method is hierarchical, that is, the items on top encompass those below them. Suppose, for example, that there is a computer with an internal hard drive. The name of this drive is "c:." On it is installed Windows, a word processor, a spreadsheet, a database, and a World Wide Web browser. All but the web browser are from the same software vendor, whose name is Carefree. The web browser is named Surfnet. When Windows was installed, using the same naming procedure as with the imaginary filing cabinet (when the name of the drive followed by a colon and a backslash and then the name of the folder was used), Windows created a folder called c:\windows. The programs from Carefree, when installed, created folders called c:\carefree, and then further divided that folder into c:\carefree\wordproc, c:\carefree\sprdsht, and c:\carefree\database. Surfnet created a folder called c:\surfnet. At present, the organization of the hard drive would be diagramed as seen in Figure 5-7. Compare this with the organization of the imaginary filing cabinet.

The names of the folders and files are derived identically to the shorthand system developed for the filing cabinet. Each starts with the name of the disk. In Figure 5-7, this is "c," which is followed by the backslash (\), then the names of each lower level of folders separated with a slash. The final name in this shorthand, or path as it is called, is the name of the folder or the file. It can be deduced whether the name is a file or folder by the context in which the term is used. If a file is in c:\carefree\ wordproc, it can be concluded that the term is referring to a folder. If on the other

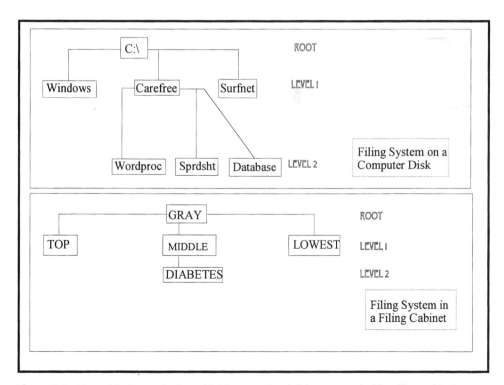

Figure 5-7 • Hierarchical organization of folders on a hard disk compared with a filing cabinet.

hand, c:\carefree\wordproc\nurse, is to be retrieved, this must be a file. If, however, c:\carefree\wordproc\ is seen or a path name with a final slash, this is in reference to a folder, not a file. Files never have a slash after their name.

When the Carefree programs were installed, they created the first-level folder "Carefree" and second-level folders "Wordproc," "Sprdsht," and "Database." When Windows was installed, it created a first-level folder called "Windows" (and several second-level folders, which because of paper limitations, are not shown). Programs, however, are not the only thing that can create folders; users can do this, too.

In creating a level-one folder and several subfolders for the files a user creates using Carefree application programs, a user might create a first-level folder called c:\myfiles. Although files from any type of application program can be put into a folder, separate second-level folders are initially created for the files with each of the three applications programs. The user decided to name them c:\myfiles\wp (the folder for word processing files), c:\myfiles\ss (spreadsheet files), and c:\myfiles\db (database files). Third-level folders are needed under the spreadsheet folder because the spreadsheet will be used to create a budget and a decision model. At this point, the folders on the hard disk look like those in Figure 5-8.

Diskettes can also be organized by creating folders. Unless a Zip™ or Jaz™ drive is used, or a number of small folders are backed up, this is not often done. The way files are organized on an external diskette is identical to that on the hard drive. The only difference is that the path name will start with the letter assigned to the external drive into which it is placed. With 3.5-inch diskettes this usually is a: or b:.

The name of a file is not simply the name given when it is saved. Its real name consists of the pathway to it from the root of the disk, plus the name the user assigned to

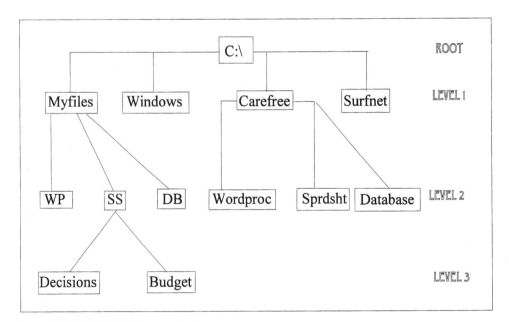

Figure 5-8 • Hard disk folder organization.

it. This makes it possible for a user to assign an identical name to a file, as long as it is in a different folder. For example, on the hard disk named c:, in the folder c:\myfiles\wp, the user decides to create two third-level folders called "papers" and "projects." In both third-level folders, the user has saved a file named "todo." Although the name assigned to both files is the same, these two files have different names. The one in c:\myfiles\wp\papers is named c:\myfiles\wp\papers\todo, and the one in c:\myfiles\wp\projects is named c:\myfiles\wp\projects\todo.

THE WORKING FOLDER

The folder into which a file goes when saved, or the folder where the computer will look for a file, is not a random choice. When using the "open file" icon, the files seen are the ones in the current working folder. When the user saves a file, they either enter the full path name of the file, or it arbitrarily goes to the "open" or "working" folder. Or, the user may "browse" and select another folder.

COPYING OR MOVING FILES

The name given to backing up files is copying. How this is accomplished differs among programs and operating systems, but it is not difficult to learn. Although some programs provide copy options, copying a file can always be done from either the File Manager (versions of Windows prior to 95) or Explore. Use the help option if instructions are needed.

Access to the World Wide Web

With the popularity of accessing information on the WWW, many application programs today provide the ability to place a "link" in a document. This area is visible by the use of different attributes. It may be a different color, underlined, or both. When a user clicks on the link, if the computer on which the program is being used is connected to the Internet, an Internet browser takes the user directly to the address specified in the link.

Another function many programs provide is publishing to the WWW. If a documents is to be readable on the WWW, it needs to be formatted in a given way. This formatting involves adding what are called "tags" to various parts of the document. This can be done manually, but is a tedious job, and like programming, it is prone to human error. To prevent these headaches, most programs today provide a function that allow the document to be formatted so that web browsers can read them. It is often called publishing to the WWW. The exact procedure is different for programs from various vendors, but usually it is available.

Summary

The first computer application a person learns is generally difficult because the user is learning not only the application program, but many computer conventions. Concepts such as the use of delete and backspace are universal in computer programs, as are cut, copy, paste, and word wrap. If one is using a computer with a GUI, the screen layout, the contents of many options on menus, and the results that occur when certain icons are clicked will be similar in all programs.

All modern programs have help available. This help function is useful to both beginners and experts. When it is known what a program can do, the help option is the logical place to start trying to learn how to perform a function. Similarities are also found in graphical objects, which behave similarly in all application programs, whether they are clip art, a drawing, an object that has been scanned in, or the result of a screen capture. All programs allow the user to create files. File organization on a disk pertains to all programs, as does backing up important files. Saving a file follows the same principles in all programs. For this reason, each new application program becomes easier to learn because more and more similarities become apparent.

EXERCISES

1. Open several programs at the same time. Compare the options found in the File, Edit, and View menus. Briefly describe the concept on which the options in each menu are focused.

2. Experiment with the help option:
   a. In the operating system that you are using
   b. In an application program

3. Copy a file to another disk.

4. When you learn a second program, list some of the similarities between the two programs. List the differences.

CHAPTER 6

Working With Numbers

Numbers are often part of the information nurses need to manage. Computers, together with specialized software, provide freedom from the drudgery of manual calculations and make managing numerical information much easier. The first spreadsheet, developed in 1979, gave calculating power to individuals and greatly accelerated the acceptance of computers in the business world. What is most remarkable about the first spreadsheet is that the design is so functional that few changes have been made to it over the years. Instead, many more features have been added, such as graphs and features that make it easier to enter formulas. Because the design is so intuitive, there is probably the least variation in performing functions in different vendors' spreadsheets than in any other application program.

Spreadsheets are not the only type of application program that simplify managing numerical data. There are programs, called financial managers, that allow checkbooks to be balanced and the management of a personal budget, including providing help in categorizing items to facilitate tax preparation. There are also programs that use imputed data and bring in data from a financial manager or spreadsheet to create and print tax returns. Another type of number manager is statistical packages.

 Spreadsheets

One reason electronic spreadsheets caught on so quickly is that they were an electronic representation of something with which all business people were familiar: the multicolumn analysis paper (Fig. 6-1). Learning to enter

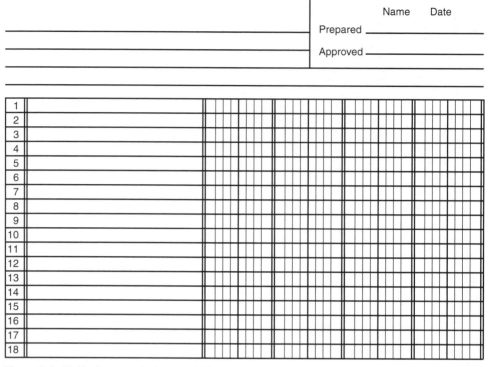

Figure 6-1 • Multicolumn analysis paper before electronic spreadsheets.

data on a computerized multicolumn screen was no harder than learning to use an old calculator, and those with the responsibility of working with numbers gladly adopted this invention to free themselves from the tedium of manual arithmetic.

A spreadsheet is a table whose rectangles, or cells, are capable of containing data or a formula to produce information or knowledge from the data in other cells. In Figure 6-2, notice the top row consists of letters in alphabetical order and the first column contains numbers that increase in increments of one. The cells are named by the letter at the top of the column and the number of the row.

SPREADSHEET SCREENS

The screens for spreadsheets resemble other GUI products. At first glance, the main difference between a spreadsheet and a word processor is that the document screen in a spreadsheet is a table. Many of the familiar icons used in word processing are in

	A	B	C	D	E
1	A1	B1	C1	D1	E1
2	A2	B2	C2	D2	E2
3	A3	B3	C2	D3	E3

Figure 6-2 • Spreadsheet cells labeled with their names.

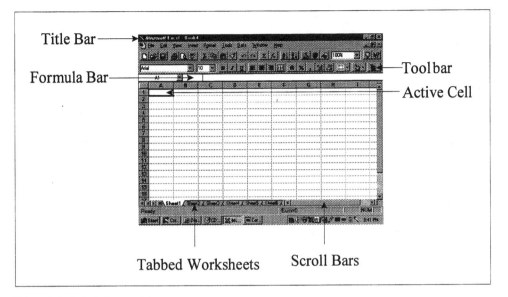

Figure 6-3 • Labeled spreadsheet screen.

their usual place, such as the title bar (Fig. 6-3). There are, however, some differences. For instance, there is a formula bar under the toolbar. At the bottom of the screen there are tabs.[1] For behavioral similarities between word processors and spreadsheets, see Table 6-1.

VOCABULARY

The vocabulary of spreadsheets is not very complex. A *cell* is the name given to the rectangles in the table. A *row* is a horizontal group of cells, and a *column* is a vertical group of cells. *Cell address* is the name given to a cell, and it is derived from the letter of the column and the number of the row where it is located. The *active cell* is analogous to the insertion point in other programs. It is the location where any information entered will be placed. Besides being visible in the table by bold lines (see cell A1 in Figure 6-3, or B2 in Figure 6-4), the contents of the active cell are mirrored on the formula bar line. A *range of cells* is a group of contiguous cells, for example, cells C1 to E3. The range of C1 to E3 in Figure 6-5 would be expressed as C1:E3 or C1..E3, depending on the spreadsheet vendor. Users can name ranges of cells and use this name in commands instead of the cell location.

Two terms that may at first seem a little confusing are worksheet and workbook. A *worksheet* refers to one table, whereas a *workbook* consists of one or more worksheets. On one worksheet, there is room for 256 columns and 16,384 rows. When

---

[1]In GUI interface, a tab is a *bump* shaped like the protrusion on manilla folders used for labeling a folder. Clicking on them gives access to the contents of the folder.

TABLE 6-1 ● *Similarities Between Word Processing Programs and Spreadsheets*

Function	Characteristics special to spreadsheet
Resizing and moving windows and graphics	No differences; select object or window and drag to resize
Toolbars	Like most application products, they can be edited to suit your working preferences
Drop down boxes and dialog boxes	Identical to word processors
Editing	Delete will delete the entire cell contents unless you are entering or editing data Backspace works identically to other programs Data can be entered with the numeric keypad
Enter key	Moves the active cell to the one beneath the current active cell
Selecting Cut, copy, and paste	Can select, cut, copy, and paste pieces of text, a cell, a group of contiguous cells known as a range, or graphical objects
Click and drag	Identical to word processors
Undo and redo	Can undo only the last change
Create files	Files are a workbook; workbooks can contain many worksheets
Automatic backups	Identical to word processors
More than one document open at the same time	Can have several workbooks and worksheets within a workbook open at one time (like all programs, if you open more than the RAM in your computer can support you will notice that all actions are slowed)
Navigation	Similar to tables in word processing, except for enter key. Enter key moves down one row. Tab key moves active cell to the right, Shift-Tab moves active cell to the left. Arrow keys and page up and page down work identically. Ctrl-Home goes to the beginning of worksheet and Ctrl-End to the end.
Navigating with the mouse	The horizontal scroll bar is on the rifght side of the bottom of the screen to make room for the tabs for the different worksheets in a workbook.

Formatting
  Attributes including changing the appearance, size or type of font
  Text justification
	Can also format the contents of the cell, i.e., specify that numbers in selected cells should contain decimals, dollar signs, and so forth. Otherwise identical to word processing.

Graphics	Graphics, besides clip art or drawings, can consist of charts. Spreadsheet tools are excelent for creating charts (graphs).
Printing	If the table will not fit horizontally on one page, the columns will be printed on another page. This may break up the continuity of the table. The best results occur when you designate a range of cells to be printed. Keeping the size of a worksheet to a printable size is another option. The print option will let you print selected cells, the current worksheet, or the whole workbook.
Speller	Works almost identically to word processor
Templates	Same principles
WWW access	Like word processing, you can link to the WWW or publish a table, chart, graphic, or any combination to the WWW.
Record macros	Same principles. Be careful if you receive a macro from another source, it is possible for macros to contain viruses. Check it with an up to date virus checker before using it.

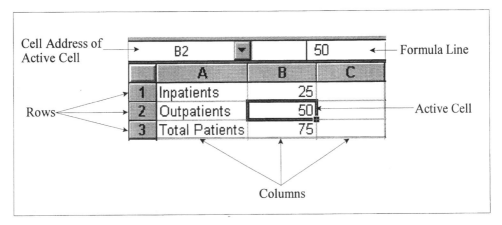

Figure 6-4 • Vocabulary.

working on a project, however, it is advisable to keep the size of a worksheet smaller than this. A spreadsheet that is using 256 columns, unless it is used for research data, may be more manageable if several worksheets are created. The worksheets are indicated by the tabs on the bottom of the screen. A user moves between the worksheets by clicking on the tab. To name a worksheet, double click on the tab and enter text. When they are saved, worksheets create a workbook.[2] Spreadsheets also allow users to have several workbooks, each containing many worksheets, open at one time.

The contents of a spreadsheet are not confined to a table. It is possible to add graphics or charts to any worksheet.[3] These items can be positioned next to the data in the table to which they apply, or they can be placed on a separate worksheet. A separate worksheet can also be used for documentation for the workbook. Documentation helps the user remember the assumptions on which various items are based. It is also useful when others need to see the worksheets. Worksheets do not need to remain in the order in which they were created. They can be placed in any order in the workbook by dragging the tab for that worksheet to the desired location.

[2]The term *notebook* is used by some spreadsheets to denote this same concept.

[3]*Chart* is the name computer programs give to a graph, such as a bar or line graph.

	A	B	C	D	E
1	Inpatients	25			
2	Outpatients	50			
3	Total Patients	75			

Figure 6-5 • The cells C1:E3 are a range of cells. They can be given a name and treated as an object.

USES FOR SPREADSHEETS

Although spreadsheets are used extensively for budgets and the management of financial records, they are useful whenever calculations are needed. For example, a nursing information system could link to a spreadsheet that had ready-made drug calculation formulas available. To ensure accuracy of the output, this system should leave the full equation visible on the screen with the results. This would allow the nurse to check the input for accuracy, a "mission critical" factor in producing correct output.

The real power of a spreadsheet is not so much in its ability to organize and edit data but in its ability to recalculate when a number in a referenced cell is changed. A *referenced cell* is one that is included in a formula in another cell. For example, in Figure 6-6A, the cell F3 contains a formula. It references the cells B3, G3, and C3. Any changes made to the contents of any of these cells will cause the number in cell F3 to change. In a real spreadsheet, the result of the calculation, as shown in Figure 6-6B, would be apparent. The formula, however, would still be visible on the formula line.

CALCULATION CONSTANTS

The principles and symbols of formula calculation are identical in all computer programs. The characters used to communicate to the computer to perform a specific calculation, such as multiplying or dividing, are not, however, always the same as the ones used on paper. An asterisk (*), is used to denote multiplication. If the familiar × were used, the computer would be unable to distinguish whether the keystroke refers to a single precision variable or a symbol for multiplication. A command for the multiplication of 5 times 50 becomes 5*50. Assuming the numbers were in cells C3 and C5, the command becomes (C3*C5). To write this formula in a spreadsheet, enter the formula, preceded by either an equal sign (=), or the (@), depending on the vendor of the spreadsheet, for example, (=C3*C5) or (@C3*C5).

	A	B	C	D	E	F	G	H
1								
2		Desired Dose:	Have on Hand	=		Needed Volume	Volume on Hand	
3		80	100			= (B3 * G3) / C3	2	
4								

A

	A	B	C	D	E	F	G	H
1								
2		Desired Dose:	Have on Hand	=		Needed Volume	Volume on Hand	
3		80	100			1.6	2	
4								

B

Figure 6-6 • Referenced cells and formulas.

TABLE 6-2 • *Dividing in Spreadsheet*				
			Results	
Divide the number	**By**	**As an integer**	**Round to two decimals**	**Round to zero decimals**
29	5	5	5.80	6
32	6	5	5.33	5
Spreadsheet formula		INT (Formula)	ROUND (Formula, 2)	ROUND (Formula, 0)
Example		INT (B3*B5)	ROUND ((B3*B5), 2)	ROUND ((B3*B5), 0)

There is no divide key on the computer. To signal division, the computer uses the forward slash (/) (located under the question mark). For example, in telling the computer to divide 10 by 5, the command becomes 10/5. A formula entered for division looks like (=C3/B2) or (@C3/B2).

The results of division are not always an integer or whole number (Table 6-2). In a formula, specify whether the result is to be the integer (whole number) or to be rounded to a specified decimal place. Asking for just the integer or rounding to a given decimal place are two different operations, because the integer truncates or cuts off the fractional part of the answer and shows the largest whole number that is the result of dividing the two cells. Rounding produces accuracy to the decimal point specified.

To raise a number to another power, called *exponentiation*, use the caret (^), which is located over the 6. In telling the computer to raise 2 to the power of 4, the command looks like 2^4 (Table 6-3).

PRIORITY OF MATHEMATICAL OPERATIONS

In performing arithmetical computations, computers do not follow a strict left-to-right order. There are three factors that determine the order in which mathematical procedures will be performed:

▼ The kind of computation required
▼ Left-to-right placement of the expressions in the command
▼ Nesting, or the placing of an expression within parentheses

TABLE 6-3 • *Mathematical Operators*			
Symbol	**Function**	**Alternate**	**Example of formula***
-	Subtraction		= B3 - A1
+	Addition	SUM	= B2 + D5
*	Multiplication	PRODUCT	= D4 * A3
/	Division		= INT(C2/B1)
			= ROUND(C2/B1,2)
^	Exponentiation		= B4^2

*In some spreadsheets, the symbol @ is used instead of the = sign.

TABLE 6-4 ● *Acronym to Remember the Order in Which Computers Perform Calculations*					
Please	Excuse	My	Dear	Aunt	Sally
		Equal		Equal	
Parentheses	Exponentiation	Multiplication	Divison	Addition	Subtraction

The computer arbitrarily performs mathematical operations in the following order, regardless of where they are placed in a statement.

- ▼ Anything in parentheses is performed first
- ▼ Exponentiation is done next
- ▼ Multiplication and division follow
- ▼ Addition and subtraction are performed last

If there are ties (two commands to multiply, or one to multiply and one to divide), a left-to-right order prevails (Table 6-4). For example, in the expression 5+18–10, the 5 and 18 are added and then 10 is subtracted from the 23, for a result of 13. In the command 5+4*3, the multiplication of 4 by 3 would precede the addition of the 5. The result of this statement would be 17, not 27. But, if the expression employed parentheses, for instance, (5+4)*3, the operation inside the parentheses of 5+4 would be performed first, then the result of 9 would be multiplied by 3, for a result of 27. Additionally, parentheses can be nested if the rule that the procedure in the most inner set of parentheses will be performed first is followed. In the expression (3*(4+6))/2, the first thing the computer will do is add the 4 and 6, then multiply 10 by 3, divide the resulting 30 by 2, for an answer of 15.

These rules, which follow algebraic custom, are used in all application packages that allow calculations such as spreadsheets, statistical packages, and databases.

FORMULAS

Formulas in a spreadsheet are either relative or absolute (Fig. 6-7). A relative formula, which is the default, when copied to another cell, adjusts to the move by changing the referenced cells. An absolute formula retains the original cells when moved.

Errors can creep into a spreadsheet when entering cell addresses in a formula. To prevent this, spreadsheets provide a point-and-click method of entering cell addresses. After entering the symbol indicating that a formula is about to be entered, put the mouse pointer on the cell whose cell address is needed and click once with the left mouse button. The cell address appears in the formula. Enter the necessary mathematical symbol, then point and click at the next cell needed. When the formula is complete, tap the enter key.

To simplify the use of some common formulas, spreadsheets provide many that are already constructed. These are called *functions*.[4] When reading about functions,

---

[4]Be careful when entering functions. If a space is not placed after the function name and before the open parentheses, the function may not work.

	A	B	C	D
1				
2	·	24	48	B2 + C2
3		64	36	B3 + C3
4				

	A	B	C	D
1				
2		24	48	B2 + C2
3		64	36	B2 + C2
4				

A. Relative formula **B.** Absolute formula

Figure 6-7 ● In *A*, the formula in cell D2 was copied to cell D3. Because it was a relative formula, it automatically changed its contents from B2 + C2 to B3 + C3. In *B*, the formula in cell D2 has been designated an absolute formula. When copied to cell D3, the contents did not change.

the word argument is used. *Argument*, in computer instructions, means the data the user furnishes on which the program will perform the stated function. While setting up formulas to average some numbers, for instance, instructions in the help menu might read AVERAGE (argument1, argument2,...). This means that the user substitutes the numbers, or cells, wanted to average for argument 1, argument 2, and so on. The argument can be a number, a cell, or even a range. The parentheses are an integral part of the formula, and must not be omitted. Spreadsheets have many preprogrammed functions, including a wide variety that are statistical. The statistical functions beyond simple descriptive statistics are not as easy to use as those in a statistical package.

SOME ADDITIONAL FEATURES

Besides the normal functions that can be applied across the board in most Windows™ programs, spreadsheets possess some unique characteristics that require specialized functions.

Formatting Cells With Type of Contents

There are generally two different types of contents in a spreadsheet cell: text or numbers. Numbers, depending on what they reference, can be formatted in different ways. If a number represents a dollar amount, a dollar sign ($) may be added to the number. If the number is the result of division, it may be rounded to a given number of decimals. Or, the number may be represented as a percent (%). It is possible to have the computer automatically represent numbers the way the user desires. How this is done varies with vendors, but all require the cells to be formatted to be selected, then the attribute applied. Search the help menu with the word format to discover how to perform this task.

Freezing Headings

When the rows in a spreadsheet become too numerous to be viewed on one screen, it becomes difficult to know what the numbers in each cell represent. Spreadsheets provide a way to freeze the headings so they are always on the top of the screen. To learn how to accomplish this task, use help and search under the term windows, then depending on the vendor, select freeze windows or split window panes.

Automatic Entry of Data

In constructing a spreadsheet, there are times a user needs to have column headings that are used sequentially, such as the days of the week. Spreadsheets have a feature that allows the user to make a few entries and then have the computer complete the series. This function also works with numbers. It will even enter numbers that are not next to each other if the sequence increases or decreases by the same number (e.g., 2,4,6). This function is indexed in the help menu under automatic fill.

Database Functions

Spreadsheets are also capable of some database functions. A user can resort the order of a range of cells or the entire database, ask questions of the data, filter out unwanted items, and find specific items. As would be expected, none of the database functions are as robust as those in a true database, but they are functional for many noncomplicated operations. A spreadsheet, or any range of cells, is also easily exported to the companion database (program that is part of the same suite) for more extensive data manipulation. Any data that are structured in a table format, whether in a spreadsheet, a table in a word processor, a statistical package, or a database, can be easily passed from program to program.

Linking Cells From Other Sources

There are times when a value a user wants to include as part of a spreadsheet is in another workbook or another worksheet within the same workbook. It is very easy to use a cell as a value in another sheet or workbook, and this method is much less prone to error than trying to check the other sheet, copying the value, and entering it into a formula. When cells are linked, if the value in the linked cell changes, the change will be visible in the worksheet containing a reference to that cell. To use information from other worksheets or workbooks, check the help menu for linking.

Other Features

There are many other spreadsheet functions, such as data entry forms. When data need to be entered into a spreadsheet, a user can create a data entry form that will show only one row, called a *record*, at a time. Spreadsheet forms, however, compared with database forms, are minimally functional. In addition, printouts can be dressed up with headers, page numbers, and page breaks in printouts, just like in word processing.

SPREADSHEETS AS DECISION MODELS

A natural tendency with spreadsheets is to regard them as an elaborate calculator and forget that the power of having all referenced cells recalculate after a change permits one to test different theories. Spreadsheets also provide other features to allow testing theories or solving problems. A cell with a formula, for instance, can be set so the value in a referenced cell will change to produce a given value. This is useful when the answer needed is known but requires working backwards to find it.

TIPS FOR BETTER SPREADSHEETS

Designing a spreadsheet that effectively communicates does not happen with a casual approach. If spreadsheets are to be useful, they need to be well organized. If one is designing a complex sheet, a table of contents should be included. Explanations of any logic or assumptions can also be included on the first worksheet. If others will be using the spreadsheet, clear instructions and labels are imperative. Users of computer items rarely have the same viewpoint as the creator. For complex formulas, especially those that reference the results of formulas, test the formula with simple numbers, particularly if the spreadsheet will be used with many different values.

Another helpful organizing trick is always to start different blocks or sections on a worksheet at the right lower corner of the previous block or place it on another worksheet. This allows rows and columns to be inserted within a block without changing any other block. Above all, keep the spreadsheet as simple as possible. Organize work by using different worksheets in a workbook instead of placing everything on the same sheet. Probably the most helpful tool is to spend time planning a spreadsheet before the computer is even turned on. It is easier to make changes before any data has been entered than after a user has laboriously worked something through.

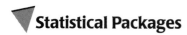 Statistical Packages

A statistical package takes data and performs the math required for a statistical test in a fraction of the time that it would take a user to write down the formula. Statistical packages allow users to manipulate data, such as reversing the data for a variable—for example, taking all fives and making them ones while making all ones into fives. It is also possible to write formulas that make other data changes.

STATISTICAL PACKAGE SCREENS

There are two screens in statistical software: the data screen and the output screen (Fig. 6-8). The data screen resembles a spreadsheet. The toolbar does not have the new document icon because a statistical package only allows one file to be open at a time. When a statistical test is performed, a document is created that is visible on the output screen. The document is cumulative, or in other words, the results of each statistical test are added to the document. The document in the output file can be printed, or it can be saved to a file. It is also possible to edit this file by selecting and deleting items. In some packages, although the file itself is in a proprietary format, it can be exported to an ASCII format, in which case it can be opened and edited by any word processor or text editor.

VOCABULARY

The vocabulary of statistical packages is identical to that for research. Before doing statistics, whether manually or with a computer, the user must be clear about the difference between independent and dependent variables. The user also must know

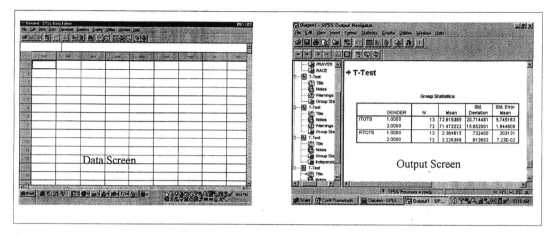

Figure 6-8 • Data and output screens for SPSS, a statistical package.

what statistical tests are appropriate for the level of data, as well as the probability level that will satisfy the hypothesis.

TIPS FOR BEST USE

A statistical package will perform a given test when it believes that it has the appropriate information regardless of whether that test is a valid or invalid test for the hypothesis the user is testing. For example, if asked, a statistical test will provide an average, standard deviation, and variance for identification numbers, as well as test for differences or correlation if the user gives it another variable that meets the conditions of the test. The results, however, will be meaningless. There is no substitute for understanding the requirements of the statistical test needed and the assumptions.

▼ Charts

A chart is a graphical presentation of a set of numbers. Charts are used to communicate meaning that can be difficult to surmise from a raw set of numbers. Creating charts with a computer is relatively easy. Like statistical packages, a computer will produce any type of chart, whether it communicates anything meaningful or not. Using charts appropriately involves knowing what is meant to be communicated and selecting the type of chart that best accomplishes this aim.

Although word processors, databases, presentation packages, and spreadsheets all facilitate the creation of charts, spreadsheets in many cases, have the most powerful tools. Perhaps the biggest plus for creating charts in a spreadsheet is that if the numbers in the cells used to create the chart change, the chart automatically reflects this change.

VOCABULARY

To construct a meaningful chart, it is necessary to understand the vocabulary. Table 6-5 and Figure 6-11 can assist in this task.

TABLE 6-5 • *Chart Vocabulary*	
Term	**Meaning**
X axis	The horizontal axis (line) of a bar, line, or scatter graph; generally represents time values, categories, or divisions
Y axis	The vertical axis (line) of a bar, line, or scatter graph; most often used to represent amounts
Data	A number without meaning; one that is unprocessed
Data series or set	A set of numbers that will be represented in the chart, usually on the y axis, or a group of items that will be represented on the X axis
Axis title	The title for the information displayed on an axis
Graph title	A description of the graph used to title the graph
Legend	The visual representation of the data series. May be a color, shape, or both
Data point	The point where a number is plotted. It is the intersection of its value on the X and Y axis.
Data labels	Labels that show the actual value of a specific data, or the data points
Two-dimensional charts	A chart that represents data on the X and Y axis. (See Fig. 6-9)
Three-dimensional charts	A chart that adds a third axis, referred to as the Z axis. Can be very misleading; use only when it communicates an added dimension. (See Fig. 6-10)

TYPES AND THEIR USES

Computer application programs allow the creation of many different types of charts. The first task in creating any chart is to select the cells that represent the data to be charted.

Once the appropriate cells have been selected, click on the chart tool, place the mouse pointer on the cell in the spreadsheet where the chart is to start, and drag until an area is created that is large enough for the chart. The size can always be changed later, so the exact dimensions chosen are unimportant. In fact, it may need to be resized to allow all of the labels to be visible. Once an area for the chart is se-

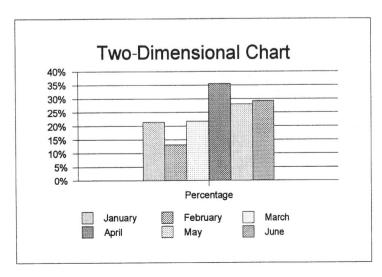

Figure 6-9 • Two-dimensional chart.

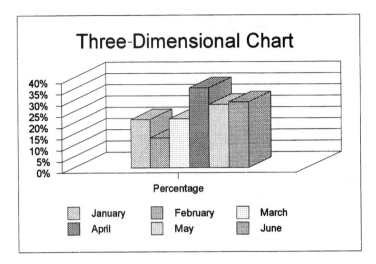

Figure 6-10 • Three-dimensional chart.

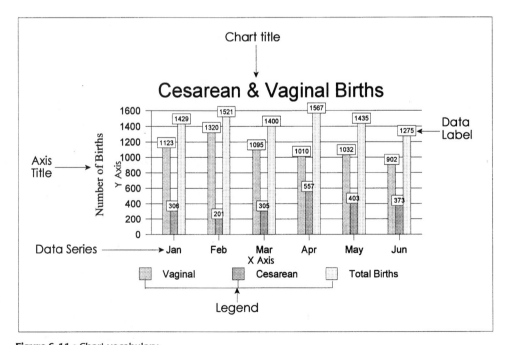

Figure 6-11 • Chart vocabulary.

lected, the next steps depend on the program. All, however, allow the selection of types of charts, placement of labels on the axis, and editing.

Pies

Pie graphs are used to communicate the proportion of various items in relation to the whole. They are designed to show percentages, not amounts. A pie may also be used to show a proportional relationship between a slice and the whole. The different pies in Figure 6-12 were designed to show what percentage of care was being delivered by each of three categories of nursing personnel—RNs, LPNs, and NAs. Notice that the numbers represent percentages, not numerical amounts.

There are variations that can be used in all charts. They do not, however, always add to communication. Look at the three-dimensional chart in Figure 6-12. The bottom wedge appears to be the most important, as does the wedge that is exploded in the right most pie (Jones, 1995). If one is using these variations, be certain that they reflect the point to be communicated. If one is reading these charts, be aware that distortions can be produced by pies that are either three dimensional or have a wedge exploded.

Donut Charts

A close cousin of the pie chart is a donut chart. The donut chart allows the comparison of percentages for one item against those of another. In Figure 6-13, the donut chart shows the percentage of births each month that were cesarean or vaginal deliveries. The inside loop is January, and the outside loop is June.

XY Charts

Charts constructed with an X and a Y axis are the most common types. The most common types of XY charts are bar and line charts. No matter which type is used, there are conventions that, when they are adhered to, create the best charts. Placing amounts on the Y axis meets the common expectation that an upward movement is associated with an increase in amount, whereas down movement indicates a decrease. When the X axis is used for the passage of time, the best communication is achieved when the earliest time is placed on the left and followed to the right. To pre-

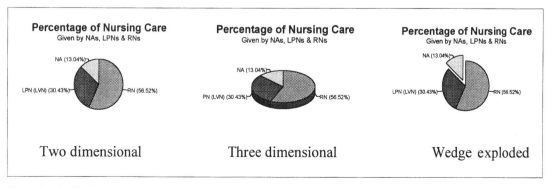

Figure 6-12 ● Pie charts.

	Vaginal	Cesarean	Total Births
Jan	1223	282	1505
Feb	1372	197	1569
Mar	1205	287	1492
Apr	1010	623	1633
May	1032	502	1534
Jun	902	402	1304

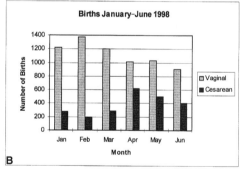

Figure 6-13 • Donut chart of data.

vent a distortion of value, it is best if the Y axis starts with a zero. If this approach is not followed, include an explanation with the chart.

Bar Charts. Bar charts are generally associated with comparisons of amounts. Figure 6-14*A* is a bar chart that uses data to depict the total number of births in each month for the first 6 months of 1998. The goal was to compare the number of births each month with other months. If instead of comparisons of totals a user wanted to show

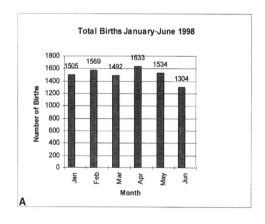

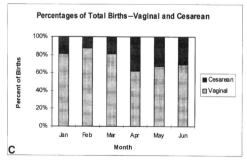

Figure 6-14 • *A*, a simple bar chart. *B*, bar chart showing comparisons. *C*, 100% bar chart.

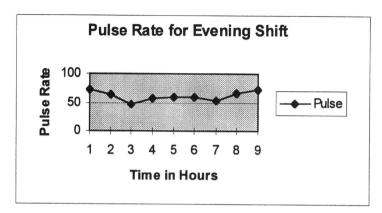

Figure 6-15 ● Line chart of pulse rate.

comparisons between the percentage of vaginal and cesarean births for each month, a 100% bar chart (Fig. 6-14C) would be the appropriate choice. Although a pie graph would clearly show these percentages for 1 month, when making comparisons with different months, a 100% bar chart is superior to a series of pie graphs. Like the donut, the 100% bar chart allots a space on the bar proportional to the percentage of the whole that the item represents.

Line Charts. Line charts also show amounts, but their emphasis is on communicating changes in data over a time period, as opposed to comparisons represented by a bar chart. Vital signs plotted on a graphics sheet is an example of a line chart. Figure 6-15 is an example of the use of a simple line chart to depict the pulse rate of a patient over a period of 9 hours.

It is also possible to place more than one series of data on a line. Figure 6-16 contains a data set that is the result of three tests that were performed on the same subject. Also contained in this figure is a line graph depicting these sets. Which do you think communicates the rise in test scores best, the table or the line graph?

CASE	TEST 1	TEST 2	TEST 3
A	46	57	64
B	38	64	70
C	53	69	82
D	43	57	70
E	54	72	86
F	43	62	81
G	47	66	81
H	49	66	76
I	57	65	72
J	31	40	49

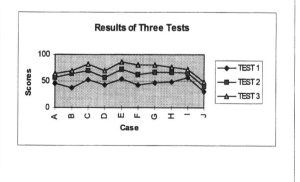

Figure 6-16 ● Line graphs of three data sets.

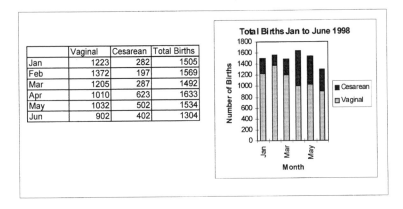

	Vaginal	Cesarean	Total Births
Jan	1223	282	1505
Feb	1372	197	1569
Mar	1205	287	1492
Apr	1010	623	1633
May	1032	502	1534
Jun	902	402	1304

Figure 6-17 • Stacked bars.

Stacked Charts. In a stacked chart, as seen in Figure 6-17, only the first data set starts at zero. The next data set uses the previous one as its baseline. Stacked bar charts (Fig. 6-18) and area charts (Fig. 6-19) are both examples of stacked charts.

If there is no understanding of how the chart is constructed, or if it is used for the wrong purpose, misconceptions will result. Figure 6-18, constructed from the salary data in the figure, could give the impression that RNs start at $37 an hour instead of $17. Instead of providing information on individual salaries, the chart emphasizes totals for each level and as a whole. It is not very helpful because it has little relationship to anything, unless the mix of nursing staff per hour is one level-1 RN to one level-1 LPN to one level-1 NA, an uncommon situation. In this case, it would depict costs per hour for this team.

If area graphs show more than one data set, they are usually stacked. Figure 6-19 shows a stacked area graph of the data in the figure. If there is no understanding that this is a stacked graph, it may be concluded that the number of cesareans exceeds the number of vaginal births for each month. If it is interpreted correctly, the number of cesareans is seen as increased from April to June, but the 100% area graph probably

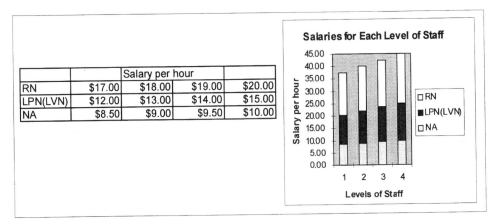

		Salary per hour		
RN	$17.00	$18.00	$19.00	$20.00
LPN(LVN)	$12.00	$13.00	$14.00	$15.00
NA	$8.50	$9.00	$9.50	$10.00

Figure 6-18 • Data and stacked chart for salary levels.

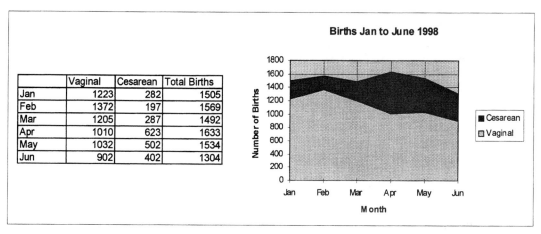

	Vaginal	Cesarean	Total Births
Jan	1223	282	1505
Feb	1372	197	1569
Mar	1205	287	1492
Apr	1010	623	1633
May	1032	502	1534
Jun	902	402	1304

Figure 6-19 • Area graph of births per month.

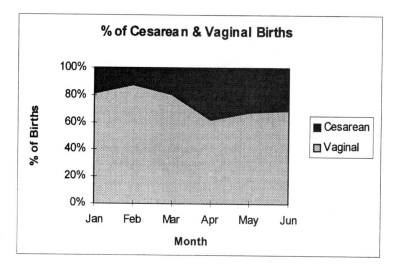

Figure 6-20 • 100% Area line graph.

depicts this more eloquently (Fig 6-20). Like the 100% bar chart, a 100% area graph is analogous to a pie graph, in that it shows percentages.

▼ Summary

Although they make it easy to do calculations, computers can also perform miscalculations. When using a spreadsheet, it is crucial that the user check formulas and input data. A small error in one place can result in a massive error in another.

Spreadsheets have many uses outside of accounting. Their greatest advantage is their ability to recalculate when a number in a referenced cell is changed. Besides budgeting or other numerical tasks, spreadsheets are helpful in creating decision

TABLE 6-6 ● *Summary of Purposes for Charts*			
Chart	**Regular**	**Stacked/Area**	**100%**
Pie	Proportions		Is a 100% chart
Donut	Proportional comparisons		Is several 100% charts
Bar	Comparisons of amounts	Comparisons and totals of amounts	Comparisons of percentages of amounts
Line	Change over time	Comparisons of changes over time	Percentage of comparisons over time

models. When using a spreadsheet in decision making, it is important that the assumptions on which the model is based be known. Like entering erroneous numbers, incorrect assumptions can also create massive errors.

Statistical packages can be used in performing statistical tests and as a learning tool in grasping the true meaning behind a statistical test. When they are well done, charts can communicate more effectively than raw numbers. The various types of charts, in addition, deliver some points better than others. Deciding the objective and selecting a chart based on this, will ensure that audiences can grasp the intended meaning (Table 6-6).

Although the programs discussed in this chapter make managing numbers easier, if they are not used carefully, they can create great misinformation. As with all computer use, nurses and other health care professionals should use common sense when interpreting computer numerical output. This includes understanding the assumptions that various models use. Given thoughtful use, software that calculates numbers can assist all health care professionals in managing information.

EXERCISES

1. In a spreadsheet, create a formula to calculate the number of intravenous (IV) drops per minute when given the IV tubing calibration rate, the time for the infusion, and the total volume to be infused.

2. Calculate the answer as a computer would to the following:
   a. 4*2+3
   b. 8+2*3
   c. 5+10/5
   d. (5+10)/5
   e. 3+22
   f. ((6+4)*3)/15
   g. 10/2*3

3. Write formulas that will
   a. Multiply 3 times the sum of 8+4
   b. Raise 2 to the power of 5, then multiply by 5 and divide by 10
   c. Multiply the sum of 4+5 times the sum of 3+6
   d. Tell you the highest whole number possible if 2020 is divided by 23.
   e. Round 25 divided by 3 to two decimals.

4. What are some ways that you see spreadsheets being used by health care professionals in
   a. Clinical practice?
   b. Administration?
   c. Education?
   d. Research?
   e. Entrepreneurial work?

5. You have data that represents the number of falls in one unit of a long-term care facility for a 6-month period and the amounts of sedatives that have been administered.
   a. You wish to communicate that the number of falls has decreased in this 6-month period. What type of chart would you select?
   b. You wish to communicate that the decrease in the number of falls parallels the decrease in the amounts of sedatives given. What type of chart will you select?

REFERENCE

Jones, G. E. (1995). *How to lie with charts.* San Francisco: Sybex.

CHAPTER 7

Presentation Software

Objectives:

After studying this chapter you should be able to:

1 State and define the features that presentation software packages provide

2 Describe some uses of presentation programs

3 Apply principles of good design in creating visuals

Nurses and students give many presentations, sometimes informally, often before a group. Feeling confident in this endeavor is something that comes with practice. Having good visuals to facilitate the understanding of your message can help this growth. Using visuals not only adds interest to a presentation but improves the retention rate. Studies have shown that visual presentations have a retention rate of 70% versus only 30% for oral presentations (Lakoumentas, 1996). Today, presentation software can help produce high-quality visuals and give the user a professional edge.

A very effective and easy way of adding visuals to a presentation is to create projected visuals, or those in which the image is broadcast onto a screen. A lighted screen has the ability to rivet the attention of an audience, making it easier for them to receive the message. Projected visuals include overhead transparencies, 35-mm slides, and computer projected slides. When using a form of projected transparency, speakers are perceived as better prepared, groups are more likely to be reach consensus, and people are more likely to act on recommendations.

Presentation software assists in communicating information by making it easier to create visuals. The software simplifies the creation of visuals by presenting the user with templates that facilitate building the major types of visuals. If one creates computer slides or visuals that are displayed using a computer and some type of computer screen projection device, it is also possible to add film clips, sound, movie-like transitions between slides, and animation, and to create a show that runs unattended. Some of the more common presentation packages are Corel's Presentations™, Lotus' Freelance™, Software Publishing Corporation's Harvard Graphics™, and Microsoft's Power Point™.

◤ Basics of Presentation Software

Each brand of presentation software, as well as specific versions within one brand, vary in how things are accomplished, yet all packages have more similarities than dissimilarities. Although the packages allow the creation of drawings, the slide show portion of the package is based on the premise that a series of visuals is being created. These visuals are referred to as *slides*, and the entire product is called a *slide show*. The series of slides creates one file, which makes up the presentation.

Despite naming the visuals slides, they are not limited to producing only slides. It is possible to develop 35-mm or computer slides, transparencies, or even a booklet. Essentially, presentation programs have many of the same graphics capabilities of other application programs, such as word processors and spreadsheets, but add many more features. To facilitate the creation of a series of visuals, presentation programs consist of different layers that the user manipulates independently. This concept differs from other application programs in which the user works with only one layer. The three layers are a background layer, a layout layer, and an editing layer, on which text or images are added (Fig. 7-1). The user can make a change to any of the layers without affecting the other two.

BACKGROUNDS

One of the first choices a user makes when creating a slide show is the background. The programs differ on what they call this layer. One may call it a template, another a master. Presentation programs come with a variety of background choices that the user can either accept as is or modify. Some of the backgrounds may have images on them that, although they are interesting, may get in the way of the message to be

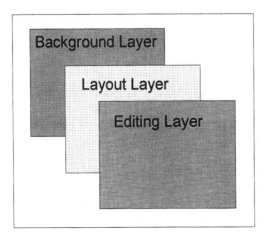

Figure 7-1 • Three layers of a slide.

communicated. There is usually a way to eliminate the objects on the background for either one slide or all the slides. Some programs make this easier than others.

When deciding about an appropriate background, select one that allows the visual to focus on the message. The effect of color combinations needs to be considered. If one is making either computer or 35-mm slides, select a dark background. For transparencies or a paper-based presentation, use white. A constant background helps hold presentations together, which is the reason the programs make it somewhat complicated to change backgrounds for only one or two slides.[1] If after creating slides, it is discovered that the background is not suitable, it can be changed for all the slides without changing any of the slide contents. Changing the background may, however, affect how the various layouts and text are positioned; therefore, it is necessary to check all slides after changing the background.

INDIVIDUAL SLIDE LAYOUT

Although in a visual production the background should be constant, the message the user wishes to convey on each individual slide often necessitates a different positioning of the objects (pieces of text and images) that make up the slide. For example, the first slide in a visual presentation is often a title slide. On this slide, the title should predominate, although one's name and credentials may also be included. A slide with bullet points pertaining to the presentation may be next. To facilitate the construction of such slides, presentation software provides a set of ready made templates, or layouts, from which the user selects. The variety of different layouts varies from program to program, but there are generally preformatted layouts for a title slide, bulleted slide, text slide, and organizational slide (Fig. 7-2). There is also the ability to select a slide with no preformatting and to remove the background.

Once a layout is selected, directions for entering text appears on the screen. Text is usually entered into rectangles or what is known as a *text box*. Although you see the rectangles while creating the slide, you may leave any of them blank; these rectangles will not be seen when the slide is shown or printed (Fig. 7-3). Each layout has a preselected text font and size, but these features are modifiable.

EDITING THE SLIDE

Using the preformatted layout does not preclude the user from adding additional text or images anywhere on the slide. When adding objects, remember that the point of visuals is to communicate a message to the audience. A little variety, especially when it adds to the message can be helpful, but be careful not to distract the audience.

If entering text without making any changes to the preformatted layout, use the *outline view*, which depicts a screen with the text for several slides. Some programs let the user select the type of layout for the outline format; others have predetermined that all slides created with the outline view will be in the bulleted format. The outline

---

[1]It is relatively easy, however, to have no background, which is something you may wish to do when you are displaying a picture or other image.

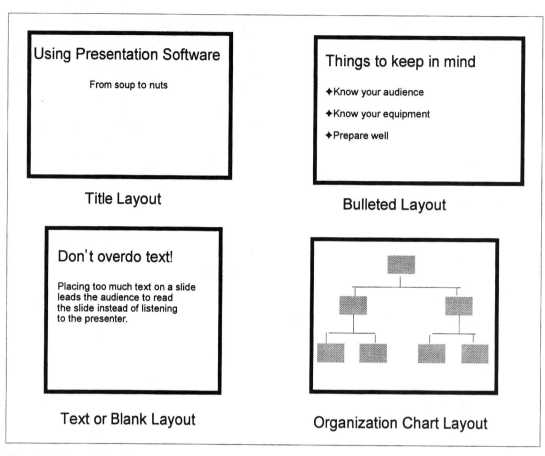

Figure 7-2 • Layouts for slides.

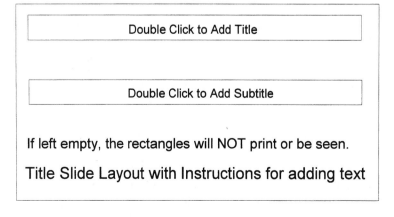

Figure 7-3 • Title layout as it appears when creating a slide.

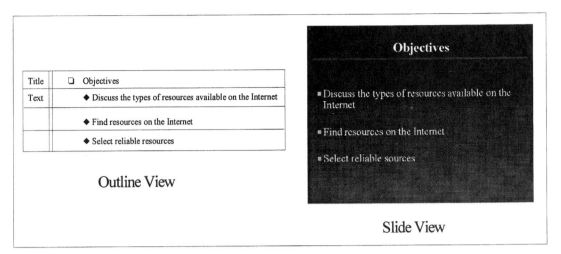

Figure 7-4 • Outline and slide views of same slide.

view does not limit the amount of text that can be entered. When entering text in the outline view, switch to the *full screen view* to be sure all of the text fits on the screen. The full slide view displays slides for the entire presentation (Fig. 7-4).

Entering the text for slides in the outline view follows the same principles as using the outline function in a word processing program. Tapping the enter key allows the user to enter the next point, tapping the tab key will create the appropriate mark for the next lower level, and tapping shift-tab creates the appropriate delineation for the next highest level. Using the outline view does not preclude one from using the full slide view to either adding objects or editing the slide.

SPECIAL EFFECTS

Although one can add special effects independent of the visuals, those that are made possible by presentation software are generally available only when the computer is used for the presentation. In this format, it is possible to add sound, video, animation, and transitions. A show can also be planned in which the slides are not displayed in a given order. When doing a computer slide show, especially when using special effects such as sound and video clips, the complete presentation should be tested using the equipment that will be used during the actual presentation.

Sound

Sound can be added by recording it using a microphone attached to the computer and special software, or through a *sound file*.[2] Some sound files can be found on the

---

[2]A sound file is sound that is recorded. Creating a sound file is done similarly to recording sound on a tape recorder, except that the sound is recorded on a computer disk as a file.

Internet, whereas others can be purchased in a software package. Once the file is selected, follow the directions prescribed by the presentation package you are using to attach the sound to a slide.

Video

Video clips are equally easy to insert. The video, however, must be in digital format instead of the analog of ordinary video tape. Conversions of analog tape can be done, or cameras that record directly to the computer can be used. If one is planning to add video, limit its length to 45 to 60 seconds; more than that distracts the audience. As with sound, before using video in a presentation, check the equipment. Have a copy of the presentation without video in case the video portion of the presentation equipment fails on the day of the presentation.

Transitions

A transition is the way a slide makes its entrance. There are many different types of transitions. Some scenes fade in, some appear first at the center, then expand the view, and others sweep across the screen. These types of transitions and more are available in presentation software. Transitions can be dramatic, enhance your message, or distract the audience. The best rule is to use them sparingly.

Animation

The term animation is used somewhat optimistically in the more well-known presentation software. Generally, animation takes the form of progressive disclosure. Progressive disclosure is a technique in which you reveal one item on a slide at a time until all the items are displayed. When revealing bulleted points, for instance, those that have been discussed can be dimmed or converted to a different color while the current point has center stage.

There are also many options for how items will be revealed. Some of these options are for the item to slide in from any direction, bounce in, fade in, or even curve in. Like all the options, this feature should be used judiciously. Progressive disclosure can be used with 35-mm slides and transparencies but requires a different slide for each point.

NONLINEAR PRESENTATION ON THE COMPUTER

When giving a presentation, it is necessary to be somewhat flexible. Some audiences may ask questions, whereas others do not. A presenter can also misjudge the time. If using the computer for a presentation, these eventualities can be handled easily. Depending on the program, the presenter can prepare a hidden slide to show if a specific question is asked or if there is extra time.

CHARTS AND TABLES

A table or chart is often more explicit in communicating meaning than text. Presentation software provides the ability to create or import a chart from other programs. Some also allow the creation of a table. Additionally, presentation software provides the ability to import data directly from a spreadsheet.

SPEAKER NOTES

Speaker notes are text entered while designing the slide. Although the notes are not seen on the slide, they are connected to the slide in a way that allows them to be printed for use either as notes during the presentation, when rehearsing, or for handouts.

VIEWING THE PRESENTATION

In addition to the outline view and the full slide view, another helpful way of seeing the presentation as a whole is the *slide sorter view* (Fig. 7-5). With this function, several slides can be seen at the same time. In the slide sorter view you can move, insert, copy, edit, or delete slides. Playing the slide show and printing the slide show are other ways to review the presentation.

THE FINISHED SHOW

Once the slide show is completed, there are several alternatives. If it is a 35-mm slide show, there are many ways the file can be transferred to slides. Which method is used depends on the options available. Some institutions provide an in-house slide devel-

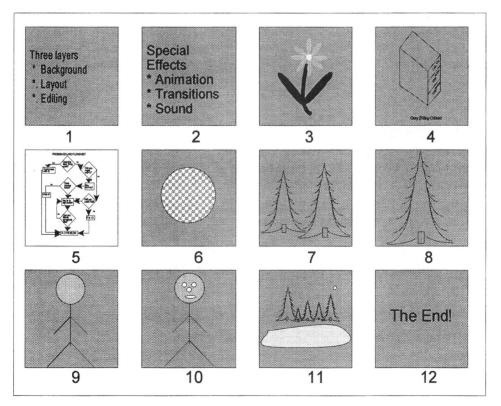

Figure 7-5 • Slide sorter view.

opment service that take the file and create the slides. Commercial slide services are also available. They may even accept the file by modem.

If one is planning to show the slides as a computer show, presentation programs provide two options. First, open the program and play the slides, or second, compile the show so it will play on a computer that does not have the program that was used to create the show installed. If one is planning to present the slide show on a different computer, be certain that the file does not get too big to move. The size of the file varies with the number of slides, but it varies even more so with their contents. Adding images of any size increases the size of a slide. Additionally, if one is compiling a show, the resulting file can be two or three times the size of the original file. The size of the file a user can move is depends on the mode of transfer. If using 1.4-megabyte, 3.5-inch diskettes, the file size must be less than 1.4 megabytes. If using a Zip™ or Jaz™ drive, a problem is not likely to occur.

SPECIAL FEATURES OF USING THE COMPUTER FOR A PRESENTATION

If you show the slides on a computer, there is the option of using the mouse to write on your slides during the presentation. This writing only shows as long as the slide is viewed. If in the presentation you return again to this slide, the writing will not appear. Some programs also provide the ability to use the mouse pointer as an arrow.

Depending on your purpose, the slides can be designed so that the presenter advances them while speaking. They can also be set to advance after a stated time length, or to start again when the slide show is finished. The latter type of presentation may be used in waiting rooms, or under conditions in which the audience is expected to view and move on.

▼ Projection Equipment

The biggest limitation to your decision on what type of visuals to make is the equipment available for the presentation. Overhead projectors are almost standard equipment, whereas slide projectors are a harder to obtain. Although they becoming more common, projectors for computer screens are less familiar.

Computer projectors are devices connected to the monitor output of the computer. This connection is easy to make; the cables are designed so that the user cannot attach the computer and projector incorrectly.[3] Most laptops today are designed so one can toggle between having the image only on the computer screen, only on the projector, or in both places. Some projectors allow remote control of the slide show. Two things that need to be considered when selecting a means of projection are the light source and the resolution of the projector. Most projectors have a standard 640 by 480 dot resolution, although high-resolution projectors with 1024 by

---

[3]It is possible, however, to mistake output for input on the projector, the result of which is that you will be informed that there is no signal. Just unplug the device, and move it to the input port.

768 dot resolution can be purchased. Many monitors now use a higher resolution, which can create a problem when used with a lower resolution projector. Some can transform an 800 by 600 dot resolution to a 640 by 480, and some cannot.

LCD PROJECTORS

The least expensive computer projector is a liquid crystal display (LCD) panel. This panel is similar to the LCD screen in a laptop computer. It is about the size of a small atlas and primarily consists of two glass plates with some liquid crystal material between them. It is connected to the computer and placed on top of the stage of an overhead projector, which provides the light source. When they are connected, the computer sends visual output to the LCD, and the overhead projector casts the image just as it would an overhead transparency. Some LCD panels weigh as little as 5½ pounds, although most weigh around 8 or 9 pounds. One disadvantage to an LCD panel is lack of brightness, although this characteristic is being improved. Because the LCD panel itself absorbs some of the light, they require an overhead projector that is capable of putting out 3000 to 4000 lumens of light.

COMPUTER SCREEN PROJECTOR

A computer screen projector, sometimes called a multimedia projector, has its own built-in light source and transmits a computer screen in a manner similar to a slide projector. They are somewhat larger than a slide projector, and weigh about 10 to 20 pounds. Some are also capable of projecting from VCRs, and others have either external or built in speakers to augment any computer sound output. Some projectors, especially those with a weaker light source, do not project well in a lighted room, especially one lighted with sunlight. If the resolution of the projector is lower than the computer with which it will be used, the result may be fuzzy slides.

USING A TELEVISION PROJECTOR OR MONITOR

An overhead video projector in an auditorium or other large room may, especially if it has been purchased within the last few years, be capable of projecting computer output. Many newer television sets now have connectors for a computer. A scan converter, however, is needed to complete the transition from television set to computer screen. This solution is the least desirable, because the resulting image is not as crisp and clear as with a computer projector and it may flicker.

▼ Other Considerations in Deciding What Type of Visual to Create

The expense of creating 35-mm slides for a one-time-only presentation may be extravagant. If a user does not have access to computer projection equipment, transparencies can still do an excellent job in one time situations. If a user does have access to a computer and projector, computer slides are the least expensive visual.

If patient education is a frequent part of your job, a computer slide show may become a helpful adjunct to teaching (Table 7-1). It can be designed for use when teaching, for the client to use alone, or to run independently in a waiting room. Hard copy of the contents can also be given to the client, either as the slides alone or with a copy of the speaker notes.

PRINCIPLES OF GOOD VISUAL CONSTRUCTION

Visuals generally consist of text, images, or both. Following certain concepts ensures that visuals add to the presentation rather than detract. In designing visuals, the main goal is for the audience to grasp the meaning and for the visual to be pleasing to the eye.

Text

When placing text on visuals, include only the essential elements of concepts (Fig. 7-6). State your idea as though you were writing a headline. A visual is not meant to give the entire idea but to serve as a focus to assist the audience in following your presentation. Visuals are also helpful to the presenter as a guide to the oral presentation.

Audiences should be able to get the point of the visual within the first 5 seconds after it appears. It is argued that a presenter should be quiet for those 5 seconds to allow the audience to grasp the point (Radel, 1997). To accomplish this, it is necessary to limit the text. One way to determine whether you have too much information on a visual image is to place the information on a four by six card and try to read it from a distance of about 5 to 6 feet.

Never write the presentation on a series of slides that are intended to be read to the audience. Audiences can read faster than a speaker can talk and may become torn between reading ahead and listening (Radel, 1997). This practice also leads the speaker to pay more attention to the slides than to the audience.

Thoughts on text on visuals

1. The 5 to 7 rule
    a. Limit text to 5 to 7 lines per slide
    b. Limit words to 5 to 7 per line
2. Use sans-serif fonts
3. Font size should be at least 24 for slides, 18 for visuals
4. To emphasize a point
    a. Boldface or underline
    b. Change the color (be consistent)
5. Use upper and lower case letters; all upper case letters takes longer to read

---

Figure 7-6 • Principles for text visuals.

TABLE 7-1 • Attributes Available for Visuals

Task	Computer slides	Transparencies	35-mm slides
Number of slides	Make as many as you wish. If the slides will be shown on another computer consider how you will move the file.	Consider the cost of the transparency.	Limit number to keep costs down.
Transitions between slides	Movie-like transitions easily achieved. Consider effect on audience when using.	Not available	Not available
Progressive revelation (showing same slide, one point at a time)	Done with animation; can highlight current point	Available with the creation of extra transparencies and use of overlays.	Available with the creation of extra slides
Graphics	You can use clip art, scanned images, images from the Internet, or anything you create. (Consider copyright.)		
Colors	Be sure that there is a vivid contrast between text and background. Keep colors constant, e.g., if using yellow for highlighting in one slide, use in all for the same thing.		
	Test colors on the computer and projection device you will use to show.	Only available with a color printer. Keep text dark to allow for light background. Test with projector.	Know how the colors will translate to slides.
Sound	With sound card and speaker in either computer or projector	Only available independently	Only available independently
Video	Can be added to a slide	Only available independently	Only available independently
Font size	24-point minimum	Should be at least 1/4 of an inch (18 point for most fonts), better is 3/16 (24 point). You should be able to read from a standing position if placed on floor over a white page.	24-point minimum
Font types	One per slide; best to be consistent throughout the presentation	No more than three different types on one transparency	One per slide; best to be consistent throughout the presentation
Font attributes	Use bold to emphasize. Use italics to make audience pause; they are more difficult to read. All caps are harder to read than upper and lower case.		
Speaker notes	Can be created to match each slide. These can be printed out with the slides for your use, or as a handout.		
Preparing to show	Create a run time version. Can then be shown on any computer without the need to have the program that created it on the computer.	Print out.	The file can be taken to a slide maker as is, or a "printer" driver such as Winslide can be used to convert the file so a slide can be made from it.

An advantage and disadvantage of presentation packages is the number of fonts available, many of which are unsuitable for text in a projected visual. The templates for various visuals have preselected fonts, but it is possible to change these styles. Depending on the presentation package and the change, switching a font for one slide may or may not change the font for the entire presentation. When making a selection, remember that fonts can elicit an emotional response from the audience; thus, choose one that is not only visually appealing but one that elicits the desired response. If it is a factual presentation, keep the font simple. In a small group, you may select a font that you believe is more personal.

Some fonts have projections called serifs that are fine strokes across the ends of the main strokes of a character. Serifs create softer edges to the characters, which adds to readability on paper. When they are projected, they may have a tendency to look fuzzy (*Using fonts*, Undated). For projected visuals use a sans serif (without serifs) font such as Arial (Fig. 7-7). This font follows the basic rule in choosing a display font—that the letters be crisp and clean.

The appearance of text can be altered with attributes other than the type of font. Adding boldface text is one way to emphasize a point, as are underlining and italicizing. Italicizing, however, tends to make text more difficult to read; if you use it, give the audience more time to read the slide. If you choose to emphasize a point or points with any of the above-mentioned attributes, be consistent throughout the presentation—that is, use the same attribute for the same type of information throughout.

Text size is measured in points. Most printed documents are either 10 or 12 points. In making transparencies, do not use any font that makes the printed text smaller than ¼ inch. Thus, the smallest font that can be used in making transparencies is 18 points. For computer or 35-mm slides, the smallest readable text size is 24 points. Point size, however, is not always an accurate guide. Some fonts at 12 points, despite being one-sixth of an inch in height, are very difficult to read. This is due to what is called the *x factor*, or the height of lower case letters. The deciding criterion to use in determining font type, size, and attributes is clarity (Fig. 7-8).

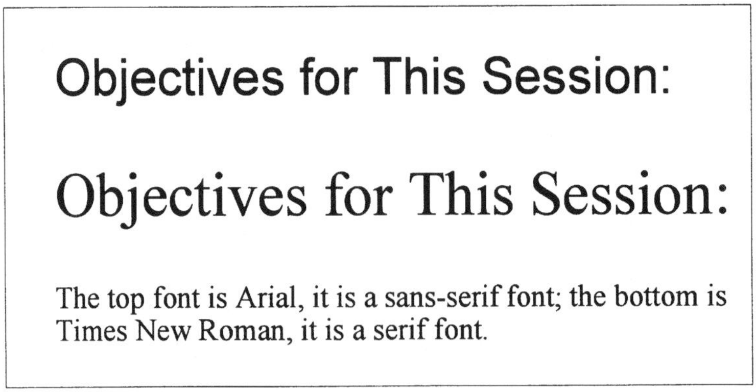

Objectives for This Session:

Objectives for This Session:

The top font is Arial, it is a sans-serif font; the bottom is Times New Roman, it is a serif font.

Figure 7-7 • Comparison of sans-serif and serif fonts.

Font	Comparison
Ribbon at 12 points Times New Roman at 12 points Arial at 12 points	*Presentation Skills* Presentation Skills Presentation Skills
Ribbon at 16 points **Times New Roman at 16 points** **Arial at 16 points**	*Presentation Skills* Presentation Skills **Presentation Skills**

Figure 7-8 • Different fonts in the same point size.

Color

Although we all like color, its use in increasing learning is inconclusive. Results favoring either monochrome or color occur with about equal frequency, although learners generally prefer the use of color (Levie & Dickie, 1973). Its use, however, in getting the attention of an audience is a different matter. To use it effectively, one needs to consider two factors—when to use different colors and what colors to use.

Different colors can be used to draw attention to a feature. When colors are combined with the progressive disclosure feature, they are especially effective. As with fonts, it is important to be consistent in using color. Once an audience grasps the meaning of a given color, the visuals are more easily comprehended. Use different colors sparingly and with a motive of drawing viewer attention.

Color, like text fonts, also has an emotional appeal. Red is exciting, whereas green is calming. Although the eye can perceive millions of colors, screen colors should be limited to about six, which are all that the eye can track at one glance (Faioloa & De-Bloois, 1988). Color should not only be used consistently but to heighten attention, as a cuing device to emphasize items, or for contrast to highlight items (Carter-Goodrum, 1996).

Color combinations should be selected that are compatible and that offer a contrast. Generally, colors on the opposite side of the color wheel offer the most contrast and an increase in reading accuracy. The highest reading accuracy was reported for blue or green on white, magenta on green or blue, red on yellow or green, and white on black (Gillingham, 1988).[4] If the background of the slide is a dark color, use a light-colored text and vice versa. A gradient background may make text difficult to read (Fig. 7-9) (Carter-Goodrum, 1996). Many of the backgrounds that are provided with the presentation programs possess this characteristic.

It is important to test color combinations. For slides, make a test slide, perhaps of a bulleted slide. If one is doing a computer projector presentation, check the readability of the slides from a distance of 5 to 6 feet. If possible, check how the slide projects

---

[4]Despite this study, the use of red on green should be avoided. About 10% of the male population has some difficulty with red-green differentiation.

with the projector. If presenting under conditions in which this is impossible, try to find out the resolution and number of colors supported by the projection unit. If it is lower than the monitor, set your video output to a lower resolution while creating the visuals. Visuals created with a higher resolution may appear unclear if they are projected at a lower rate of resolution.

Using Pictures

Many packages come with what is called *clip art*, or it can be purchased in a store or on the Internet. Clip art is a small drawing that has already been created and is in a computer file. The file is retrieved according to the dictates of the software. There is one drawback to clip art—copyright. Many types of clip art have limitations on how they can be used. If one is buying a package, be sure to read the fine print before you purchase the software.

A user can also create images by hand on the computer. All of the presentation packages provide this option in rudimentary form. There are also more advanced drawing packages that give much more help in this endeavor. Optical scanners can also import a picture into the computer.

As mentioned earlier, it is also possible to acquire pictures or clip art from the Internet. To download an image from the World Wide Web (WWW), place the mouse pointer over the image and click the right mouse button. A menu appears from which you select save image as. Another screen then pops up that gives the name of the image and tells you where the image will be saved. Read this information, and note the folder into which the image will be placed; if you do not,the image may become lost in your computer.

Occasionally when one is using visuals, an image may not translate into the desired finished product. To prevent this problem, check the appearance of the slide in play mode before committing to using the visual. If one is using a computer projection device, it is also a good idea, if possible, to check how it projects. Generally, if an image looks good in playback mode, it will project well.

Although using a scanner, clip art, or images from the Internet makes it possible to include very detailed pictures, these images can sometimes be confusing to the learner. For example, in presenting information about circulation through the heart,

Figure 7-9 ● A gradient background.

a detailed picture would probably not aid understanding as much as a schematic drawing that just depicted the four chambers and the veins and arteries leading into and out of the heart. To emphasize a point, one can use the principle of progressive disclosure with visuals. Presentation programs provide a way for objects to appear one by one, as well as bulleted text points.

Organizing the Presentation

Creating good visuals does not alone ensure a good presentation. The visuals and the presentation must reinforce one another. Start with an introduction that includes main points or goals, provide the content, and conclude by summarizing the information. It is an accepted fact that most people attending a presentation will remember no more than five key points (Feierman, Undated). To ensure that important points are remembered, start planning for the presentation by stating the five key points that the audience should retain. Build an outline around these points.

STORYBOARDING

Once the outline is completed, the presenter should create a storyboard. A storyboard is a drawing of the outline that is coordinated with notes about the oral presentation (Brown, 1997). Storyboarding forces the presenter to organize his or her thoughts. It helps to determine where the presentation is weak, thus making it easier to make corrections.

Advantages to storyboarding are that it

▼ Organizes the details of the presentation (Wadley, 1997)
▼ Forces a logical and efficient creation process
▼ Gives a plan to follow in creating your visuals
▼ Helps to see the presentation as a whole
▼ Helps limit the amount of information on a slide

To create a storyboard, roughly create a sketch of each visual you will need and add notes about what you intend to say when each visual is seen. Create your storyboard with 4- by 5-inch cards. They are about the same size as a computer screen or a slide, and they can easily be rearranged if there is a need to reorganize the presentation. When the cards are turned 90 degrees, they can mimic the size of a transparency. The visual can be sketched on one side, while notes can be put on the other.

CREATING AND USING A VISUAL PRESENTATION

With your storyboard in hand and the presentation package of your choice on the screen, the presenter is ready to create visuals. In deciding which features of the package to use, keep the objective of getting a message across to the audience uppermost. Once the visuals are finished, rehearse the presentation by using them in computer format. Make the necessary changes, and then, if using 35 mm slides or transparencies, "print" these. Make any necessary handouts or notes, and rehearse before the actual presentation.

TABLE 7-2 • *Basic Rules for Creating Visuals*	
Designing visuals	
Text	Limit to 6 to 7 words in a line and 6 lines on a slide
Fonts	Choose a sans-serif for projected visuals; limit number of different fonts
Font size	Transparencies, 18 points; Slides, 24 points
Colors	
Text and background	Contrasting—opposite sides of wheel
For emphasis	Be consistent
Number	5 to 6

Most of the presentation packages allow the slide show to be converted to a file that can be used on the WWW. In order to do this, the presenter may need to redo the slides. Most slide shows are highlights of a talk and do not stand alone well. Also, when a slide show is put on the WWW, each slide downloads separately (and often slowly), which may exhaust the patience of a viewer. Use this practice sparingly if at all.

▼ Summary

Although several vendors make presentation packages, they have similarities. Basically, these packages facilitate the job of creating good visuals by providing a constant background for the visual and tailored layouts. It is possible to modify any of these things at any time. Although there are many options available, such as adding images or special effects such as sound, video clips, animation, and progressive disclosure, they should be used only to enhance the message. In the same vein, select colors, fonts, backgrounds, and layouts to enrich a message (Table 7-2).

Even a small presentation given to a group of colleagues will be better received if the appropriate visuals are used. As a nurse progresses up the career ladder, knowing how to make impressive presentations is an aid to advancement. Professional, effective communication is the key to a successful career.

EXERCISES

1. Experiment with different backgrounds and decide why or why not they would be desirable in a specific type of presentation, such as a research report, a class project, or a welcoming speech. If they are not appropriate, how could they be modified to be more useful for your purpose?

2. How could you use a cartoon in a visual? What are some of the things you would have to consider if you choose to do so.

3. You need to teach a class about the physiology of the kidney. What visuals would you use?

4. What are some ways you see presentation software being used by health care professionals in

   a. Clinical practice?

   b. Administration?

   c. Education?

   d. Research?

   e. Entrepreneurial work?

REFERENCES

Brown, A. (1997). Using storyboards as visual guide for powerful presentations. *Presentations, 11*(8), 33–34; 36.

Carter-Goodrum, M. (1996). *Design tips for presentations.* Available: http://www.bus.indiana.edu/isweb/techn/design.htm.

Feierman, A. (Undated). *The art of communicating effectively.* Available: http://www.presentingsolutions.com/effectivepresentations.html.

Gillingham, M. G. (1988). Computer-based instruction: what the research says. *Journal of Computer Based Instruction, 15*(1), 1–6.

Lakoumentas, C. (1996). *Great presentations made easy.* Available: http://www.promedia-systems.com/proavll.htm.

Levie, W. H. & Dickie, K. E. (1973). The analysis and application of media. In R. Travers (Ed.), *The second handbook of research in teaching* (pp. 858–882). Chicago: Rand McNally.

Radel, J. (1997). *Effective presentations.* Available: http://www.kumc.edu/SAH/OTEd/jradel/effective.html.

Wadley, E. (1997). Storyboarding your educational multimedia project. *Syllabis, 11*(3), 22–23.

Using fonts effectively in your multimedia presentation. (Undated). Available: http://www.presentersuniversity.com/cgi/course.cgi?site=fonts.html&list=visaids.html.

CHAPTER 8

Multitasking and Sharing Data Between Programs

Objectives:

After studying this chapter you should be able to:

1 Differentiate between multitasking and having several files open in the same program

2 Explain embedding and linking

3 Understand computer viruses

4 State safe computing practices

*H*ealth care professionals and students are very familiar with multitasking. Throughout the day, everyone takes information used in one setting and uses it in another. It should not be surprising, therefore, that computers can be directed to do the same thing. Called multitasking, this feature is very helpful in managing the information that health care professionals need to synthesize and share.

Multitasking

Multitasking, or task switching, is a very convenient feature of Windows™ but one that beginners are often reluctant to use. It can prove to be invaluable when faced with a project. For example, a nurse may be asked to devise a plan to increase the number of mothers that deliver in a hospital who are still nursing their baby after 6 weeks. The first step may be to find out what is known about this subject, both in the literature and from the Internet. The nurse uses a computer to do a literature search. The literature search can either be downloaded to a bibliographic reference manager, or using cut and copy, be placed in a word processor. The nurse is also using the word processor to create a plan for the study.

During this time, the nurse is also obtaining data on the subject for baseline information, and entering this data into a spreadsheet or database. To analyze the data, it is moved into a statistical package. Because the nurse needs to make a presentation about the results, the spreadsheet and a statistical package is used to create graphs, and a presentation program is used to develop slides. Results are written up on the word processor. Multitasking allows all the programs needed for this project to be open at the same time. It is easy for the nurse to switch among programs and copy and paste.

DIFFERENTIATING BETWEEN MULTITASKING AND DIFFERENT FILES IN ONE PROGRAM

Although the term multitasking generally refers to being able to have more than one program open at the same time, it is often confused with having more than one file open in the same program. In Figure 8-1, the large square represents the graphical user interface (GUI) program. Within it, four programs are open—a word processor, a spreadsheet, a presentation program, and a statistical package. Within each of these programs, there are at least two open files. The figure is a graphical representation of a computer when a user is multitasking and using a program's ability to support more than one open file.

Neither multitasking nor having many files open in one program limits the functions that can be performed with any program. The only limiting factor is the amount

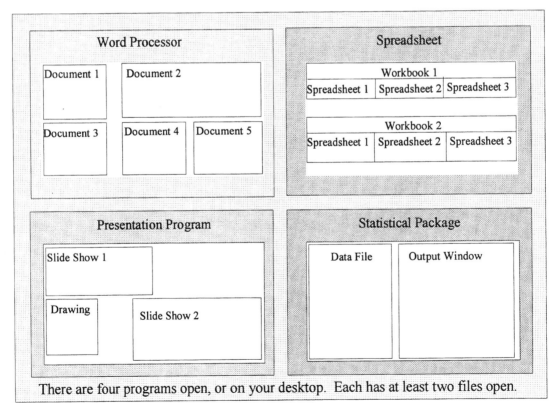

Figure 8-1 • Windows within windows.

of RAM available. Too little RAM may cause a slower reaction time. This can be solved by closing some programs or large files, or purchasing more RAM.

USEFULNESS

Multitasking is a very helpful feature, one that can save time. Before Windows, if a user was working in a word processor and received a phone call in which someone asked a question that required accessing the database, the user had to save the document, close the word processor, open the database, find the answer, relate it to the caller, close the database, reopen the word processor, retrieve the document, find their place, and resume working.

In Windows, when the user is working in the word processor and needs information from the database, he or she simply leaves the word processor running, opens up the database (or switch to it if it is already open), retrieves the information, switches back to the word processor, and resumes working. A user can cut and paste from one application to another. Although he or she is probably not aware of it, a user is already multitasking when running Windows and an application program. Windows is always in the background waiting for a request.

▼Embedding and Linking

Information can be exchanged within programs and between different applications by cutting and pasting, and also by embedding and linking. For example, a chart in a spreadsheet can be linked to a document in a word processor (Fig. 8-2). A program that supports these connections is said to support object linking and embedding (OLE). Embedding means the object is placed as is into another program or document. Linking means the object is directly linked to the original, and any changes made to the object in either place will be reflected in each location. This is also known as *hot linking*.

Selecting between embedding or linking is based on need. If the information in the chart in the second location is permanent, that is, it will not change even if the data supporting it change, embed the chart. If the chart should always reflect the current data, link it.

For example, an infection control nurse needs to make a report each month based not only on the monthly statistics but the year to date. This report is written and presented to the staff each month, so charts in word processor and on a slide in the presentation program are needed. The nurse wants to *embed* the chart for the information for the month because that will not change, however wants to *link* the chart of the yearly information because that data will change each month. Once the two items are linked, any editing changes made to the object in any location—the spreadsheet, presentation program, or word processor—will be reflected in all three programs. This includes changes that might be automatically made to a chart when the figures on which it is based change.

There are a few things to keep in mind when linking or embedding an object. When a *hot* link is made, the receiving program has a record of the full file name that

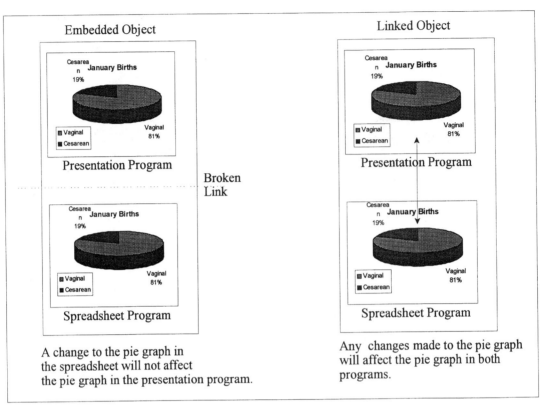

Figure 8-2 • Embedded and linked objects.

holds the original object. If the file name is changed, either by renaming the file or moving it to another folder, the hot link is broken. Additionally, if the program with which either an embedded or linked object was created is not open when a user attempts to open the file containing the embedded or linked object, the result may be a computer crash.

Moving Data From One Program to Another

Once a block of data is entered into the computer, it should never have to be entered again. When the data are entered properly, it can be transferred between programs. The ease with which data can be moved between programs depends on the type of data. Structured data in a spreadsheet, statistical package, or database can be easily transferred from one program to another. Data from word processing programs can also be moved between programs, but the usefulness of this maneuver depends on how the information was entered and the use to which it is put in the second program.

One thing that can be done with most files, except graphical files, is to save them in an ASCII format. Except for graphical and some statistical programs, most applications will create (export to) and open (import) an ASCII file. To create an ASCII file, select save as from the edit menu. On the save screen, in the rectangle labeled file type, select ASCII DOS or TEXT (these are identical terms), then save the file. This is called exporting a file to ASCII format. Opening an ASCII file, or other file type that is different from the one that is specific to the program, is called importing a file.

The most common reason for exporting or importing data to another program is that the program in which the data resides cannot manipulate it to meet a given need. For example, a user may have data in a spreadsheet that needs statistical analysis or data in a spreadsheet that requires manipulation that is more easily accomplished in a database.

Planning for many uses when entering data into a computer is necessary to preserve the one data entry principle. If because data entry is easier in a database, you are using it to enter data for manipulation in a statistical package, know the rules of the statistical package about length of fields and field names and enter the data accordingly. The most inflexible data format is that of a word processor, because the text is usually *free text*, that is, there is no structure to it. The exceptions to this are data that are in a word processing table, which can often be copied to a spreadsheet, and data that are in the data format for a mail merge.

One example where preplanning is necessary is the process of entering data for the purpose of creating a list of names or addresses, or both. If this information is entered into the computer as free text, that is, not in a table structure or mail merge format, it will be difficult to use in other ways. If instead of using a word processor this information is entered into a database, the list can be sorted by name, city, state, and zip, and can be used again for many purposes as well as to create the list, which was the original purpose of the data entry.[1] This scenario applies when any list is created on a computer, although if each entry consists of different items separated by the same character (called a delimiter), such as a comma or a tab and then saved as an ASCII file, the list can be imported into a spreadsheet or database. Note that any spaces in the entry before or after the delimiter are considered part of the data.

Data can also be imported into a computer through the use of scanners. Often tests or the answers to research questionnaires are bubbled onto special (optical mark scan) paper for the purpose of being scanned. The output, besides being printed, can be used to create an ASCII file. This ASCII file can then be imported into a database, spreadsheet, or statistical package for further manipulation.

▼ Sharing That Should not Occur

Sharing information is vital to the global health care system. Unfortunately, a small percentage of sharing can cause problems. Computer viruses and undocumented sources fall into this category.

---

[1] It is easier to convert a database file to word processing data file format than the other way around.

VIRUSES

Similar to viruses that cause disease in humans, computer viruses replicate using the resources of the host without the consent of the host. Unlike disease-causing viruses, computer viruses do not generate spontaneously; they are made by humans. Besides good antiviral software, the best defense against viruses is to understand what they are, what they are not, and how they are spread.

A *virus* is a piece of code that is written to attach itself where it does not belong and perform its functions without permission. It attaches either to other programs, such as a word processor or spreadsheet, or to the section of a diskette that the computer accesses when it boots. Essentially, viruses have two functions—to spread and to implement the desires of the perpetrator (Symantec, 1997). Viruses can be benign or malignant. A benign virus is not intended to do real damage to a computer, though in some situations it may. Instead the perpetuator designed it to make itself known when given conditions are met, such as a specified date, by displaying some sort of message, or creating a noise. Malignant viruses are those that are destructive to your computer. They might cause changes in programs so they do not perform properly, alter information about where files are stored, or erase files.

There are only a few types of viruses—those that infect programs, those that infect the boot sector of a disk, and those that are a combination of both. A virus that affects files is called a file infector. It only affects what are called executable files. An executable file is not data but a program that runs and performs a function such as allowing a user to word process. When the infected program is run, the virus activates itself and infects other executable files. These viruses are activated only when an infected program is run. If a user has an infected program on a computer and does not run it, the virus will not be activated. Using a virus checker before using any new program will protect users from this type of virus.

Unfortunately, macros are executable programs. As such, they, too, can be infected with a virus. Like other file infectors, macro viruses are spread by running the infected macro. Word processing or other application program files can contain macros that run when a file is opened. Therefore one should check all files received by email or other users with a virus checker before opening.

The second type, a boot sector virus, infects the boot sector of a disk. Every disk, whether a hard drive or a diskette, contains what is called a boot sector. This sector contains information needed by the computer when it boots. The boot sector on nonbootable diskettes contains the information that displays the message, nonsystem disk when a user attempts to boot with a diskette in the drive. This type of virus is spread by booting the computer with an infected disk in the a: drive. When the computer is booted, the virus enters into the computer's memory and infects the boot sector of the hard drive. Once the boot sector of the hard drive is infected, any disk used with this computer, whether at the same session that the hard drive was infected or later, will have its boot sector infected.

There are many antivirus programs on the market. Purchasing and installing one is the first step in virus protection. The next step is to create a clean, write-protected bootable system diskette. If a hard disk has a virus, before it can be eliminated with a virus protection program, the user needs to boot the computer without activating the virus. This diskette will accomplish this task. Most antivirus programs assist in creating these diskettes. Once this procedure is done, write-protect the diskette or diskettes and place them in a safe place.

SAFE COMPUTING PRACTICES

1. Obtain a good antiviral software package, install it, and update it frequently
2. Make a clean, write-protected, bootable diskette
3. Use only software from a know producer obtained from a reliable source
4. When you receive a file, whether downloaded from the Internet, received via email, or given to you, scan it with the antivirus program before using it
5. Never turn on the computer with a diskette in the a: drive. This will protect you from a boot sector virus

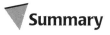

Summary

Multitasking, or having more than one program immediately available for use either for informational purposes or for reusing the same piece of data, is an important computer feature. Cutting and pasting between programs and embedding or linking data make the tasks of reusing and updating information easier. It is far more simple to have correct information when data in only one place need updating.

Although they are a real threat, computer viruses are controllable. There are a few basic viruses—file infectors, boot sector viruses, and those that combine these characteristics. Using safe computing practices along with a good antivirus program and a clean, write-protected, bootable diskette keeps a user relatively safe.

EXERCISES

1. Describe the difference between multitasking and having several files open in the same program.
2. In your work, what are advantages to having several programs open at the same time?
3. Describe some situations when you would
   a. Embed an object
   b. Link an object
4. Describe how a computer can contract a file infector and a boot sector virus. How would you protect yourself against viruses?
5. What are some ways that you see multitasking being used by health care professionals in
   a. Clinical practice?
   b. Administration?
   c. Education?
   d. Research?
   e. Entrepreneurial work?

REFERENCES

Kanish, B. (1997). *An overview of computer viruses and antivirus software.* Available: http://www.hicom.net/%7Eoedipus/virus32.html#what.

Symantec. (1997). *General virus information.* Available: http://www.symantec.com/avcenter/vinfodb.html.

Databases

Some patient care information is filed in patient records, and some information health care professionals simply internalize. If nurses wish to use this data to gain a broader understanding of a condition, the idea is generally discarded because the data recorded are in a format that makes this type of information retrieval difficult. When patient care data are structured in a database (instead of in individual medical records), the information can still provide an individualized picture of a patient. However the information can also permit health care workers to make comparisons among patients with like conditions (Display 9-1). To use this wealth of knowledge requires an understanding of what databases are, how they are structured, and some basic querying concepts.

Nursing and Databases

A database is a collection of data that is organized or structured in such a way that pieces are easily retrievable, either singly or as a group. Database concepts, such as how to structure a database, query a database, or create reports, apply to any database: a small database such as an address book, or a large clinical database.

Nursing and Information

Nursing is information intensive. The amount of time nurses spend in handling information varies from 28% to 40% (Zielstorff, Hudgings, & Grobe 1993). Collecting the data that are part of this information is the most

●▼●▲●▼●▲●▼●▲●▼●▲●▼●▲●▼●▲●

Display 9-1 ● STRUCTURED DATA

Data is structured when it is organized into a table format. When data are structured, it is possible to pull out separate pieces for many records; for example, all the cities in the table below. Or, we could pull out only the data for one or more records, such as all three pieces of data for Mark Time. It is also possible to make comparisons between records.

Name	Address	City
Will Coyote	2233 Forest Glen	Sherwood Forest
Mark Time	45 Big Ben Drive	London
Sea Shore	45 Ocean View Lane	Charleston

expensive part of any information system, yet we continue to squander this resource by recording it in a way that makes retrieving any of the data very difficult.

Nurses use data from many sources every day. In planning care for a patient, a nurse processes data about the policies of the agency, information known about his condition, and data about the patient. In this processing, a nurse may also add data from other resources such as a colleague, drug reference, or an article. When making a decision about how to care for the patient, the nurse is transforming data to information, information to knowledge, and acting using a synthesis of all the data, information, and knowledge. After taking care of the patient, as the nurse reflects on what was learned, this experience may be combined with other experiences to increase a personal knowledge bank. The nurse is putting together similar data from different experiences and coming to conclusions that are used to update his or her personal knowledge database. The next time the nurse takes care of a similar patient, this personal database will be called on, along with anything new learned since then. All of this information is synthesized and used in patient care.

Everyone has these personal databases; without them, we would be unable to function. When we find ourselves in a strange situation in which we are uncomfortable, the feeling of discomfort is often generated from the insufficiency of our present personal database to cope with the situation. When we gain the needed data and transform it to information and then knowledge, we are again comfortable. We know what to do because our personal database now provides us with the information to allow us to act in the appropriate manner.

The human mind, however, is limited in the amount of data it can hold or work with at one time. The data that we in health care need to recall and synthesize is both prodigious and complex. Living in the Information Age as we do, it is impossible to effectively manage this information manually. Computer databases are needed for some of these responsibilities.

Bibliographical Databases

One form of database with which many are familiar is the bibliographical database. This type of database has references to books, audiovisual programs, and journal articles. Most of these databases are now *online*, or available electronically. In fact, many libraries no longer have print versions of these databases. Knowing how to use this type of database effectively is important to a professional. Understanding how a database is constructed makes understanding how to use bibliographical databases easier.

Clinical Needs

Databases that help in patient care are not limited to bibliographical databases. In order to improve practice, nurses need data from clinical practice. Knowledge comes not only from what is learned in nursing school but from scientific studies and reflections on personal experience, which is informal, personal research. All professionals whose practice improves with time are engaged in research, whether personal, informal, or formal.

This personal knowledge database, although it may be shared with colleagues and new nurses, is not in a format in which it can be used to promote quality nursing care for others. Nor is it in a format that can be used objectively to determine whether one's experiences are similar to those of other nurses in other institutions and geographical areas. In most cases, even the data recorded is not in a format that permits its use in improving patient care. Retrieval of data from most written records requires wading through many pages and manually recording the data on another form. Additionally, in many agencies, even if someone is willing to do the work, he or she would be limited in this endeavor because few agencies keep a record of nursing observations or care plans (Gassert, 1997; Milholland, 1997).

Databases: Structuring the Data

Making this information available so that decisions can be based on data instead of suppositions requires that patient records be computerized. The information that can be derived from a database is dependent on how it is designed. Simply computerizing a patient record will not permit data manipulation. Thought must be given to what data to collect and how to structure it. In a well-designed system, information is received from the patient once, entered into a database once, and is then available for different uses. This avoids asking the patient the same questions many times and recording the data in different places to meet the needs of the different health care disciplines. The key to an efficient database is to adhere to the following maxim: one piece of data, many uses. When the personnel in the admitting department ask the patient a question and enter it into a database, it can be made available to all disciplines in any format that is needed.

What allows us to manipulate data in a database is the structure. When it is examined closely, a database resembles a spreadsheet. The data are organized horizontally and vertically. Each row is a record, and each column is a *field*. Unlike a spreadsheet, individual field entries cannot be isolated by an address, such as A3; instead, they must be specified by either their contents or the field name.

Table 9-1 is a fictitious flat database for clients who have had some type of hip surgery. The labels across the top are called field names. The first record, which has record number 1122, is for the patient Forest Green. In that record, Forest is the field entry for the field First Name. The field entry for the field Age is 23. All of the field entries in the first record are data elements that are specific to Forest Green. They are part of Forest Green's record. The fields, or columns, however, contain data representing the same element for many patients. The entire set of records is a table. All of the tables involved in the project are called a *database*. The software used to manage databases is called a *database management system (DBMS)*.

When examining a table, data are seen in the aggregate. In this format, it is possible to learn things about patient experiences as a whole. Nurses can learn the minimum, maximum, and average length of stay (LOS) for patients who have had a left hip arthroplasty, they can count the numbers of patients for each type of surgery, or average the LOS for all clients for all surgeries. With a small number of patients, this could be done manually. In real patient care situations, however, the number of patients makes this impractical. When the data are computerized, however, nurses not only can perform the above calculations, but can reorder the records to look for patterns in each type of surgery as in Table 9-2. In Table 9-2, all clients with the same type of surgery are grouped together, and in the grouping for the same type of surgery, the records are ordered by LOS.

TABLE 9-1 ● *Client Database*

Rec #	First name	Last name	Age	Sex	Surgery	LOS	
							← Field Names
1122	Forest	Green	23	M	ORIF - Rt hip	4	← Record
1212	Summer	Day	78	F	Rt hip arthroplasty	4	← Record
1234	Sea	Shore	65	F	Lt hip arthroplasty	3	← Record
1331	Will	Coyote	82	M	Lt hip arthroplasty	7	← Record
1357	Jersey	Farmer	55	M	ORIF - Rt hip	3	← Record
1441	Storm	Wave	68	M	Rt hip arthroplasty	4	← Record
2121	Star	Bright	33	F	ORIF - Rt hip	6	← Record
2211	Glen	Springs	70	M	Lt hip arthroplasty	3	← Record
2323	Tuesday	Night	77	F	ORIF - Lt hip	4	← Record
3113	Spring	Flower	73	F	ORIF - Lt hip	3	← Record
3232	Pearl	White	81	F	Rt hip arthroplasty	4	← Record
4114	Tiffany	Light	69	F	Lt hip arthroplasty	3	← Record
4321	Misty	Mountain	72	F	Rt hip arthroplasty	6	← Record
4567	Caspar	White	59	M	Rt hip arthroplasty	3	← Record
7654	Mark	Time	70	M	Lt hip arthroplasty	4	← Record
↑ Field	↑ Field	↑ Field	↑ Field	↑ Field	↑ Field	↑ Field	

Rec #	First name	Last name	Age	Sex	Surgery	LOS
1331	Will	Coyote	82	M	Lt hip arthroplasty	7
7654	Mark	Time	70	M	Lt hip arthroplasty	4
1234	Sea	Shore	65	F	Lt hip arthroplasty	3
2211	Glen	Springs	70	M	Lt hip arthroplasty	3
4114	Tiffany	Light	69	F	Lt hip arthroplasty	3
2121	Star	Bright	33	F	ORIF - Rt hip	6
2323	Tuesday	Night	77	F	ORIF - Lt hip	4
1122	Forest	Green	23	M	ORIF - Rt hip	4
1357	Jersey	Farmer	55	M	ORIF - Rt hip	3
3113	Spring	Flower	73	F	ORIF - Lt hip	3
4321	Misty	Mountain	72	F	Rt hip arthroplasty	6
1212	Summer	Day	78	F	Rt hip arthroplasty	4
1441	Storm	Wave	68	M	Rt hip arthroplasty	4
3232	Pearl	White	81	F	Rt hip arthroplasty	4
4567	Caspar	White	59	M	Rt hip arthroplasty	3

TABLE 9-2 ● *Primary Sort (Surgery) and Secondary Sort (LOS) of Records From Table 9-1*

WHAT ARE DATA?

In designing databases, it is important that the fields consist of atomic level data, that is data that has not been interpreted or data at its smallest level. Notice in the database in Table 9-1 that there is a separate field for both the first and last name. When data are not at the atomic level, flexibility in using and transforming the data is lost. The more complex the data, the more important is the thought that is given to designating field structure.

TYPES OF DATABASE ORGANIZATION

There are three main types of database—flat, relational, and hierarchical.

Flat Database

The databases in Tables 9-1 and 9-2 are flat databases. That is, all the data are contained in one file, which is really the complete database. Flat databases are very simple to construct and use, but they have limitations (Display 9-2).

Relational Database

A relational database is one that allows data to be used from more than one table to produce information. All that is required is that each table have at least one field in which the data in both tables is identical.[1] Full-scale database programs for personal

---

[1]It is also possible to relate tables on the uniqueness of combined fields.

●▼●▲●▼●▲●▼●▲●▼●▲●▼●▲●▼●▲●▼●▲●

Display 9-2 ● FLAT DATABASE

A flat database is a collection of specific pieces of information organized in such a manner that the data are easy to retrieve and can be transformed into information using such procedures as:

1. Reporting on different fields.
2. Grouping of like records to determine similarities and differences.
3. Comparisons between data in different records.

computers are relational databases. If a project requires only one table, a relational database program can be used as a flat database. A flat database, however, such as the address book that comes with many word processors, cannot be used as a relational database.

Refer again to Table 9-2. Do you notice that for each surgery, there is one patient whose LOS is noticeably greater than that of the others? Is there any way to discover why that might have occurred from the data in this table? Not at this point; to do that more data are needed. One way to investigate this question is to see whether the nursing diagnoses for each client could have an effect on this issue. How could this database be expanded to include nursing diagnosis?

The only solution that will preserve all the functions of a database is to create another table that is related to the first table. This table will have two fields—record number and nursing diagnosis. The record number field will allow us to match the data in this table with the data in Table 9-1. Using this table structure, if a patient has more than one nursing diagnosis, another record will be created in the second table. To illustrate, look at the data in the database in Table 9-3. There are four nursing diagnoses for record number 1122. Using the record number 1122, one can refer to Table 9-1 and locate the record that has 1122 in the record number field. Once that record is found, the user has access to the other data about that patient that is contained in that table.

In this case, we performed this procedure manually. The computer automates this process. The file in Table 9-1 is known as the *master* or *parent table*. It contains the base information for the database and is organized, or indexed, by record number. The file in Table 9-3 is a *detail* or *child table*. It contains data that is related to data in the master table. (Table 9-2 is a transformation of the master table.) In this example, the tables have been related in what is called a one-to-many view. That is, the master table has one record that is related to many in the detail table. In a one-to-many relationship, the master table is always the table that contains one, but never more than one, match for each record in another table. The detail table may contain no matching records or hundreds. The key in relational tables is that there be an identical field or fields that can be used to locate the desired information in the other tables.

TABLE 9-3 ● *Nursing Diagnoses*

Rec #	Nursing diagnosis	Etiology	*Resolved
1122	Fear	Anticipated postoperative dependence	
1122	Impaired physical mobility—Level 1	Pain	4
1122	Ineffective management of therapeutic regimen	Insufficient knowledge of activity restriction	2
1122	Powerlessness—Low	Perceived interpersonal control by others	
1212	Colonic constipation	Immobility	
1212	Impaired home maintenance management	Support system deficit	4
1212	Impaired physical mobility—Level 3	Pain	4
1234	Impaired home maintenance management	Support system deficit	3
1234	Impaired physical mobility—Level 3	Pain	3
1331	Colonic constipation	Immobility	5
1331	Impaired physical mobility—Level 4	Pain	7
1331	Pain	Ineffective pain management	7
1357	Altered role performance—work	Change in physical capacity to resume role	
1357	Impaired physical mobility—Level 1	Pain	3
1357	Powerlessness—Low	Perceived interpersonal control by others	
1441	Colonic constipation	Immobility	
1441	Impaired physical mobility—Level 3	Pain	3
1441	Ineffective breathing pattern	Decreased energy	3
2121	Impaired home maintenance management	Insufficient family organization	4
2121	Impaired physical mobility—Level 1	Pain	5
2121	Pain	Ineffective pain management	5
2121	Risk for altered parenting	Physical disability	
2211	Impaired physical mobility—Level 3	Pain	2
2211	Pain	Ineffective pain management	2
2323	Impaired physical mobility—Level 3	Pain	3
2323	Ineffective breathing pattern	Inability to clear secretions	3
2323	Potential for impaired tissue integrity	Altered circulation	
3113	Impaired physical mobility—Level 3	Pain	3
3113	Ineffective breathing pattern	Knowledge deficit	1
3232	Impaired physical mobility—Level 4	Pain	2
3232	Ineffective breathing pattern	Increased bronchial secretions	2
3232	Potential impaired tissue integrity	Immobility	
4114	Colonic constipation	Immobility	3
4114	Impaired physical mobility—Level 3	Pain	3
4321	Impaired physical mobility—Level 3	Pain	5
4321	Pain	Ineffective pain management	5
4567	Impaired physical mobility—Level 1	Pain	2
4567	Ineffective breathing pattern	Anxiety	1
7654	Altered tissue perfusion	Interruption of venous flow	2
7654	Impaired physical mobility—Level 3	Pain	3
7654	Potential impaired tissue integrity	Altered circulation	3

The field resolved contains the day after surgery that the nursing diagnosis was resolved. If the field is blank, the client was discharged with that nursing diagnosis unresolved.

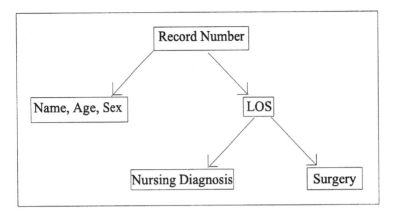

Figure 9-1 • Hierarchical database.

Hierarchical

A hierarchical database (Fig. 9-1) is a database whose structure is organized in the shape of a pyramid, much like the file organization described in Chapter 6. In this organizational plan, often called a tree structure, records are linked to a base, or root, but through successive layers. For example, for the data in Table 9-1, the root might contain the record number of a patient, which would link to the record with the name, age, sex, and also, LOS. The LOS would link to surgery and nursing diagnosis. The difficulty with the hierarchical structure is that it is hard to link one branch of the tree, for example, the LOS branch, with the name branch. When it is used, it is important to consider the challenge of multiple relationships.

Transforming Data Into Information

Structuring data properly in a database is only one step in making it useful. Humans must use ingenuity when transforming raw data into information and knowledge. If aggregate data are to be used for making data-driven decisions, an individual must have the vision to conceive of the information a given set of data can produce. One way to do this was already seen when the records were stored in the database in Table 9-1, using surgery as the primary sort and LOS as the secondary sort. When the re-sorted data were examined, it was seen that for each surgery, there was one patient whose LOS was beyond the usual range (see Table 9-2).

QUERYING A DATABASE

Another way we can use databases to produce information, is to *query* the data, or ask questions of the database. To illustrate, consider the hypothesis that the nursing diagnoses for each client may have affected the LOS. To produce only the data needed, in the query, we will ask to see only the information in the LOS, nursing diagnosis, and etiology fields. We will also tell the computer to retrieve only those records in which the LOS exceeds 4 days and to sort the results by nursing diagnosis. The data are seen

TABLE 9-4 ● Query to Find Nursing Diagnosis for Clients With Higher Than Normal LOS				
Rec #	LOS	Nursing diagnosis	Etiology	Resolved
1331	7	Colonic constipation	Immobility	5
2121	6	Impaired physical mobility—Level 3	Pain	5
4321	6	Impaired physical mobility—Level 3	Pain	5
1331	7	Impaired physical mobility—Level 4	Pain	7
2121	6	Pain	Ineffective pain management	5
4321	6	Pain	Ineffective pain management	5
1331	7	Pain	Ineffective pain management	7
2121	6	Risk for altered parenting	Physical disability	

in Table 9-4. Interestingly, pain with the etiology of ineffective pain management shows up in connection with three clients, as does impaired physical mobility.

Using our personal knowledge base, we realize that all the patients who had hip surgery have a diagnosis of impaired physical mobility. However, they do not all have the nursing diagnosis of pain due to ineffective pain management. We also wonder if any patients who did not have a diagnosis of pain due to ineffective pain management, stayed longer than 4 days. With this thought, we ask the computer to produce the records for patients who have either stayed longer than 4 days or who had a nursing diagnosis of pain due to ineffective pain management. The result can be seen in Table 9-5. We find that all the patients whose pain was due to ineffective pain management stayed more than 4 days, and all patients with the diagnosis of pain due to ineffective pain management had an LOS exceeding 4 days. Using a database, we identified a practice problem. Even with 15 patients, it is unlikely that this information would have been gleaned without the help of a database. The computer, however, did not perform these feats without human intelligence.

BASIC CONCEPTS IN TRANSFORMING DATA

Transforming the data in these two tables into the knowledge that the LOS is greatly impacted by ineffective pain management required that we were able to envision the information or knowledge that could be derived from the data. This ability is even more important than knowing how to perform the computer skills necessary to design the query. Learning these skills for a database, however, may help a user gain the

TABLE 9-5 ● Ineffective Pain Management and LOS				
Rec #	LOS	Nursing diagnosis	Etiology	Resolved
1331	7	Pain	Ineffective pain management	7
2121	6	Pain	Ineffective pain management	5
4321	6	Pain	Ineffective pain management	5

TABLE 9-6 ● *Symbols Used to Designate Criteria*			
Symbol	**Meaning**	**Example**	**Translation**
>	Greater than	> 4	Find the records in which the field entry is greater than 4
<	Less than	< 4	Find the records in which the field entry is less than 4
>=	Greater than OR equal to	>= 4	Find the records in which the field entry is greater than OR equal to 4
<=	Less than OR equal to	<= 4	Find the records in which the field entry is less than OR equal to 4
=	Equal to	4	Find the records in which the field entry is 4

conceptual tools necessary to design the questions. The exact method of conducting the queries and the name given to various functions varies from program to program, but the concepts are the same.

In essence, the records a user wishes to see can be pinpointed by any criteria in any of the fields. In the last query, it was specified that we wanted to see only records that had pain in the nursing diagnosis field or in which the patient stayed longer than 4 days. Although in the queries performed so far we asked for exact matches, we could also request partial matches. These could be requested by telling the computer that the criteria for the records we wish to see should resemble the field entry, be part of the field entry, or be greater than, less than, or more than the field entry. In asking for matches by numerical criteria, there are universal symbols that are used (Table 9-6). These operators are also used in spreadsheet formulas.

The mathematical signs in Table 9-6 can also be used with text. If a user wants to see all the patients in the database table in Table 9-1 whose last names started with W, the equal sign and the syntax would be used. The user could also ask to see all the records for those whose last names start with letters that are contiguous in the alphabet, for example, all the names that start with the letters A to N. The computer locates this information by translating the letters to ASCII numbers. Because each letter in the alphabet has an ASCII code higher than the last, A is 65, B is 66, this request would be specified by using the less than (<) rather than the greater than (>) sign with the letter. The request would be worded as <=N.

In searching, we can also use *wild cards*. For example, suppose we wanted to find all the clients in the master table that had an arthroplasty. The data are entered in the database as Lt hip arthroplasty and Rt hip arthroplasty. To find all the records that contained arthroplasty in the surgery field, we would use the symbol for a wild card used by the specific application program to tell the computer to find the records that contained the word arthroplasty in the surgery field.[2]

[2]In application programs, wild cards generally have one symbol or wild card to designate one character and another to designate one or more characters. Wild cards, however, are used differently when searching bibliographical databases. There, you enter the first letters of the word, followed by the wild card symbol. This symbol takes the place of one or many characters.

Boolean Logic

Boolean refers to a type of logic named after the 19th century mathematician George Boole, who recognized that any mathematical expression could be stated as either true or false. When the records that had pain in the nursing diagnosis field were requested, the computer translated the request into nursing diagnosis field entry = pain. It then looked at each record. When it found pain in the nursing diagnosis field, it flagged the record as true. Those that did not have this entry were flagged as false. All the records in which the equation was true were then shown.

Keep in mind that in database queries, equal is translated to mean identical to. In other words, all of the characters, including spaces, must be the same. If the entry in the nursing diagnosis field were designated as some pain instead of pain, the match would not have been made. To find records with both pain and some pain in the nursing diagnosis field, wild cards would have to be used, telling the database that we were looking for the characters "pain" anywhere in the field entry.

The symbols in Table 9-6 are called Boolean operators. When a user wants to find records that have matches in more than one field, the additional Boolean operators "and," "or," and "not" are employed. To select the records seen in Table 9-5, we asked the computer to find all those records in which the entry in the nursing diagnosis field was pain or the entry in the LOS field was greater than four. When the operator "and" is used, both conditions must be true for the record to be selected. When the operator "or" is used, only one of the conditions needs to be true. The operator "not" is fairly clear, it means the entry in the record should not match the stated criteria. What can be confusing when trying to use the Boolean operators is that we often use the word "and" when we mean "or." Constructing a request using the chart in Table 9-7 may help.

As can be seen, querying is a way of filtering out items in which we have no interest so the data that we need to make a decision can be seen more clearly. Database programs also permit queries that mimic those found in a spreadsheet, such as counting the number of times a specific field entry is in a table and calculating averages, sums, minimums, and maximums. Some programs also allow a query to be used to change the entries in a field.

		Actual values in fields A and B		
Operator	Values of the variables to test	A = 2	B = 1	Record shown?
And	A = 2 and B = 1	True	True	Yes
	A = 2 and B = 2	True	False	No
	A = 3 and B = 2	False	False	No
Or	A = 2 or B = 1	True	True	Yes
	A = 2 or B = 2	True	False	Yes
	A = 3 or B = 2	False	False	No
Not	A = 2	True		No
	A = 1	False		Yes

TABLE 9-7 ● *More Boolean Operators*

Keep in mind that computers return whatever they are told. They do not evaluate whether the criteria entered provide the answer to a question; they just return the records that meet the conditions that are stated. When constructing any query beyond a simple query, the way the query is stated should be tested with a small, known set of data to be certain that the right question is being asked. Even experienced users have to stop and think when constructing involved queries. As with all computer tools, there is no substitute for thinking.

▼Reports

Reports are the method of presenting information in a database. What the report includes depends on the needs of the person receiving it. A report can be based on just the information in one record, on selected fields in records, or from multiple tables or any combination of these items. Reports can also be generated from queries. They can be simple or involved. Figure 9-2 shows a report designed from Table 9-4 that groups the records by nursing diagnosis. In this report, it is easy to see that although these patients all had some level of impaired physical mobility, the only nursing diagnosis that those whose length of stay was greater than 4 days had in common was pain due to ineffective pain management. Thus, the data in a table can be used to produce reports that show the data in many different ways, allowing us to see relationships that otherwise would probably remain hidden.

Once a report is designed, it can be used many times. Each time the report is used, it retrieves the current data in a table to produce a report that reflects the current content. Thus, the same report will differ each time the data in the table is changed. For example, if every month we use the same report that produced the output seen in Figure 9-2, the results will differ depending on the data in the database. They will either lend more support to the hypothesis that ineffective pain management leads to an increased LOS, or they will show the fallacy of this hypothesis.

These features could be used by a nurse who needs both to report the incidence of wound infections every month and to produce a yearly report. The nurse would design one report and each month tell the computer to use only the records for that month in the report. At the end of the year, the nurse would use the same report but query the database for the entire year. Most database application programs also provide a way to summarize the data by month or any other time period.

A report can be on screen or printed. It is the ability to construct a report by using data from various tables such as the one in Figure 9-2 that enables the one piece of data many uses concept to be a reality. By using screen reports, data entered in the admitting department or any other department can be retrieved and shown in the format that is most useful to the discipline requesting the information. The reports need not be the same. For example, nursing may need to see all the pieces except insurance but might also require information from other sources in that report. This outcome is accomplished by designing reports that contain the necessary data in a format that is useful to those who request the information. Whether on screen or in hard copy, creating reports that are useful to a given discipline can be done only with cooperation among those in the discipline who use the report and the programming

Nursing Diagnosis: <u>Colonic constipation</u>

> Rec #:   1331   LOS: 7
> Etiology: Immobility

Nursing Diagnosis: <u>Impaired home maintenance management</u>

> Rec #:   2121   LOS: 6
> Etiology: Insufficient family
>   organization

Nursing Diagnosis: <u>Impaired physical mobility - Level 1</u>

> Rec #:   2121   LOS: 6
> Etiology: Pain

Nursing Diagnosis: <u>Impaired physical mobility - Level 3</u>

> Rec #:   4321   LOS: 6
> Etiology: Pain

Nursing Diagnosis: <u>Impaired physical mobility - Level 4</u>

> Rec #:   1331   LOS: 7
> Etiology: Pain

Nursing Diagnosis: <u>Pain</u>

> Rec #: 1331 LOS: 7   Rec #: 2121 LOS: 6   Rec #: 4321 LOS: 6
> Etiology: Ineffective pain   Etiology: Ineffective pain   Etiology: Ineffective pain
>   management   management   management

Nursing Diagnosis: <u>Risk for altered parenting</u>

> Rec #:   2121   LOS: 6
> Etiology: Physical disability

Figure 9-2 • Report of nursing diagnoses and etiologies for patients with a length of stay (LOS) of more than 4 days.

staff. The screen design of a report, or the way in which the data are printed, can either hinder or help those who need information.

Data Mining and Warehousing

Data mining is a way to discover useful, previously unknown information that is hidden in large databases. For example, data mining software may allow the discovery of patterns of use of an emergency department that are previously unknown. Querying data brings to light only requested relationships. Data mining software, however, makes comparisons that users do not consider.

Data mining is usually performed with data from large warehouses that contain information from many sources. Data warehouses are data archives that preserve data. Data in warehouses is integrated. In other words, the same terminology is used to denote the same phenomena (Inmon, 1995). To illustrate, although different organizations may use different terms to denote fever, the data would need to be transformed so that one term was always used. Integration is also applied in units of measurement. For example, decisions are made as to whether data representing temperature will be stored in Celsius or Fahrenheit. Any data representing a temperature is converted to the selected measurement scale before being stored.

Data in a warehouse covers a long time period. In an ongoing clinical information system, the time horizon may be 30 or 60 days. In a warehouse, it can be 5 to 10 years. Additionally, data in a warehouse cannot be updated unless a serious mistake has been made in filing the data.

Accuracy, privacy, and confidentiality are factors that must be considered when warehousing data.

Data, Information, Knowledge, Wisdom

In general language, the terms *data, information,* and *knowledge* tend to be used interchangeably. When discussing databases, however, the word *data* denotes discrete elements that have not been interpreted. Information is data that has some type of interpretation or structure, and knowledge is a synthesis of information. Wisdom, on the other hand, is knowing when and how to use knowledge (Joos, Whitman, Smith, & Nelson, 1992). As an example, the number 37 representing a patient's temperature is a piece of data. It is transformed into information with the fact that 37 is a normal body temperature. To make it knowledge, it is synthesized with the patient's condition. It becomes wisdom when we combine this information with other knowledge and use it as a basis for our actions. The computer can be programmed to make many of the transformations, with the exception of wisdom. That needs to be done by health care professionals.

How data are transformed into information and knowledge is determined by one's world view. If a diabetic patient walks into a health clinic and has a blood sugar of 350, the number 350 is a data element. This data element is interpreted differently by different disciplines within the health care framework. A physician will take this data and synthesize it with her or his knowledge base about the type of insulin and the dosage to prescribe for the patient. On the other hand, the nurse will take the data and synthesize it with her or his knowledge base and attempt to treat the behavior that may have caused the high blood sugar level. At the same time, a dietician will use this piece of data to incorporate into dietary teaching. Each is a vital use of the data, and each professional combines it with different information and knowledge to create the wisdom to act. Databases can provide us with data that can be transformed to information and even knowledge. How this information or knowledge is interpreted and transformed to wisdom is a human act.

 Output Determinations

Useful and easily interpreted information can be produced from properly created databases. Those creating databases, however, must keep in mind several principles.

STRUCTURE AND CONTENTS DETERMINE OUTPUT

The structure and contents of a database determine the output. Obviously, if a piece of data is not recorded, it cannot be used. If hair color is not recorded in a database, it will be impossible to use the data to determine if red-haired women are more likely to have a postpartum hemorrhage than brunettes. Another factor, which was addressed earlier, is that the data in each field determines the usage. In the database in Table 9-1, the patient's name was broken into two fields to permit each field to be used separately.

Databases present problems to individuals who use a first initial and a middle name. Many databases are structured on the assumption that everyone has a first name, then a middle initial, and last name. Under this assumption, the middle initial field only has room for one character.

When structuring fields, always opt for data flexibility, even if the need does not seem obvious at the time.

FIELDS MUST CONTAIN LIKE INFORMATION TO DENOTE THE SAME THING

In the example database seen in Table 9-1, arthroplasty and open reduction internal fixation (ORIF) are entered using either left or right. As seen when Table 9-1 was sorted to produce Table 9-2, this factor complicated the result. As far as the computer was concerned, a lt hip arthroplasty was a different entity from a rt hip arthroplasty, and an ORIF-Lt hip was different from an ORIF-Rt hip. Although wild cards can be used to pull out all of those patients who have had arthroplasties, or ORIFs, there is nothing that can be done to make them sort as the same piece of data. Notice, however, that the records for those patients who had left and right ORIFs were at least sorted one after the other because the field started with the name of the surgery. (This factor still would create a problem if a secondary sort was performed.) The records of patients who had arthroplasties, however, were in different areas, because the field entries were made with Lt or Rt as the first characters.

There are several solutions to this situation. One would be to have a separate field for right or left. This could create problems if surgeries were entered that were not

```
┌────────────────────────────────────────────┐
│                                            │
│  Record Number: 1122  LOS: 4   Surgery: ORIF - Rt hip │
│                                            │
│  First Name: Forest   Last Name: Green     │
│                                            │
│  Age: 23       Sex: M                      │
│                                            │
└────────────────────────────────────────────┘
```

```
┌──────────────────────────────────┐
│                                  │
│  # 1122          ORIF - Rt hip   │
│                                  │
│  Forest Green     23     M       │
│                                  │
└──────────────────────────────────┘
```

Figure 9-3 ● Some form views for a record.

designated as right or left, but that problem could be solved by designating an entry for that field when it is not applicable. A better choice would be to eliminate left and right. To make databases useful, nurses and other health care professionals need to evaluate what information they need so only data that are necessary to these ends are recorded yet nothing vital is omitted. The terminology that is to be used for various conditions also needs to be determined.

VALIDITY CHECKS ON DATA

To prevent different forms of the same phenomena being entered as data, good systems provide a method of validating new entries. One of the most common methods is to present a list of options to the person entering the data. This list is accessed when data are being entered into the field. For example, if one were entering pathogens into an infection database, they would be presented with a list that would contain the acceptable text for each pathogen. Without this list, one might see entries of S. aureus, Staph, and Staphylococcus aureus for the same pathogen, making it impossible to sort the records by pathogen.

▼ Forms for Data Entry

In Tables 9-1 to 9-5, the data were presented in what is called a table view, which is similar to a spreadsheet format. Data can also be looked at in a form view. In this view, it is possible to look at all the data for only one record.[3] Forms are similar to reports. They can be designed to show all fields or only the fields the user wishes to have on the screen. They can be used to view data or to enter data. Figure 9-3 (top) is a form view of all the data for Mr. Green. Note that the term record number instead of rec # was used to precede the record number. A form can be designed using names for fields that give the exact meaning instead of the field name, or the field name can be completely omitted. Other information can also be added to aid the individual

---

[3]Forms can also be designed to show multiple records. The design preference depends on their intended use.

who is using the form. Figure 9-3 *(bottom)* is another form view of Mr. Green's record. This one omits the LOS field and does not show field names.

When designing a form (or screen report), the prime consideration should be how individuals will use the data. Forms in which a user has to search for what she or he needs reduce productivity. It is possible to design many different forms (or reports) for the same data, thus making it easy to provide the appropriate screen design for all who need the data.

▼ Creating a Small Database

The physical creation of a database is simple. The more complicated steps involve deciding what the database will be used for, what fields are needed, and how these fields should be placed in tables.

PLANNING

The first step in creating a database is planning. Developing a useful database with a minimum of effort involves a number of criteria:

- ▼ Deciding on the output
- ▼ Determining what data are needed to create this output
- ▼ Normalizing the data into the needed tables
- ▼ Planning the flow of information through the database
- ▼ Creating tables, forms for data entry, and reports

Perhaps every semester, a nursing student has to produce a list of the institutions in which she or he has clinical experience, another for procedures performed in the clinical area, and another for the interventions done for specific nursing diagnoses that includes the primary medical diagnosis and the etiology of the nursing diagnosis. The nursing student decides to experiment with using a database for this assignment. The first step is to plan. The nursing student concludes that she or he will require the following reports:

- ▼ The procedures performed in clinical situations, the date on which they were performed, and the institution and clinical unit in which they were done
- ▼ The institutions and units where clinical experience was obtained
- ▼ The nursing diagnoses for which an intervention was provided, the primary etiology for each nursing diagnosis, and the primary intervention performed for each nursing diagnosis. This report should also have the medical diagnosis of the client

Now that the nursing student has determined the information needed from the database, the data required to produce this information must be stated (Table 9-8).

Knowing the information necessary for reports, the nurse can now determine what data must be in the database. The following information is required:

- ▼ Date of care
- ▼ Institution where it was given

Procedures	**Institutions**	**Nursing diagnosis and interventions**
1. Date	1. Institution	1. Nursing diagnosis
2. Institution	2. Unit	2. Primary etiology
3. Unit		3. Primary medical diagnosis
4. Procedure		4. Intervention

TABLE 9-8 ● *Data Needed on Each Report*

▼ Unit in that institution
▼ Primary medical diagnosis
▼ Procedure
▼ Nursing diagnoses
▼ Primary etiology for each nursing diagnosis
▼ Primary intervention for each nursing diagnosis

The nurse now must structure the information so it can be easily retrieved. Structuring involves a process called *normalization*. Technically, there are five levels of normalization. The first level is to eliminate *repeating groups*, or a group of fields with duplicate information in records. For example, when different nursing diagnoses are recorded for the same client, unless the tables are normalized, the nurse would be repeating all of the other information about the client. Normalizing tables involves creating a parent (master) and at least one child (detail) table. In the database of orthopedic surgeries, when a separate table was created for nursing diagnoses, instead of duplicating the information in the other fields, the database was normalized (see Tables 9-1 and 9-3) by creating a child table of nursing diagnoses.

In the list of data compiled so far, there is no one unique piece of data or a field around which all the other data can revolve. The nursing student decides that for the purpose of this database that the most appropriate central piece of data would be the client. In a desire to preserve patient confidentiality, the nursing student also decides to devise a code consisting of the first three letters of the month, with a different number for each patient in that month. For example, the first patient for whom care was provided in January is coded as jan1, the second jan2, and so on. This adds an additional field to the database, which is then named client code.

In normalizing the data, the nursing student determines that client, date, institution, unit, and primary medical diagnosis are the fields that can have only one possible entry for each client. It would be possible, however, to perform two procedures on the same date and for a client to have two different nursing diagnosis. Thus, he or she decides to create the tables as seen in Table 9-9.

The nurse decides to name the parent table Clients, and the child tables Procedure and Nxdx. Knowing that memory can sometimes fail, the nurse keeps a data dictionary that will allow matching the field name with its contents. The nurse also decides what to call each field and what the key fields will be.

A key field or fields are what make each record unique. That is, no two records will have the same entry in this field. In the client table, each client will have a differ-

TABLE 9-9 ● *Fields and Definitions for Each Table*	
Client table	
Field Name	*Contents*
Client*	The code for the client
Institution	Institution where the client was cared for
Unit	Unit in that institution where the client was cared for
Medical	Primary medical diagnosis for the client
Procedure table	
Client*	The code for the client
Date*	Date on which care was given*
Procedure*	Procedure that was performed
Nxdx table	
Client*	The code for the client
Date*	Date on which the intervention was performed
Nxdx*	Nursing diagnosis for an intervention was provided
Etiology	The primary etiology for this diagnosis
Intervention	The main intervention provided for this nursing diagnosis

*Indicates a key field.

ent client number, so that field can be used for a key. In the procedure and nxdx tables, the client number field will not be unique in each record because more than one procedure can be performed on a client or the client may have more than one nursing diagnosis for which interventions were performed. To give these tables a unique key, the nurse creates what is called a *composite key*, or one that is composed of more than one field. For those tables, the nurse keys both the client's name and the date. To be sure that each record is unique, in the procedure table, the nurse also keys the procedure and, in the nxdx table, the nursing diagnosis.

Before constructing the tables, the nurse has to decide what transformations or manipulations will be needed to allow the creation of needed reports. A data flow diagram (DFD) could be made in order to visualize how data will flow in the database.

A DFD is a tool that allows one to visualize how data will flow through a system and where processing or analyzing of the data has to occur. DFDs can be at a very abstract level, such as for an entire system, or at a basic level, detailing what data are required for a specific function and how it should be manipulated. There are many variations on constructing a DFD. The objective of all of them is to permit the visualization of how data needs to flow through a system. Data flow diagrams must represent four entities—data flow, where the data are stored, how it is processed, and its eventual destination (Kozar, 1997). The symbols used to represent these entities may vary from DFD to DFD. In creating the DFD, the nurse decides to use the following symbols:

▼ Input—a rounded rectangle
▼ Data flows—movement of data in the system—arrows (→)
▼ Data stores—data repositories for data that is not moving (a table in our situation)—a rectangle that is open on the top
▼ Processes—transformation of data, a circle (○)
▼ External entities—sources or destinations outside the specified system boundary—a rectangle (□)

The DFD for this database is represented in Figure 9-4.

With these tools, the code book, and DFD, the nursing student is ready to go to the computer to construct the database. Using the table structure she or he created (see Table 9-9), three tables are created. She or he then makes a form for data entry. To take advantage of the one piece of data/many uses principle, an integrated form that hot links all the tables is created. With this type of form, when the client code is entered into the client or master table, this information will automatically be entered into the other two tables. Hence the information will only be entered once.

In these reports, the only transformation will be moving data from tables to a report. It is very possible to do other things with the data. The database could be asked to count the number of different procedures or interventions performed. Some other

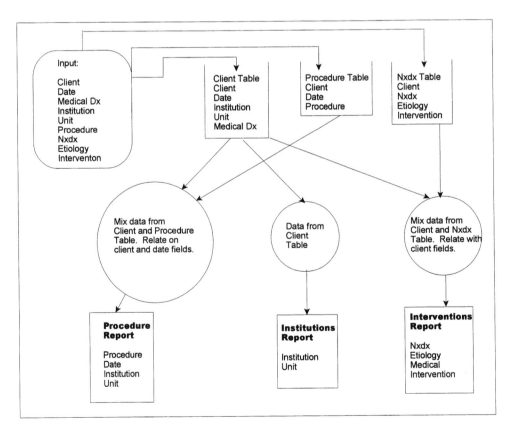

Figure 9-4 • Data flow diagram.

transformations of data to information that a database can be asked to perform include averages and sorting.

▼Assumptions in Databases

If the database just discussed was actually created, some interesting things would be discovered. When an attempt is made to record a procedure, such as taking a blood pressure more than once for a given client and date, it will be rejected by the procedure table, because it will duplicate another entry, which the key fields in the database will not permit. The assumption on which this database was created was that the user would only record more complex procedures that would be performed only once a day. If these aims are different, the problem could be solved by adding a time field to the procedure table and creating a five-field composite key.[4] The same assumption is at work in the nxdx table.

In this instance, it is easy to add another field. In clinical databases, it is not always practical to capture all data. Thus, those who design databases must make decisions. What data are captured, what is ignored determines what information the database can produce. The view of health care held by the people deciding on what a health care information system will produce determines what information is captured and what is ignored. Assumptions in themselves are not bad, but they should be acknowledged. The information from a database is only as objective as the data that it contains. To rely on output from a database without an understanding of the data that was used to create the information is to make decisions with inadequate knowledge.

▼Databases in Patient Care

Gaining information from data about falls, medication errors, or other data is facilitated when a computerized database is used. In an ideal situation, all needed data would be downloaded from the larger hospital information system. When this is not possible, it may be necessary to collect the data at the unit level. Regardless of the source of the data, the concepts of querying data and creating reports are important in managing information for patient care, whether the goal is to ascertain quality and effectiveness of care or to create educational records for staff.

▼Summary

Databases are the underpinning of all health care information systems. When designing a database, there are several criteria to keep in mind. Because the structure of a database determines the output, efforts should be made to keep the data at the atomic level or as small a piece of data as can be reasonably collected, even if output demands do not require this at present. Databases have a way of expanding once users see their potential. Using data for other purposes is best accomplished when the fields are designed with expansion in mind.

---

[4]Or create a time/date field into which both the time and the date can be entered. Then you would only need a four-field composite key.

In health care databases, as in all databases in which personal information is collected, security is a significant issue. Those who need the information must have access, yet those who are just curious must be kept out. As with database design, there are always trade-offs. The more secure a system is, the less available the data are for producing information and knowledge. The easier the access to the data, the less secure the system becomes.

Databases do not necessarily mirror reality 100%. The data that are collected and the structure are based on assumptions that represent the world view of those responsible for the database. Thus, if nursing is going to be able to support the contention that nurses add value to health care, nurses must be a part of deciding what data are captured, how data are structured, and the vocabulary used.

In many health care institutions, cost-cutting efforts turn to labor. Nursing is one of the biggest labor costs in health care institutions. Among those responsible for budgets, there is often a belief that nurses can be replaced with lower paid workers who can be quickly trained to do procedures. It would be easy to support this belief in a database by capturing only the procedure, without any indication of the outcome or the critical thinking needed to perform it safely. If nurses are to be truly valued as professionals, they need to document the knowledge they add to elements of care.

EXERCISES

1. Define the terms field, record, table, and database as they are used in a database
2. Describe the difference between a flat and relational databases
3. What are some ways you see databases being used by health care professionals in
   a. Clinical practice?
   b. Administration?
   c. Education?
   d. Research?
   e. Entrepreneurial work?
4. You have a database that contains over 1000 records. The fields in this database are Client ID, Primary Medical Diagnosis, Length of Stay (LOS), Nursing Diagnoses, Client Age, and Gender. What questions can you ask of this database?

REFERENCES

Gassert, C. A. (1997, July). Professional practice trends and issues. Paper presented at the Nursing Informatics Practice Review, Baltimore, MD.

Graves, J. R., & Corcoran, S. (1989). The study of nursing informatics. *Image, 21*(4), 227–231.

Inmon, W. H. (1995). What is a data warehouse. *Prism 1*(1). Available: http://www.cait.wustl.edu/papers/prism/vol1_no1/.

Joos, I., Whitman, N. I., Smith, M. J., & Nelson, R. (1992). *Computer in small bytes.* New York: National League for Nursing Press.

Kozar, K. F. (1997). *Systems with data flow diagrams.* Available: http://spot.colorado.edu/kozar/DFD.html.

Milholland, D. K., (1997, July). Computerized patient care systems. Paper presented at the 7th Annual Summer Institute in Nursing Informatics.

Zielstorff, R. D., Hudgings, C. I., & Grobe, S. J. (1993). *Next-generation nursing information systems: Essential characteristics for professional practice.* (Pub No. NP-83). Washington, D.C.: American Nurses Association.

CHAPTER 10

Nursing Knowledge:
Access Via Bibliographic Databases

Margaret Allen, MLS-AHIP[1]

Objectives:

After studying this chapter you should be able to:

1 Access nursing knowledge via bibliographic databases

2 Identify bibliographic databases useful to nursing

3 Understand the structure of a bibliographic database record

4 Select appropriate databases for a variety of information needs

5 Search bibliographic databases using thesaurus terms and limit functions

6 Plan a literature search strategy for a complex question

7 Describe the use of reference management software

Given the vast amount of published information, it is impossible to know everything applicable to nursing practice. According to one author, "[to read] everything of possible importance to medicine, one would need to read 6,000 articles each day" (Arndt, 1992). In order to help find the information resources needed, librarians have created indexes that serve as guides to the literature. Originally developed in print formats, such as the card catalog and annual indexes of the periodical literature, these systems are now produced as databases that can be searched electronically. Electronic databases are more flexible than print indexes and often contain more information. They are compiled by developing a database record for every item indexed in the database. Many resources are indexed in databases, such as the online catalog MEDLINE, the International Nursing Index, and CINAHL (Cumulative Index to Nursing & Allied Health Literature), found in libraries. Library and Internet databases can be searched for information, and the user can develop bibliographic databases using reference management software.

Earlier, the development of a database to track clinical information on a group of patients, namely those hospitalized for a hip arthroplasty, was explored. It was discovered that not all patients recover from this surgery in a standard fashion, yet the goal of the hospital is to reduce the standard length of stay. Much more specific

[1]Library/Information Consultant; Resource Librarian Consultant for Cinahl Information Systems, Inc.; Project Director, Northwoods HealthNet, Northern Wisconsin AHEC, Inc.

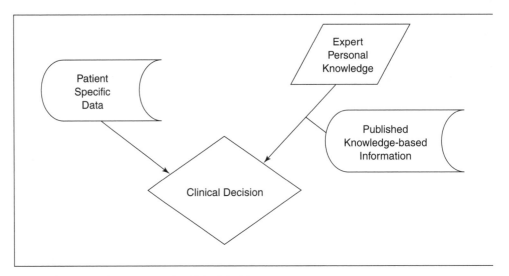

Figure 10-1 • Knowledge sources for clinical decisions.

data can be retrieved on this subject. Perhaps a supervisor now asks a nurse to develop a critical path for hip replacement patients. Information needs to be gathered in order to develop this critical path. In the model developed by Graves and Corcoran (1988), sources of information for a clinical decision are shown as coming from patient-specific information found in the patient record and from two sources of knowledge—expert knowledge possessed by the nurse and his or her colleagues or published information resources (Fig. 10-1).

Searching the literature is an important tool for improving the quality of patient care. Research has shown that the information provided by literature searches changes clinical decisions (King, 1987; Marshall, 1992). Other researchers have found that when searches were done early in a hospitalization, the results lead to decreased length of stay (Klein, Ross, Adams, & Gilbert, 1994). A study conducted in the United Kingdom demonstrated that information from searches was applied not only to immediate clinical decisions but also to the evaluation of practice outcomes and the design of practice guidelines and educational offerings (Urquhart & Davies, 1997).

▼ Bibliographic Databases

Electronic knowledge databases may be provided via a local area network, an Intranet, or networked access to Internet resources. For example, a collection of reference books on CD-ROM may be networked on your hospital information network. Other indexes and databases will be found in the library.

Some indexing tools include full-text information as well as the indexing data, so the distinction between bibliographic databases and full-text databases is becoming blurred. Bibliographic databases contain citations and indexing information that lead to the actual information resources, whereas full-text database means that the database includes both the citation and the complete text of the indexed document.

Online library catalogs are databases with a record for every title owned by a library or a group of libraries. To search an online catalog, you can choose to search by author, title, or subject heading, just as you would in the old card catalog. Some systems allow searching in additional fields, such as the call number. In addition, you can usually search by keyword, so that you do not need to know the first word in a title you want to find. Many online catalogs are accessible via the Internet, using either Telnet or web search engines. For example, the National Library of Medicine (NLM) holdings are online. They are found on the NLM home page at http://www.nlm.nih.gov/. At the time this chapter was written, NLM Locator served as the online catalog, using a Telnet search engine. Three separate catalogs were maintained for books, audiovisual programs, and periodical holdings. However, NLM had just announced the purchase of a new integrated library system, which may be in place by the time you read this chapter (National Library, 1998a). As technology and budgets allow, libraries will change the system they use to provide more sophisticated search options and features. With the basic record format well defined and standardized, records can be transferred from one system to another without corruption.

▼Key Databases for Nursing Knowledge

The NLM has the mission of making the knowledge derived from biomedical research accessible to all health professionals. With funding from the U.S. Government, NLM developed the online MEDical Literature Analysis and Retrieval System (MEDLARS®), and produced MEDLINE® (MEDlars onLINE), the first online database indexing journal articles (National Library, 1998b). MEDLINE records begin with 1966 journals, with experimental records from 1964 and 1965 now available as OLDMEDLINE.

The MEDLINE database was initially planned to include all journals indexed for *Index Medicus,* which included just six nursing journals in the early 1960s. When MEDLINE was in the planning stages, both the American Nurses Association and the American Dental Association were invited to participate in its development, increasing the journal coverage for these professions. MEDLINE has evolved from a fee-for-service database searched only by librarians to its current widespread availability. In 1997, NLM announced free access to MEDLINE via the World Wide Web (WWW). Free MEDLINE is one of the choices on the main NLM home page at http://www.nlm.nih.gov/.

International Nursing Index (INI), now published by Lippincott Williams & Wilkins, is based on the nursing subset of MEDLINE. A comprehensive international index, the print version of INI includes additional material not in MEDLINE, such as a list of doctoral dissertations in nursing. For access to the journal literature, INI includes the MEDLINE indexing for approximately 300 nursing journals, including the 43 nursing journals now included in *Index Medicus.* INI also includes any articles with nursing content from any of the 3900 periodical titles indexed in MEDLINE and any of the additional titles included in the *Hospital Administration and Planning Index.* Produced by the American Hospital Association in cooperation with NLM, this latter index is available online from NLM and other vendors as the HealthSTAR database. The diagram in Figure 10-2 illustrates the relationship of these key databases and their print index counterparts.

MEDLINE: *Index Medicus*
            Index to Dental Literature
            International Nursing Index

HealthSTAR: *Hospital and Health Administration Index*

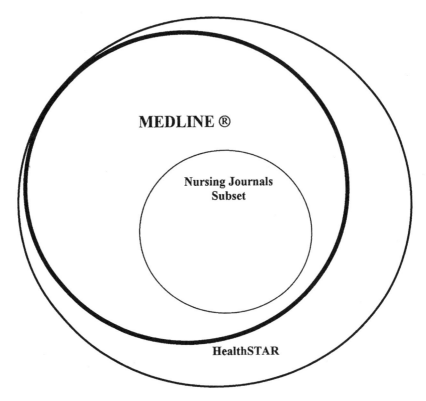

International Nursing Index = Nursing Journals Subset plus selected articles from
all of MEDLINE and HealthSTAR

Figure 10-2 • Relationship of MEDLARS databases to each other and print products.

NLM offers other online databases, including CATLINE for books, AVLINE for audiovisual programs, AIDSLINE for comprehensive coverage of information related to acquired immunodeficiency syndrome (AIDS), HealthSTAR for health care management, and BIOETHICSLINE for information on health-related ethical topics. These subject-specific indexes include all relevant MEDLINE journal article records, plus records for pertinent articles from additional journal titles and other information formats—including books, proceedings, and technical reports. NLM databases are available directly from NLM and from other online vendors who license the database records from NLM and design their own search software for retrieving document records. Future plans call for the merging of many of the NLM databases into the PubMed database.

The *Cumulative Index to Nursing and Allied Health Literature* (CINAHL) is a comprehensive database for nursing. Like the NLM databases, CINAHL is available from multiple online vendors. CINAHL is considered an integrated database because it indexes multiple information formats.

Examples of other specialized subject databases include PsychINFO, CANCERLIT and Physicians Data Query (PDQ®). These databases and others are described in the Selecting Databases section, which appears later in this chapter.

Full-Text Databases

In addition to bibliographic citation databases that help find information resources, some databases include the (full-text information) resources. Because of copyright laws, database producers must either obtain permission to include copyrighted information resources or create original content for inclusion in the database. CINAHL includes a limited amount of full-text information, such as

- ▼ Articles from a few nursing journals, particularly state nursing journals
- ▼ Critical paths
- ▼ Government publications in the public domain
- ▼ Research instruments
- ▼ Original documents written for Cinahl Information Systems

Other databases may either include full-text articles as part of the indexed content, or link to a collection of full-text journals.

Internet Databases

Two types of databases are available through the Internet—factual databases and bibliographic databases. Examples of factual databases include the Sigma Theta Tau Registry of Nursing Research, and other online directories, encyclopedias, and reference works, such as drug information databases. Many of these databases limit access to subscribers or members of the sponsoring organization and thus require a password. Databases are expensive to produce and require income from subscribers or sponsors to support their development. This is also true for full-text journal databases. Many universities and several states subscribe to factual and full-text databases that can be used by authorized individuals.

Bibliographic Database Structure

The record structure of a bibliographic database includes fields for both descriptive and subjective data. It is helpful to review the record format used in library catalogs. In the book record format, the author, title, edition, publisher and date, and description fields are used to describe the information resource. Recording this information is considered descriptive cataloging. Subjective data fields include those for subjects and the call number. A cataloger assigns subject headings and a call number by examining the book and determining the main subject or subjects covered in the book.

This number is determined by the classification scheme used by the library, such as the Dewey Decimal system, used by most public and school libraries; the Library of Congress scheme, used by most academic and special purpose libraries; or the NLM classification, used by most hospital and health science libraries.

SUBJECT HEADINGS

Subject headings are also standardized. Again, the library chooses a single standard authority for all its cataloging. Libraries using the NLM classification use the subject headings found in NLM's Medical Subject Headings (MeSH®), which is the controlled vocabulary NLM uses for cataloging books and other holdings and for indexing articles, including MEDLINE (National Library of Medicine, 1998c). MeSH differs from other subject heading lists, in that it is based on a hierarchical structure. Because of this factor, searches on a broad subject can be constructed to include the narrower subjects in the MeSH tree structure for the broader term.

ORGANIZATION OF THE SUBJECT HEADINGS

Both MeSH and the CINAHL thesaurus use a hierarchical tree structure. See Figure 10-3 for an example. Each indent indicates a lower level of specificity. MeSH subject headings can be found online in the MeSH Browser on the left side of the PubMed search screen at http://www.ncbi.nlm.nih.gov/PubMed/ or by using the Find MeSH

Anatomy (MeSH Category)
    Body Regions (Non MeSH)
        Extremities
            Amputation Stumps
            Arm (+ more specific terms)
            Leg
                Ankle
                Foot
                    Forefoot, Human
                        Metatarsus
                            Toes
                                Hallux
                    Heel
                        Tarsus
                Hip
                Knee
                Thigh

Figure 10-3 • MeSH tree.

feature in Internet Grateful Med (IGM) at http://igm.nlm.nih.gov/. The Find MeSH feature uses the UMLS (United Medical Language System) Metathesaurus, which includes terms from nursing and other medical classification systems.

DATABASE INDEXING

When a journal article or other information resource is included in a database, a record is created using a standard format for the type of information. The database record has fields to describe the document and index the content using subject headings. Most of the information in the database record can be entered by data entry clerks or even transferred electronically from the publisher. Human indexers are responsible for adding information in the publication type, instrumentation, and subject heading fields. Like subject headings, publication types are selected from lists specific to the database. The instrumentation field is unique to nursing databases.

Subject indexing varies based on the differences in the thesauri and individual human variation. The first consideration is that the indexer must choose terms from the database thesaurus, MeSH for MEDLINE indexing, and the *CINAHL Subject Heading List* for CINAHL indexing. Indexers are expected to use the most specific term available, and they may select as many subject headings as are required to describe the content of the article. Both major and minor subject headings are selected. The print version of the index lists the article citation under each main subject heading. Minor headings cannot be used for searching in the print index but can be used in online searching. Minor subject headings include common terms referred to as *checktags*, which indicate the populations studied (age groups and others), as well as additional subjects addressed in the article. Subheadings may be used with both major and minor headings to describe the content of the article better. In the MEDLINE record, major headings are indicated by the addition of an asterisk in front of the term. The CINAHL record has separate fields for major and minor headings, often abbreviated MJ and MN.

Given the multiple options, it is not surprising to discover that indexing is an art, not an exact science. Given the same article, indexers will often differ in their selection of subject headings. Most of the time, however, they will agree on the key concepts in the article. Figure 10-4 compares MEDLINE and CINAHL indexing for one article. For more detail on the indexing process, see "Selecting key words: Helping others find your article" (Allen, 1998, Winter).

▼Performing a Literature Review

Literature searches are a vital step in developing research-based practice. Understanding subject headings is a key factor in developing search strategies that will lead you to the most useful information on your topic. Titler and others (1994) describe the role of the literature search in their article presenting the Iowa Model of Research in Practice. Although ideas for change may come from regular reading of the literature, the search is critical in determining whether the published research warrants a change. In their model, the Iowa group also notes the importance of critical review of the research literature found in a literature search. For more on this step, see articles on reading research such as "How to assess a research study" (Rankin & Esteves, 1996).

Author: Gammon J. Mulholland CW.
Title: Effect of preparatory information prior to elective total hip
replacement on post-operative physical coping outcomes
Source: International Journal of Nursing Studies 1996 Dec; 33(6): 589-604

MEDLINE	CINAHL
Major MeSH: Hip Prosthesis/ *rehabilitation *Patient Education	Major Headings: Coping Hip Surgery Joint Replacement Postoperative Period Preoperative Education
Minor MeSH: Adult Aged Aged, 80 and over Analgesia Evaluation Studies Exercise Therapy Female Hip Prosthesis/psychology Human Length of Stay Male Middle Age Movement Outcome Assessment (Health Care) Postoperative Complications Postoperative Period Surgical Procedures, Elective	Minor Headings: Aged Aged 80 and Over Ambulation. Data Analysis Software Descriptive Statistics Female Length of Stay Male Middle Age Outcomes of Education. Postoperative Complications Postoperative Pain Quasi Experimental Studies Recovery Research Instruments T-Tests United Kingdom

Figure 10-4 ● Sample subject indexing comparison.

DEFINING YOUR TOPIC

The first step in developing a search strategy is to define the topic. It usually helps to write out the search question. As an example, to develop a research-based critical path for the care of patients undergoing a hip arthroplasty, research articles from the biomedical and nursing literature must be found, as well as examples of critical paths from other organizations. The question might be, "What factors affect the recovery of patients undergoing hip replacement surgery?" The major concept in this question is hip replacement surgery. Other concepts could include age group or groups, length of stay, preoperative care, postoperative care, and rehabilitation.

SELECTING DATABASES

For most searches on clinical topics, a researcher will want to use the library catalog and the MEDLINE and CINAHL databases. Searches on nonclinical topics often require the use of other databases such as BIOETHICSLINE or HealthSTAR.

Another database for the nursing periodical literature is RNdex®, which is available from the Information Resources Group (1998). Although the database is limited to just 150 leading nursing and case management journals, it includes original abstracts when author abstracts are not available for inclusion in the database. For a comparison of the index coverage and research content of key nursing journals, see the online chart Key Nursing Journals: Characteristics and Database Coverage (Allen, 1998).

PsychINFO

Because nursing is a holistic profession, some questions may best answered by adding searches of psychosocial databases such as PsycINFO and Sociological Abstracts. PsycINFO is produced by the American Psychological Association (APA). Libraries may subscribe to the complete collection of PsycINFO databases, or subsets, including the ClinPSYC® CD-ROM database for coverage of the clinical literature indexed by PsycINFO. PsycLIT® is the name for the CD-ROM version of Psychological Abstracts online, which is available in many academic libraries.

Sociological Abstracts

Sociological Abstracts, Inc. (SAI) is the producer of three databases—Sociological Abstracts, Social Planning/Policy & Development Abstracts (SOPODA), and Linguistics and Language Behavior Abstracts. These databases offer abstracts of information from more than 2000 journals from sociology and related social sciences, as well as citations to books and book chapters, conference papers, dissertations, and reviews of books and other media (SAI, 1998).

Oncology Questions

For oncology questions, search CINAHL and CANCERLITR or MEDLINE for literature and use the Physician's Data Query (PDQ®) system for additional information. Produced in cooperation with the National Cancer Institute, CANCERLIT and PDQ are linked from the NLM home page under the database menu. PDQ is an example of an authoritative full-text database. The registries and directories can help patients as well as health professionals find cancer centers working with the latest research and drugs specific to their treatment needs (National Cancer Institute, 1988).

Practice Guidelines

For practice guidelines, the HSTAT database from NLM provides access to the full-text of practice guidelines from a wide variety of U.S. Government agencies (NLM, 1998d).

Management Topics

A business database may be added to a search. Business methods are often applied in health care, with the latest research and innovations coming from outside the health care sector. Ask librarians about business database availability. Many are produced with a large proportion of full-text articles, so that the information is readily available. When searching HealthSTAR for management topics, note that a MEDLINE search does not need to be done, because HealthSTAR includes all management-related citations from the MEDLINE database (see Figure 10-2). HealthSTAR is available free from NLM, using the IGM search engine at http://igm.nlm.nih.gov. HealthSTAR is also available from many other database vendors. For background information on HealthSTAR, see the factsheet at http://www.nlm.nih.gov/pubs/factsheets/healthstar.html (NLM, 1998e).

Education Topics

For education topics, searching ERIC (Educational Resources and Information Clearinghouse) can also be useful. ERIC is an online index of articles, books, and reports related to education. Most academic libraries offer ERIC access using the search software from their primary database vendor. For free access, use the AskERIC™ program based at Syracuse University (AskERIC, 1998). Go to http://ericir.syr.edu/ and select the Search button to search the ERIC database, 1989 to date. Because it is produced with government funding, the ERIC database subscription cost is relatively low.

Patient Teaching

Patient and consumer teaching resources can be found in a wide variety of databases. Both MEDLINE and CINAHL index selected consumer health information resources. In CINAHL, some documents, particularly government publications, are available in full-text format. Because CINAHL has publication types for teaching materials and consumer/patient teaching materials (the latter beginning with 1997 indexing), it is easy to limit searches to this type of information. When information produced for the consumer cannot be found, articles in the nursing and allied health literature can be located that will help you with patient teaching.

Several other commercial databases also index the consumer health literature, including EBSCO's *HealthSource*, the *Health Reference Center* from Information Access, and *MDX.Health Digest*, which is produced by Medical Data Exchange. These databases contain both bibliographic and full-text information. Ask your librarian about availability—these databases are primarily marketed to organizations, not individuals.

A free source worth searching is *CHID: Combined Health Information Database*, which contains records for pamphlets, kits, videos, articles, books, and book chapters on 18 major health care topics. CHID is a database constructed by health-related agencies of the Federal Government (CHID Online, 1998). CHID is available at http://chid.nih.gov/.

In addition to bibliographic databases for consumer and patient health information, several publishers produce full-text patient education databases that can be licensed for access by organizations through CD-ROM or the Internet. Examples include Clinical Reference Systems (1998) and the Micromedex CareNotes™ System (Micromedex, 1998). Both of these products feature patient education materials written in both English and Spanish.

Web-accessible resources from government organizations and nonprofit organizations are often free. The problem with relying on the WWW for consumer and patient health information is that the information must be evaluated before using it in patient teaching. There are some reliable web sites that review and index selected consumer health web sites. Developed by libraries and government organizations, they offer a filtered road map to quality health information on the web. Examples include the following:

▼ Healthfinder, sponsored by U.S. Government agencies at http://www. healthfinder.gov/

▼ HealthWeb Consumer Health, at http://www.uic.edu/depts/lib/health/hw/ consumer/. This is keyword searchable from the main HealthWeb page at http://healthweb.org/

▼ MEL (Michigan Electronic Library) Health Information Resources, at http://mel.lib.mi.us/health/health-index.html

▼ NOAH: New York Online Access to Health at http://www.noah.cuny.edu/ —unique for providing its original information in both English and Spanish versions.

▼ Health Care Information Resources, for patients, their families, friends and health care workers, from McMaster University in Hamilton, Ontario, at http://www-hsl.mcmaster.ca/tomflem/top.html—offers an international selection of information resources.

MAKING THE SELECTION

From the listing of databases in this section, realize that selecting the most appropriate database is just as important as the search strategy. If one is looking for peer-reviewed professional literature, use the catalogs for libraries serving populations engaged in health care and education, and search databases and indexes such as MEDLINE, CINAHL, and the International Nursing Index. The important thing to remember is that a comprehensive search cannot be limited to online resources. Although a wide range of information resources may be found online, libraries, librarians, and bookstores are vital to help borrow or purchase the knowledge-based resources needed for nursing education and practice.

SEARCH STRATEGY DEVELOPMENT

Once the databases are selected, the key to a successful search strategy is understanding how the software works in tandem with database features to help focus a search on the most relevant information resources available in the database. Software for searching is often referred to as a *search engine*. Just when a particular search engine is mastered, the software typically will be upgraded or changed. The basic principles of database searching will have to be employed again to learn how to use the new search engine. If the following questions can be answered, search engine mastery will not be a problem:

1. What is the default search mode? Some database search engines open with a screen that maps the user to thesaurus terms, whereas the default in most is keyword searching. Mapping to subject headings is the default when using CINAHL*direct*®, Ovid, and PaperChase software. When subject mapping is not the default, some search engines offer an online thesaurus for finding thesaurus terms. Examples include IGM, the PubMed MeSH browser for use with the Entrez search engine, and SilverPlatter.

2. How does a user switch from the default search option to other search modes?

3. Can you use Boolean operators in your search? If yes, must AND and OR be capitalized? Is this done by filling out a form that automatically ANDs or ORs the information on each line or by typing these operators between terms? Remember that AND narrows a search, whereas OR broadens. In the diagram shown in Figure 10-5, use of AND will retrieve documents containing the condition specified in each circle, resulting in a relatively small group of records represented by the intersection of all three circles. Using OR will retrieve the records from all three circles—all of the records represented by circles A, B, and C.

4. Can separate search statements be combined with Boolean operators? If yes, how is this done? Example: S1 represents the first search request, and S2 the second in CINAHLdirect. S1 AND S2 narrows, whereas S1 OR S2 broadens. Search statements can be combined within parentheses: (S1 OR S2) AND S3.

5. When searching databases with subject headings arranged in hierarchical trees (NLM and CINAHL databases), can subject headings explode to retrieve all the narrower terms included under a broader term? If yes, is this automatic, or can this feature be invoked when the user decides it is needed?

6. Is phrase searching available? If yes, are operators such as ADJ needed for adjacent, or must the phrase be enclosed in quotes? Many search engines surpris-

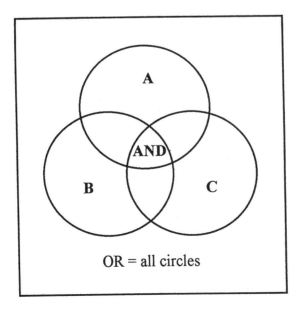

Figure 10-5 ● AND, OR.

ingly do not allow phrase searching. Instead, the words typed are automatically linked with an OR, broadening instead of narrowing the search.

7. Can terms be truncated to search on the root of a word? If yes, what symbol is used to indicate truncation? In many cases, but not all, an asterisk is used at the end of a root word, like psycholog* for psychology, psychological, and any other words beginning with psycholog. Although this system is useful for plurals and other word variations, be careful when truncating common medical terms because an unmanageable number of documents will be retrieved.

8. When using keyword searching, are all fields searched in the database record, or only fields predetermined by the database vendor?

9. Can specified fields be searched? For example, how does a user search by author or title? Can an author and title search be combined?

10. Can searches be limited to particular populations, year or years of publication, publication types, language, or subsets? If yes, how?

11. How are display and print records used?

12. Can records be downloaded or emailed for use in word processor or reference management software?

To learn about the search engines for the databases to be searched, look for tip sheets in libraries or on their web page. Also look for online help files that are part of most search software. For limiting searches, it is helpful to know the age groups and publication types for the databases, particularly when the search engine does not list the options as part of a special limit function.

SEARCH EXAMPLES

To illustrate the search process, some sample strategies are outlined below. Italics indicate field names, and bold type indicates use of a formal subject heading. Unless otherwise noted, the MEDLINE searches were done with the Entrez search engine for PubMed at http://www.ncbi.nlm.nih.gov/PubMed/, and the CINAHL database searches were done using the CINAHL*direct* web search engine, available online at http://www.cinahl.com.

Example: Care of Hip Replacement Patient

For the search question on care of the patient with a hip replacement, it was decided to search a library catalog and the MEDLINE and CINAHL databases.

In PubMed MEDLINE (Advanced Search), look up hip replacement in the MeSH browser, which suggests using these MeSH terms: **arthroplasty, replacement, hip** or **hip prosthesis.** Combining these two terms with an OR leads to more than 9000 citations. The next step is to search for the terms as major MeSH headings. It is always a good idea to search for the main concept as a major subject. In some systems, this process is referred to as limit to focus. The user can then use AND with the result with a search for English in the *Language* field. The number of citations retrieved, although reduced, is more than 5000. The next step is to use AND with the term **aged** in the *MeSH* field to limit the search to this population. Age groups should not be searched as major MeSH terms. Some software includes limit functions for population or age group, language, publication type, subset, and year or years of publication searches. With more than 3000 citations from the last search, change the display request to 5 years, which limits the result to just under 500 citations.

At this point, combine with other subject headings such as **length of stay,** or try the clinical queries feature in PubMed. This helps narrow a search to quality studies, particularly clinical trials. Using this feature, type the MeSH heading **arthroplasty, replacement, hip,** and limit the search retrieval to the past 5 years. This strategy leads to a manageable retrieval of 85 citations, including several articles related to the prevention of deep vein thrombosis. The majority of the articles retrieved were from medical journals, which is to be expected in a MEDLINE search.

In CINAHL, hip replacement is not a subject heading. Review of the CINAHL subject headings suggests the two subjects can be combined:

S1: Explode **joint replacement** (to include the narrower term **joint prosthesis**)
S2: **hip surgery**
S3: S1 AND S2 results in 173 articles.

This is a large retrieval, so review the first citations (usually the most recently published), or limit the search to certain publication types, such as research.

Example: Research, Protocols, and Guidelines Related to Hip Replacement

In MEDLINE, one can search on **clinical protocols** as a MeSH term and guidelines as a publication type, but there is no option for limiting to research articles. With some search engines, a search can be limited to articles with abstracts, but that strategy may eliminate some excellent possibilities. In PubMed, **arthroplasty, replacement, hip** [Major MeSH] AND **clinical protocols** [MeSH] narrowed the retrieval to 16 documents. Combining the subject with the word guideline in the *Publication Type* field produced just two citations.

In CINAHL database searches, the publication types can be limited. Using publication type limits with the search result from the first strategy, the following hits were produced:

S3 and *Publication Type* = Critical Path—11 citations
S3 and *Publication Type* = Clinical Guideline—0 citations
S3 and *Publication Type* = Protocol—6 citations
S3 and *Publication Type* = Research—65 citations

The research *Publication Type* is useful in nursing, in which not all studies are clinical trials. It allows relevant research to be identified, including potential research instruments to use in research replication or similar studies. To determine whether or not a study used a research instrument, review the *Instrumentation* field, which lists the research instruments used in a study.

Example: Research on Postoperative Pain

After reviewing the literature found in the searches for information on care of the patient undergoing hip replacement surgery, it is determined that postoperative pain is a major factor affecting length of stay. It is decided that the search should be broadened by looking for research articles on postoperative pain.

To do this search in MEDLINE, the official subject heading is Pain, Postoperative. Because a search on this term retrieves more than 8000 citations, use the Clinical Query feature in PubMed (an alternative for other search engines would be to combine with the therapy subheading, explode the search, and limit to Publication Type = Clinical Trial). With this strategy, the retrieval is more than 1800 citations. Adding AND with the phrase hip surgery reduced the retrieval to 25 citations.

Example: Age-Specific Pain Control

Instead of the hip or orthopedic surgery limit to the postoperative pain search, one might want to try limiting the pain search to a specific population, such as the elderly. It is important to use the identical age group designations used in the indexing. Both databases use the same terms for age groups, but CINAHL uses **child** for ages 6 to 12, whereas MEDLINE uses **child** for the entire age range from birth to 18 (exploding the term Child retrieves all the smaller age ranges listed under Child). In MEDLINE, adding AND **aged** AND **English** [Language] to the Clinical Query on **pain, postoperative** retrieved more than 500 citations, 230 of which were published in the last 5 years. For effective review of this topic, consider how the result might be limited to surgical procedures related to hip surgery but without making the strategy too narrow. One possibility would be to look for articles in English on **arthroplasty, replacement, pain, postoperative** and **aged**. This strategy retrieved 112 citations, 49 of which were published in the past 5 years. An alternate strategy is to combine with a second MeSH term, **length of stay**, which retrieved 63 citations, 41 of which were published in the last 5 years.

In CINAHL, limiting the **postoperative pain** search to **aged** and *publication type =* research retrieved 97 citations. Combining with the additional subject heading **length of stay** reduced the retrieval to only three citations.

Example: Nursing Classifications: Impaired Physical Mobility

In thinking about patients undergoing hip replacement, searches may be included on potential nursing diagnoses and interventions to consider in the critical path. A search on **Impaired Physical Ability (NANDA)** in CINAHL is relatively successful, retrieving 46 citations. Unfortunately, combining this subject heading with **hip surgery** results in no references, because nothing on this combination of topics had been indexed at the time the search was done.

In broadening the nursing search to include the biomedical literature or the earlier years covered by MEDLINE (1966 to date versus 1983 to date in CINAHL), try using the Find MeSH feature in IGM. This feature is based on the Unified Medical Language System (UMLS®) developed by NLM. The UMLS Metathesaurus includes terms from about 40 medical vocabularies, including nursing classifications (NLM, 1998f). When it is used with IGM, the UMLS Metathesaurus offers suggestions for finding MeSH terms most closely related to the terms from all of these vocabularies.

Example: Patient Education Resources Related to Pain

Limit a CINAHL search to the publication types Teaching Materials and Consumer/Patient Teaching Materials. Both publication types are needed because the latter publication type is relatively new. Search statements need OR to retrieve the documents indexed with the older basic publication type:

S1: **hip surgery**—292 citations
S2: S1 and Publication Type = Consumer/Patient Teaching Materials—one citation
S3: S1 and Publication Type = Teaching Materials—three citations
S4: S2 OR S3—four citations

In this example, one of the three older citations was actually relevant.

For this question, search other consumer and patient health information databases, as described earlier in this chapter.

FINDING ARTICLES SIMILAR TO A SPECIFIC ARTICLE

When a good article is found, more information on the same topic may be desired. A good way to do this is to search for the article using the author and key words from the title. For these searches, be sure you are searching the author field for the author's last name (MEDLINE and CINAHL use only first initials, so using first names will be counterproductive) AND the title field for words from the title. After finding the online record, choose a display format that allows how the article was indexed—this approach helps identify subject headings, which can be used to find other articles indexed with the same or similar subject headings.

The Entrez search engine for PubMed and IGM MEDLINE has a built-in shortcut to finding articles similar to the one you selected. After conducting an author-title search, you can select Related Articles and retrieve a list of citations to articles indexed with the same or similar subject headings.

AUDIOVISUALS ON NURSING THEORY

To search CINAHL for audiovisual programs on any of the nursing theorists, the best strategy includes these steps:

S1: Explode **nursing theory**; limit to focus (major heading) = 2232 citations
S2: Limit to *Publication Type* = Audiovisuals—17 citations

A similar strategy can be used to find research based on a particular nursing model. Because the model is usually not the main focus of the research, do not limit to focus for this type of search.

SEARCH STRATEGY REVIEW

In these examples, strategies used in broad searches were refined to limit retrieval to the most relevant citations. This method saves the time required to look at hundreds of citations and abstracts, so there is more time for the next steps of retrieving and reviewing the documents found in your searches. As the articles and other information resources are read, additional database searches may be needed. Bibliographies can also be used for finding important citations missed in your database search. Perhaps the indexer did not assign the subject headings chosen for the search, or the journal was not indexed in the databases you searched. Sometimes, older, classic articles are included in bibliographies, which can be used in a clinical practice or research project.

BROADER SEARCHES

Sometimes, searches will not retrieve enough citations. A question may be very narrow, or there simply may not be a lot of research published on the topic. When searching for an in-depth research project, comprehensive literature searches must be performed to be sure any significant research has not been missed. In these cases, broaden your search strategy. This procedured can be done by searching additional databases or using broader or related search terms. For medical topics, there are other databases that your librarian can recommend. One example is EMBASE, which indexes a different selection of journals than MEDLINE, including more European and pharmacology titles. Although MEDLINE indexes approximately 3900 journal titles (3200 current), NLM estimates that 13,000 to 14,000 biomedical journals are published each year (NLM, 1997).

To find broader or related terms for searching, use the thesaurus function provided by the search engine or engines used for searches. The thesaurus will show where the term you select fits in the hierarchical tree structure so that a broader term can be selected. This is how the term Arthroplasty, Replacement was found for the postoperative pain search in MEDLINE. The online thesaurus often includes a *scope note*, which defines the term. It may also include see related references that point to other terms. Sometimes, it is easier to select search terms from a print version of the thesaurus because related terms and cross-references can be viewed for a whole page of terms. The thesauri should be located in the reference section of your library—they are often kept with the print (index) version of the database. Each annual volume of *International Nursing Index* includes a very useful Nursing Thesaurus, which aids in the selection of MeSH terms for nursing topics (International Nursing Index, 1997).

▼ Building Personal Bibliographic Databases

Given the vast amount of print and online knowledge-based information resources, many health professionals have looked for tools that help organize and retrieve the information resources they encounter in the course of their ongoing reading and research. For many years, note cards were recommended for collecting information found in reading and literature reviews.

The problem with using note cards is the same problem faced by the library card catalog: a note card can only be filed in one place. Decisions have to be made on how to file cards (author, subject, or title), or multiple copies must be made for multiple points of access.

An alternative method would be for a user to create his or her own database, so they can search and retrieve information by all the access points they might want. Commercial bibliographic database management software is designed to save the trouble of designing a database that is compatible with the records from online bibliographic databases. An additional advantage is that this software can output references according to a wide variety of publication requirements, such as APA Style. Nicoll et al. (1996) reviewed five of these software packages: EndNote Plus, Library Master, Papyrus, Pro-Cite, and Reference Manager. Like any other software, these packages are constantly evolving, so it is best to check current reviews before making a purchase decision.

FEATURES OF PERSONAL BIBLIOGRAPHIC DATABASE MANAGERS

Traditional bibliographic management software packages include the following three functions:

▼ The ability to transfer bibliographic records into the personal database. This requires software filters, which may come with the package, or may be available for an additional cost. In the latter case, the user must determine which filters to acquire, because they are programmed to conform to the record structure used by the database vendor (NLM, OCLC, Ovid, PaperChase, SilverPlatter, and so on.)
▼ A database manager to develop searchable personal bibliographic databases. This usually includes the standard bibliographic fields plus a notes field for adding comments on the information resource.
▼ Tools to output bibliographies formatted according to the needed publication format, such as APA or MLA (Modern Language Association) style.

With this software, you can build a personal knowledge-based information database, which contains citations, abstracts, and—with some reference managers—links to online resources. You can choose to use call numbers and/or filing codes to link your references to a location for each of the resources you own. This systematic approach to managing knowledge-based information resources will enable you to refer back to valued information resources, without the need to remember all of the related details.

Z39.50 COMPLIANT

Some bibliographic database managers come with an interface for searching Z39.50-compliant databases and downloading the records directly into the personal database. This eliminates the need for filters in transferring downloaded records. When a program works with databases that are Z39.50 compliant, this means that they meet the requirements of this national standard for information retrieval. Officially known as ANSI/NISO Z39.50-1995—Information Retrieval (Z39.50): Application Service Definition and Protocol Specification, this standard establishes protocols for communication between two different computer systems. These protocols allow the client's software to search and retrieve records from databases residing on the server, which may be on a computer using a totally different operating system (Turner, 1997).

Most bibliographic management software also allows the user to add and edit records directly, without using the import filters or search interface. The user can copy and paste the data from any electronic document or simply type the information into the database. As a personal bibliographic database develops, the user will think of subject terms or keywords to add to the record, which will help retrieve information relevant to his or her personal interests.

BENEFITS OF PERSONAL BIBLIOGRAPHIC DATABASE MANAGERS

A major advantage of this type of software is that the record structure allows the user to develop bibliographies for papers and publications that comply with the required publication style without the need to retype the citations. This is particularly helpful if writing for a course and publications that have different style requirements. The record structure is designed to accommodate all information formats, so the databases developed are not limited to just one format, such as journal articles or books.

▼Copyright

When searching knowledge databases, it is important to realize that much of the information you retrieve is copyrighted. While downloading and storing references in a personal database for research and study is usually considered fair use, the reproduction of this information for use by others is covered by copyright law. Only the bibliographic description—author, title, and other publication data—is in the public domain. For the most part, U.S. Government information is not copyrighted, but one should check for any restrictions indicated on the actual document. Because MEDLINE is government produced, only the author abstracts are copyrighted. Otherwise, everything else you retrieve from knowledge databases is protected by copyright, including the subject indexing, abstracts, cited references, and any full-text and images. Although some copying may be allowed under the fair use doctrine, the best practice is to request permission for reproducing any copyrighted information resources.

▼Databases for the Virtual Library

As the universe of knowledge-based information resources expands to include web sites and other Internet accessible information resources, librarians and information scientists are applying subject-indexing principles to the development of databases indexing these new information formats. Web sites are now included in many online library catalogs. In the health sciences, the CINAHL database began indexing web site records in 1998. For clinical medicine, there are now web-based databases that use MeSH terms to index web sites. Some examples include

- ▼ CliniWeb from Oregon Health Sciences University at http://www.ohsu. edu/cliniweb/ uses MeSH terms from the Anatomy and Diseases tree to index more than 10,000 web sites. This database features the Saphire search engine for mapping natural language queries to MeSH terms. The web site also includes a demonstration of Saphire searching of NLM's UMLS Metathesaurus.
- ▼ Karolinska Institute Library: Diseases, Disorders and Related Topics at http://www.mic.ki.se/Diseases/index.html—MeSH based index; also in Swedish. Descriptions are from the actual web content, which are similar to those retrieved by a typical web search engine.
- ▼ Medical World Search at http://www.mwsearch.com/. From the Polytechnic Research Institute for Development and Enterprise of Polytechnic University, based in Hawthorne, NY. This site uses MeSH terms to index thousands of selected web sites. It features mapping from natural language queries to related MeSH terms, using the UMLS Metathesaurus.
- ▼ OMNI at http://omni.ac.uk/ uses MeSH to index a growing database of more than 2800 web sites. From the United Kingdom, the records include original brief descriptions of the indexed web sites.

▼Summary

A central feature of bibliographic databases is the added value provided by cataloging or indexing. In these processes, subject headings are assigned to the information resources cited in the databases. To obtain the best search results, use subject headings from the same subject heading thesaurus used by the cataloger or indexer. Specialized bibliographic databases use specialized subject heading lists, whereas general library catalogs and databases use more general subject headings. Look for and use online thesauri to help you select subject headings. Keyword searching should be reserved for situations in which subject headings do not match a need or when the user is looking for a known item.

Selecting the appropriate database or databases is just as important as devising a search strategy. Learn to match databases to information needs. The bibliographic database record includes fields for specific types of information, such as author, title, source, publication type, and subjects. Limiting searches to terms in the appropriate field or fields leads to higher quality searches. Bibliographic; database management software can help you manage the hazards of information overload.

Search engines are constantly changing and evolving. It is a time saver to become familiar with the basic search engine functions.

EXERCISES

1. Indexing an article:
   a. Find a nursing journal article, either online or in your library or personal collection
   b. Take a piece of paper and write the author, title, and source information on the top. Divide the rest of the sheet in three columns, as shown in Figure 10-6:
   c. Read the article and write the subjects you think it includes in the first column
   d. Do an author/title search in MEDLINE and write the MEDLINE subject headings in the second column
   e. Do an author/title search in CINAHL and write the CINAHL subject headings in the third column
   f. Compare and contrast the three columns

My subjects	MEDLINE	CINAHL

Figure 10-6 • Indexing worksheet.

MEDLINE	CINAHL	Website database:

Figure 10-7 • Database search terms worksheet.

2. Database searching:
   a. Choose a search topic related to a current patient care question.
   b. Plan a search strategy for MEDLINE, CINAHL, and one of the databases for web sites described in this chapter. Note the subject headings on a worksheet similar to the one used in the first exercise (Fig. 10-7):
   c. Execute the search in each of these databases
   d. Compare and contrast your results
3. Bibliographic management software:
   a. Read links on this topic on the web site for this book, including information provided by the vendor
   b. Read recent articles and reviews discussing bibliographic management software, both online and in journal articles that you retrieve through searching
   c. Investigate the availability of local workshops and support for specific products
   d. Based on your research, designate a software package that would best meet your needs and discuss the rationale for the choice

REFERENCES

Allen, M. (1998) *Key nursing journals: Characteristics and database coverage.* Stratford, WI: The author. Available: http://www.nursingcenter.com/people/nrsorgs/icirn/page1.html.

Allen, M. (1998, Winter). Selecting key words: Helping others find your article. *Nurse Author & Editor, 8,* 4, 7–9.

Arndt, K.A. (1992, September). Information excess in medicine. *Archives of Dermatology, 128,* 1249–1256.

AskERIC (1998). Available: http://ericir.syr.edu/.

CHID Online. (1998). Available: http://chid.nih.gov/.

Clinical Reference Systems. (1998). Available: http://www.patienteducation.com/.

Graves, J., & Corcoran, S. (1988, May-June). Design of Nursing Information Systems. *Journal of Professional Nursing, 4,* 168–177.

Information Resources Group. (1998). *RNdex®.* Available: http://www.rndex.com/.

International Nursing Index, 31, 1996. (1997).

King, D. N. (1987, October). The contribution of hospital library services to patient care: A study in eight hospitals. *Bulletin of the Medical Library Association, 75,* 291–301.

Klein, M. S., Ross, F. V., Adams, D. L., & Gilbert, C. M. (1994, June). Effect of online literature searching on length of stay and patient care costs. *Academic Medicine, 69,* 489–495.

Marshall J. G. (1992, April). The impact of the hospital library on clinical decision making: The Rochester study. *Bulletin of the Medical Library Association, 80,* 169–178.

Micromedex. (1998). Available: http://www.micromedex.com/.

National Cancer Institute. (1998). *PDQR—NCI's comprehensive cancer database.* Available: http://cancernet.nci.nih.gov/pdq.htm.

National Library of Medicine (1998a). NLM selects integrated library system "Voyager." Press Release February 11, 1998. Available: http://www.nlm.nih.gov/news/press_releases/voyager.html.

National Library of Medicine (1998b). *MEDLINE*®. Available: http://www.nlm.nih.gov/databases/medline.html.

National Library of Medicine (1998c). *Medical subject headings (MeSHR).* Available: http://www.nlm.nih.gov/mesh/meshhome.html.

National Library of Medicine (1998d). *Health services technology assessment texts (HSTAT).* Available: http://www.nlm.nih.gov/pubs/factsheets/hstat.html.

National Library of Medicine. (1998e). *Factsheet: HEALTHSTAR.* Available: http://www.nlm.nih.gov/pubs/factsheets/healthstar.html.

National Library of Medicine. (1998f). *Factsheet: Unified medical language system.* Available: http://www.nlm.nih.gov/pubs/factsheets/umls.html.

National Library of Medicine. (1998g). *Factsheet: Response to inquiries about journal selection for indexing at NLM.* Available online: http://www.nlm.nih.gov/pubs/factsheets/j_sel_faq.html.

Nicoll, L. H., Oulette, T. H., Bird, D. C., Harper, J., Kelley, J. (1996, January-February). Bibliography database managers: A comparative review. *Computers in Nursing, 14,* 45–56.

Rankin, M.& Esteves, M.D. (1996, December). How to assess a research study. *American Journal of Nursing, 96,* 32–37.

Sociological Abstracts, Inc. (1998). Available: http://www.accessinn.com/socabs/.

Titler, M. G., Kleiber, C., Steelman, V., Goode C., Rakel B., & Barry-Walker J. (1994, September-October). Infusing research into practice to promote quality care. *Nursing Research, 43,* 307–313.

Turner, F. (1997). An Overview of the Z39.50 Information Retrieval Standard (UDT Occasional Paper #3). Ottawa, Ontario: National Library of Canada. Available: http://www.nlc-bnc.ca/ifla/VI/5/op/udtop3.htm.

Urquhart, C. & Davies, R., (1997, June). EVINCE: The value of information in developing nursing knowledge and competence. *Health Libraries Review, 14,* 61–72.

Single Purpose Products

Not all our information retrieval, management, or communication needs fit the common application programs. The tools discussed so far are multipurpose. When information management needs arise, in many cases, users are better off adapting a regular application program to meet these needs because the skills they learn will transfer to other situations and because they will have more flexibility. Using a database or spreadsheet for grades, instead of a special grading package, is an example. There are some situations, however, in which adapting a regular application program will not provide the wealth of functions needed in the situation.

 Research Tools

Although the majority of information management needs in research are met by adapting a word processor, spreadsheet, statistical package, database, or presentation package, there are some situations in which a single purpose product adds enough value that using it is wise. One of those, a personal reference manager, was examined earlier. Anyone who accumulates a large list of resources will find that managing them is much more efficient with one of the management products.

Although a word processor, or even a database, could be adapted for creating and administering a questionnaire, there are special purpose products that assist users in these tasks. These products add value by making it easy to create any type of question—multiple choice, Likert scale, analog range, open ended, number input, and so forth (Beyea, 1996). Questionnaires can be

171

given on the computer or printed for use in situations in which a computer is not available.

Analyzing qualitative research is another instance in which a word processor or a database does not provide the sophisticated tools that a special product can. Qualitative research software allows a researcher to automate coding documents as well as to ask questions about the meaning of the data. These products can be used for small projects such as the analysis of focus groups, surveys with open-ended questions, and in constructing theories. Judy Norris maintains an excellent site at http://www.ualberta.ca/~jrnorris/qual.html, where information about these products can be found.

▼ Learning Resources

The nature of the computer leads to some special adaptations of the computer for educational purposes that cannot be met with the regular application programs. Computer-assisted instruction (CAI) is the name given to this special purpose software. It describes a great variety of programs designed to assist learners. CAI is also referred to by other terms such as computer-based instruction (CBI), computer-assisted learning (CAL), or computer-managed instruction (CMI). CAI (and any of its synonyms)[1] can be defined as any instruction in which the student uses a computer for learning. The information to be learned is not limited to knowledge about the computer; in fact, the focus of most CAI is on other topics.

In the late 1960s at the University of Illinois in Urbana, a maternity course was offered using Plato (programmed logic for automatic teaching operation), an online system designed to support CAI. Besides being the first recorded use of computers in nursing education, this CAI set a standard that even today is rarely seen. An inquiry approach in which learners had maximum control over learning was emphasized. Instead of having information delivered to them, students were led to figure things out for themselves, a process that seemed to improve the ability to retrieve information from memory (Bitzer, Boudreaux, & Avner, 1973). The results were that students using this CAI learned the content just as well as their counterparts taught in a classroom but completed their learning in 23.5 hours as compared with 66.5 hours. Additionally, the students using the CAI had excellent long-term retention of the information.

An analysis of 29 studies on computers, education, and nursing that were conducted between the years 1966 to 1991 revealed that CAI was favored over so-called traditional education (Cohen & Dacanay, 1994). Additionally, in the cases in which learner attitude was reported, learners had a more positive attitude toward CAI than traditional instruction. CAI that integrated video (known as interactive video) had the best results.

▼ One Overall Category: Many Variations

The general term CAI includes many different types of computerized instruction. It can also denote various uses of the computer, from instruction using only a stand-alone non-video-capable computer, to Internet-based distance learning using a

---

[1]CMI is sometimes used to denote a package that completely manages the entire instructional process, including presenting the instruction, grading, and reporting grades.

multimedia-capable computer. Although the various formats that CAI takes are discussed as separate entities, as the power of computers increases, the lines between categories are becoming increasingly blurred.

INTERACTIVE VIDEO

In interactive video, a computer presents instruction that integrates video, often from a laser video disk, with computer capabilities. The video segments can include regular video, slides, and other illustrations. Although integrating with video tape was the first instance of interactive video, the introduction of the laser disk allowed faster access. The laser disk did limit, however, the amount of video that could be used in a program to only 30 minutes. The laser disk is capable of storing 54,000 slides.

To use this type of software, one needs a laser disk player, a card inside the computer, and specialized software to facilitate the link. Today, video discs are being replaced by CD-ROM. CD-ROM has some of the same memory limitations that a video disk does, but most computers today have CD-ROM players and special software is not required to make it functional. As DVD-ROMs replace CD-ROMs, the memory problem will be solved. In health care, this type of CAI is referred to as computer-assisted interactive video (CAIV), or interactive videodisk (IVD). In other areas it may be referred to as IV for interactive video.

MULTIMEDIA

The only difference between interactive video and multimedia is the name. Multimedia, like interactive video, allows text, graphics, animation, and sound to be fully integrated by the computer into one educational package. Most multimedia applications are for games or other entertainment-focused goals.

VIRTUAL REALITY

The term virtual reality (VR) has many meanings, depending on the perspective of the speaker. To some, it is the use of devices, such as a head-mounted display or special gloves, whereas others stretch the term to include books or even pure imagination (Isdale, 1993). For purposes here, VR is defined as a way that humans can visualize, manipulate, and interact with complex objects. VR is more a capability that can be conveyed using multimedia than a distinctive type of CAI.

A better understanding of VR can be gained by looking at some of the ways that it is implemented. All VR is based on the concept that a *virtual world* can be created. A virtual world is a setting in which an individual interacts with objects as she or he would if she or he were in the real world. The simplest method of VR, sometimes called Desktop VR, uses the computer display screen to portray the virtual world (Isdale, 1993). Computer graphics are used to make the objects on the screen look, sound, and act real.

In another type of VR, called video mapping, a video input of the user's silhouette is merged with a two-dimensional computer graphic. On the monitor, the user sees the interaction of his or her body with the world. Another type, labeled an immersive system, completely immerses the user in the virtual world. These systems often use a head-mounted display that the user wears as a helmet or mask. This mask holds the visual and auditory displays. In a variation of immersive VR, a virtual world is simulated by multiple large projection displays that create a room called a *cave*.

In another interpretation of VR, known as telepresence, a camera is installed on a remote object that allows a user to control the object. An example is a surgeon using instruments on cables to perform surgery without making a large incision in the patient. Perhaps the most powerful and extensive type of VR uses a computer to generate inputs that are merged with telepresence or real inputs, or both, to provide the virtual world. For example, in brain surgery, images from earlier computed axial tomography scans and real-time ultrasound can be overlaid on the view of the brain. Flight simulators are another example of VR.

Virtual Reality Uses in Health Care Education

Given the practice nature of nursing and other health care education, VR may eventually come to be a very popular training method for the health care professions. One application that is under final development is a method of teaching intravenous puncture, in which *virtual tissues* are used (Merril & Barker, 1996). A virtual tissue is one that has been programmed to behave identically to real tissue when it is cut, tugged, stretched, or punctured. In this application, the tissues are programmed to resemble a rolling vein, sclerosed vein, and a vein in an obese patient.

As designed, this simulator integrates clinical decision making with learning the procedure by using various client scenarios in the program. The learner's first task is to read a client scenario and base his or her actions on this scenario. Once the scenario is assimilated, the user selects an appropriate site for the venipuncture, places the tourniquet, and manipulates the needle (Merril & Barker, 1996). Penetrating the skin produces in the user approximately the same feel as when one actually performs the procedure. The user also receives feedback that simulates how the pressure of venous wall resistance feels. During the simulation, the screen shows the user the position of the needle in relation to the vein. When the needle is inserted appropriately, blood is seen flowing from the vein into the needle.

Simulations such as this, which can be used to teach invasive procedures that need a high degree of skill if patient discomfort is to be minimized, can revolutionize how skill teaching is done. Surgical techniques are also being taught using VR. In these situations, not only do the tissues have to react normally but the circulatory systems also need to react. Such things as blood loss, heart rate, blood pressure, and cardiac output have to be integrated to produce this type of reality (Delp, Loan, Wong, & Rosen, 1996). Using this technology, a project has been developed to teach wound débridement. The scenario simulates the activities involved in this procedure, such as trimming and ligating bleeding vessels, trimming loose nerve strands, maintaining hemostasis, and detecting common errors made in the procedure.

Teaching cardiopulmonary resuscitation (CPR) can also be done by using a form of VR and interactive video. The system connects a mannequin to a computer, which records and reports the timing and effectiveness of the chest compressions and breathing. The system also includes didactic training with the use of interactive video. Although this system is not inexpensive, in situations in which CPR recertification is required frequently, it would pay for itself over a relatively short time period. The system is approved by the American Heart Association for CPR certification.

VR uses in health care are not confined to education. Researchers found that by using VR, they were able to reduce the anxiety level in student height-fearing volunteers after 2 months of treatment (Lesie, 1998). Using this technology, a therapist can control a patient's exposure to a situation while desensitizing the patient. There are, at present, four sites in the United States that use VR to treat phobias.

INTERNET-BASED INSTRUCTION

The Internet is rapidly finding a place in all types of education. Learners of all ages are using it as a library, and organizations are placing continuing education and even full courses on the Internet.

An incredible number of resources are available on the Internet. Students are using the Internet to find up-to-date information, patients use it to learn more about various disease conditions, and teachers and clinicians use it to stay updated.

Although correspondence courses are still the primary mode of distance learning in most of the world, in some areas, distance learning has gravitated to technology, such as two-way video and one-way or two-way audio. With use of the Internet, the move toward technology is continuing, especially in areas of the world that have reliable communication systems.

When describing distance learning, two terms that are frequently used are synchronous and asynchronous. In synchronous learning, class is held at set times and all participants are present, either online or with the use of microwave or other technology. This method resembles traditional education, although the students may be congregated in small groups at set locations in various places or alone at home.

Asynchronous learning means that learners use the learning resources at a time and place that is convenient for them. They may or may not have a set time for completing the learning requirements. Asynchronous learning is exemplified by correspondence courses. The Internet can also deliver asynchronous courses but with the advantage that communication between the learner and an instructor is much faster. The Internet has another advantage over correspondence courses in that it permits collaboration by learners just as if they were in a classroom. Combinations of either synchronous or asynchronous conditions are also employed, including requiring students to be physically present in one location for a given number of sessions.

A multi-user domain (MUD) is a software program that lets users interact in a virtual environment. Starting as dungeon and dragons games, MUDs and their offsprings multi-object-oriented (MOO) environments are gradually finding a place in education. The virtual environment can be a city, a university, or even a hospital. Users design the character and role they will play, and interact with other users and the environment via text. MUDs differ from chat rooms seen on the Internet in that users are able to move around, that is, they give commands to move to various places in the environment and interact with various objects found in the environment. For example, if the virtual world were a hospital, a user could command him or herself to go north. A description of what was visible would follow. Other commands would allow this same user to read a patient's chart or administer a treatment.

At present, the most common educational use for MOOs appears to be in writing classes. Students interact with one another and engage in discussion using written text. One advantage to this type of teaching environment is that all speakers respond, and conversation is not dominated by a few outspoken students. The result is that students are more involved in the discussion. In one study, despite purposely selecting students who were technophobes for these classes, students taught in the MOO environment showed more excitement and engagement in their work and generally performed better than students in regular classrooms, even when they were taught by the same instructor (Conlon, 1997).

▼ Classification of Educational Software

When considering the use of CAI, there are characteristics that need to be considered beyond the required hardware. Besides examining the content, one also needs to look at the type of program, the educational philosophy it embodies, and how well it uses the medium.

TYPES OF PRESENTATION

No matter what hardware is used in CAI, there are basically four different types of approaches to educational software. It is not unusual for one piece of software to include more than one approach and sometimes all four. Additionally, many programs can be turned into a different type by investigative learners and creative teachers. For this reason, it is often difficult to classify a program as belonging to a specific category. Examining the categories, however, presents a picture of the teaching methods that computers can emulate.

DRILL AND PRACTICE

Drill and Practice software was some of the first educational software introduced. It was relatively simple to produce, and it freed teachers from some mundane chores, mainly repetitive teaching. In one drill and practice format, the program emulates a teacher using flash cards. Other formats include multiple choice questions that students can use to review previously learned material. When they are well designed, these programs provide feedback on all of the choices. Another useful feature in this type of program is that it allows students to investigate the feedback for all answers, even when they get the right answer. This feature aids inquisitive students who want to use the program in a more tutorial mode.

The best use of drill and practice is as an aid to memorization. Although pure memorization is not a favored method of learning, there is a need to memorize such things as basic medical terminology, along with the rules for combining these terms to create other words. When selecting a pure drill and practice program, keep in mind that sometimes there are more effective ways to develop knowledge.

Tutorials

A tutorial is a program designed to impart information to learners. Most tutorials are patterned on the programmed learning model. Information is imparted, and the learner is asked questions, usually multiple choice, about the material. In one variation, if a wrong answer is given, the student is led back to the original information. In more sophisticated versions, a wrong answer branches the learner to a different approach to the information with the belief that this learner needs a different, or further explanation, before she or he will understand. Other features that may be included are an explanation for wrong answers and the use of wrong answers as a springboard for correcting misinformation.

The quality of this type of software varies from those that are merely page turners with the opportunity to answer questions, to those that meet the needs of students who need either different or more explanation. One characteristic that separates tutorials from drill and practice software is that tutorials present information. The quality of a tutorial is evident in the use the program makes of branching techniques. At the low end of the continuum are programs that only inform the learner whether an answer is correct or not. Those at the high end offer more than one explanation for the same phenomena.

Tool for Investigation

In investigative software, learners are presented with a situation, given the tools necessary to discover the answer, and allowed to proceed at their own pace. They are not evaluated on their learning but are encouraged to experiment and draw their own conclusions. In one program of this type, learners input values that the program uses to create a fetal monitor strip representing the parameters the user entered. Learners then match their diagnosis of the strip against that of the experts. This type of program tends to develop enthusiasm in the learner and lends itself well to two or three learners working together (Sweeney, 1985).

Simulations

Simulations are case studies. They are designed to allow the learner to practice a patient encounter by providing care to a simulated patient (White, 1995). The objective is to make the learner an actual participant in a patient care situation that would either be too difficult, dangerous, or time consuming to provide in a real clinical setting. The approach used with the simulation may be either tutorial, investigative, testing, or any combination of these.

An example of a very realistic simulation is one that is designed for nurses in a postanesthesia recovery room. In this simulation, the learner has all the tools available that would be available in the real situation, including monitoring equipment. When a patient arrives in the recovery room, the learner is presented with the history, then care commences. A real-time clock is started to give the learner a guide as to when various monitoring activities should occur. The nurse is expected to perform just as in a real-life situation, with no prompting from the computer. The results of all actions are seen in real time, whether it is a strip from a monitor or a readout of vital signs. The nurse is expected to base future actions on the results of assessments and standard recovery room protocols.

A simulation has many different uses. It could be used as part of an orientation for nurses, or with a computer projector in a classroom situation. There are, however, considerations that should be given when using a simulation. The simulation should match the learner's knowledge background, or at least be only slightly above it, and the philosophy of care should be similar to what is being taught.

EDUCATIONAL PHILOSOPHY

Educational software selection should take into consideration the teaching and learning philosophy expressed in the program. Most educational software follows the *behaviorist* theory of learning, although approaches that follow a more *constructivist* approach are being seen.

The behaviorist learning theory assumes that knowledge exists independently of interpretation and that learning consists of acquiring correct information (Duffy & Jonassen, 1992). It is believed that knowledge can be transferred into the mind because it can be learned out of context. The goal of a software program using this paradigm is for the learner to gain the meaning held by the teacher, not a separate interpretation of this meaning. There is an emphasis, therefore, on obtaining right answers in the most efficient manner possible. In the constructivist approach, on the other hand, learners are understood to interact with information based on their own interpretations. This philosophy holds that learning involves individuals in determining the meaning the information has for them (Bednar, Cunningham, Duffy, & Perry, 1992). Thus, instead of searching for one correct answer, learners strive for making sense of information. It is understood, however, that not all interpretations are equal and that some interpretations prove to be more useful than others. Instead of judging an answer as wrong, a constructivist would facilitate learners to discover the so-called holes in their thinking.

It is beyond the scope of this book to explore these two approaches to learning further, but they provide an anchor for thinking about methods of learning used in software.

The techniques used in software are generally somewhere on a continuum between the behaviorist and constructivist views on learning. There is merit to both perspectives, because each meets a different need. Critical thinking, however, is more often met with the constructivist method.

ROLE OF THE INSTRUCTOR

The role of an instructor who uses CAI varies. Some instructors assign a CAI program just as they would a chapter in a book. They may or may not discuss the content in class. Another approach is to integrate the CAI with another assignment, such as a short paper that helps the student to integrate the content with other information. The CAI may also be used as part of a class presentation, using a computer screen projection device.

CAI has uses outside formal education. Patient educators can design CAI to be used in a waiting room, or as part of a one-on-one or group teaching session. Staff educators have found CAI to be an excellent way to present in-service education.

Effective use of CAI requires that it be part of a total educational plan. For example, software on the behaviorist end of the continuum can be combined with critical thinking activities. Identifying the different teaching approaches used by the software, and compensating when necessary, often determines whether learners experience success or frustration.

Pros and Cons of Computer-Assisted Instruction

CAI is neither a panacea nor something that will replace teachers. Like all things, it has advantages and disadvantages. Advantages include the availability of CAI outside regular classroom hours and the patience of a computer as a teacher (Ball & Hannah, 1984). Perhaps one of the greatest advantages is that computers can be used to allow learners to participate in learning experiences that otherwise are not available outside of real life. It can also be accessed by disabled students who are physically unable to attend class. CAI can also be designed to accommodate hearing-impaired students.

CAI requires that a learner use a computer that has the software available. This can present a problem with access if there are limited numbers of computers on which the CAI is available, or if the times when these computers are available are inconvenient. This factor is starting to be solved in some places when the software is available on a network that is accessible from many locations.

High-quality educational software is expensive to create. The market for CAI is generally discipline specific, a factor that means that software developers do not often see huge returns for their efforts. The hardware needed to use the software is also a cost factor. When considering the cost of CAI, it is important to look beyond the immediate expense and factor in the costs of continuing with present educational methods.

Teachers are still searching for the most effective ways to use CAI in learning. Entrenched educational ideas, held by both students and faculty, such as believing that teachers should deliver information in a classroom rather than facilitate learning, may interfere with creative use of CAI. As more people become comfortable with computers and are able to experiment with different learning methods, CAI in its many formats will find a definite role in quality education.

Evaluation of Computer-Assisted Instruction

When evaluating CAI, the primary characteristic to be considered is whether it meets a learning need. When considering this factor, keep in mind that learners are at a different educational level than the individual selecting software and may have a different point of view. One of the best ways to evaluate CAI involves having potential users possessing three different learning abilities (low, average, and high) preview the software. Given the cost of CAI, including the hardware and the necessity of learners to be in a specific location, consideration should also be given to whether the program uses the attributes of the computer or would be better, as well as less expensive, if presented in a book.

The one characteristic that sets CAI above all other teaching mediums, with the exception of a human teacher or live experience, is interactivity. How effective an interaction is depends on the mental processing required and the nature of the learner's interaction with the content (Thede, 1995). In considering the quality of an interaction, look at both the methods used to solicit input and the way the computer handles inputs. The lowest level of user input occurs when a user answers a multiple choice question, and the highest level occurs when the user enters free text with no clues provided by questions and answers. In a simple tutorial, a high level reply includes feedback that attempts to assist the learner to correct misinterpretations. In a high quality simulation, the user sees the results of actions and needs to give input based on those results.

When evaluating CAI, examine the graphics and animation to determine whether they are used to facilitate learning a concept or as extras. Investigate if the learner is encouraged to be passive, or if the learner expected to provide input. If the learner has input, evaluate whether it is beyond answering questions: For example, can the learner determine the flow of instruction, exit the program at will, or request more information? When the student is allowed to have control, learning becomes more active (Bolwell, 1988).

▼ Sources of Computer-Aided Instruction

One of the best sources of information on nursing software is the *Directory of Educational Software* authored by Bolwell. The latest edition was published by FITNE (Fuld Institute of Technology in Nursing Education) in 1995 and includes an addendum for 1996 and 1997. The programs in the directory have a brief description and contain evaluations from those who have used the program. The directory includes programs for use in many different health care settings and disciplines. The journal *Computers in Nursing*, published bimonthly, also provides reviews of educational software. Stewart's *Interactive Healthcare Directory* is another source. It lists nearly 2000 software titles for health-related education and reference.

▼ Computers for Testing

Computers are now being used to administer the National Council Licensure Examination for Registered Nurses (NCLEX-RN). Computers can also be used in other testing situations, both to create and administer tests.

NCLEX TEST

After extensive testing, in 1994 the NCLEX exams were given for the first time on a computer. Prospective registered nurses no longer had to go to a particular site at a given time and the test no longer consisted of a certain number of questions, but instead, used a procedure known as *computer-adaptive testing* (CAT).

In CAT, the number, sequence, and content of questions is based on the responses given by the testee. For example, if a student of low ability begins to give incorrect answers to questions, the computer responds by asking easier questions until questions are answered correctly. On the other hand, students of high ability who keep answering questions correctly will find the level of questions raised until incorrect responses are given. Using a tested algorithm, the computer determines the level of achievement, which is translated to pass or fail. This process requires only 25 to 50 well-designed questions instead of the 100 or so necessary in paper and pencil tests (Educational Testing Service, 1996).

In a clinical simulation test (CST), the examinees are presented with a realistic clinical care situation and are evaluated based on their actions. The test starts by giving a brief introduction to a client, after which the examinee proceeds to the client care screen and initiates actions such as assessments and interventions, just as if the individual were working with a real client. Actions are entered as free text, without any choices being presented to the testee. Each action receives a response from the client, just as it would in the clinical area. Unlike regular tests, however, answers are not either right or wrong. Instead, credit is awarded based on the timing, sequencing, and prioritization of the responses. Credit can be given for different but equally valid patient care responses (National Council State Boards of Nursing, 1996b).

It is believed that CST evaluates clinical decision-making abilities that are not amenable to evaluation by multiple choice questions. A project is now under way to determine whether a CST should be part of the NCLEX-RN exam. In the spring of 1998, CST was pilot tested with 65 nursing schools (National Council State Boards of Nursing, 1996a). The results will be reported at the 1999 meeting of the National Council's Delegate Assembly. It is anticipated that this group will make a decision regarding future directions for CST. The earliest anticipated addition of this component to the NCLEX-RN is 2001.

ONLINE TESTING

Regular pencil and paper tests can be administered online as well. A high-quality online test allows testees do the types of things that they do when taking a paper and pencil test, such as answering questions in a nonlinear fashion, reviewing, and changing answers. A big advantage to a computerized test is that results can be learned immediately.

TEST CONSTRUCTION SOFTWARE

Test construction is a difficult and time-consuming educational activity (Kirkpatrick et al., 1996). For this reason, most instructors develop a test bank, or a collection of questions about given topics from which test questions can be selected. Some instructors use word processing or database software to construct a test bank. There is also specialized software to meet this need. Like all software, these products vary in their abilities—some permit tests to be delivered on the computer, and others permit different tests on the same topics to be constructed for administration in crowded examination rooms (Johnson, 1989).

▼ Summary

Although many information management needs can be met with typical application programs, there are some situations in which using a special purpose program adds value not found with adapting regular software. In research, a few of these situations include developing questionnaires and analyzing qualitative research.

In education, computers are used not only to manage information but as a learning tool. The use of computers in education developed over the years. CAI can be categorized by the hardware it requires, such as a laser disk player for CAIV or graphics capabilities for multimedia. It can also be categorized by the type of instructional or teaching approach used.

When selecting CAI for use, it is important to determine whether the program meets a learning need, uses computer attributes wisely, has a level of interactivity that promote the desired type of learning, and is easy enough to use that learners will not become frustrated by the technology.

Tests moderated by a computer can have characteristics that are not possible with paper and pencil. CAT permits evaluation with fewer questions, and provides a flexible testing schedule. CST permits testing of clinical decision making not possible with multiple choice tests. The use of computers in education will continue to evolve.

EXERCISES

1. What considerations would be used in deciding the format and type of CAI to use?
2. How are CAI and the Internet being used in distance education?
3. Think of some situations in nursing education in which a MOO could be useful.
4. Describe some learning situations in which CAI would be useful.
5. Evaluate an educational software program. Include information about the type of program it is and the educational approach used in the program.
6. What are some ways educational software can be used by health care professionals in
   a. Clinical practice?
   b. Administration?
   c. Education?
   d. Research?
   e. Entrepreneurial work?
7. What are some ways that software that creates questionnaires can be used by health care professionals in
   a. Clinical practice?
   b. Administration?
   c. Education?
   d. Research?
   e. Entrepreneurial work?

REFERENCES

Ball, M., & Hannah, M. J. (1984). *Using computers in nursing*. Reston, VA: Reston Publishing Company.

Bednar, A. K., Cunningham, D., Duffy, T. M., & Perry, J. D. (1992). Theory into practice: How do we link? In T. M. Duffy & D. H. Jonassen (Eds.), *Constructivism and the technology of instruction* (pp. 18–34). Hillsdale, NJ: Lawrence Erlbaum Associates, Publishers.

Beyea, S. C. (1996). Software review: NRQuery: Computer query questionnaire program. *Computers in Nursing 14*(2), 71–72.

Bitzer, M. D., Boudreaux, M., & Avner, R. A. (1973). Computer-based instruction of basic nursing utilizing inquiry approach. (CERL Report X-40). Urbana, IL: University of Illinois.

Bolwell, C. (1988). Evaluating computer assisted instruction. In T. Lochhass (Ed.), *Proceedings of the Third International Symposium on Nursing Use of Computers and Information Science* (pp. 825–830). St. Louis: C. V. Mosby Company.

Cohen, P. A. & Dacanay, L. S. (1994). A meta-analysis of computer-based instruction in Nursing Education. *Computers in Nursing 12*(2), 89–97.

Delp, S. I., Loan, J. P., Wong, A. Y., & Rosen, J. M. (1996). Surgical simulation: Practicing trauma techniques for emergency medicine. *Medical Simulation and Training 1*(1), 22–23; 30.

Duffy, T. M. & Jonassen, D. H. (1992). Constructivism: New implications for instructional technology. In T. M. Duffy & D. H. Jonassen (Eds.), *Constructivism and the technology of instruction.* (pp. 1–16). Hillsdale, NJ: Lawrence Erlbaum Associates, Publishers.

Educational Testing Service. (1996). *ETS test takers are trading pencils for computers.* Available: http://etsis1.ets.org/aboutets/z2-cbt.html.

Isdale, J. (1993).*What is virtual reality?* Available: http://www.cms.dmu.ac.uk/People/cph/VR/whatisvr.html.

Johnson, S. R. (1989). A review guide for computer assisted testing software. *Computers in Nursing, 7*(3), 119–126.

Kirkpatrick, J. M., Billings, C. M., Hodson-Carlton, K., Cummings, R. B., Hanson, A. C., Malone, J., Miller, A., Robinson, L., & Zwirn, E. (1996). Computerized test development software: A comparative review. *Computers in Nursing 14*(2), 113–125.

Lesie, M. (1998, February 26). No plane, no flying, no fear. *Cleveland Plain Dealer*, 1A, 14A.

Merril, G. L. & Barker, V. L. (1996). Virtual reality debuts in the teaching laboratory in nursing. *Journal of Intravenous Nursing 19*(4), 182–187.

National Council of State Boards of Nursing. (1996a). *Computerized clinical simulation testing (CSTR): Frequently asked questions.* Available: http://www.ncsbn.org/files/cstfaq.html.

National Council of State Boards of Nursing. (1996b, July 12). *National council selects states to participate in computerized clinical simulation testing (CSTR) pilot study.* Available: http://www.ncsbn.org/files/newsreleases/nr960712.html.

Sweeney, M. A. (1985). *The nurse's guide to computers.* New York: Macmillan Publishing Company.

Thede, L. Q. (1995). Comparison of a constructivist and objectivist framework for designing computer-aided instruction. Unpublished dissertation, Kent State University, Kent, OH.

White, J. E. (1995). Using interactive video to add physical assessment data to computer-based simulations in nursing. *Computers in Nursing, 13*(5), 233–235.

UNIT THREE

· ·

Computers as Communication Tools

▶ IN this unit, we will look at the various types of computer communications that health care professionals are using. Chapter 12 introduces computer communication and the Internet. Chapter 13 addresses the communication tools that the Internet provides. The chapters also includes suggestions for finding information on the Internet as well as evaluating this information. Unit Three ends with Chapter 14, which explores ways that the internet has changed, and is changing, health care.

Computer Communication

Objectives:

After studying this chapter you will be able to:

1 Discuss many facets of computer communication

2 Identify factors affecting speed of data transmission on the Internet

3 Identify the factor behind the development of the TCP/IP protocols

4 State factors to investigate when selecting an ISP

5 Use email etiquette

6 Differentiate between telnet and ftp

A nurse has a patient with an unfamiliar disease. From a question asked on an electronic mailing list, the nurse learns that a document on a computer in another country has information about caring for patients with this disease. Within 60 seconds of logging on to the Internet, the nurse is printing out the document. This ability to exchange information on a global scale is changing the world. No longer do health care professionals have to wait for information to become available in a journal in the country in which they live. Nurses and other health care professionals can and do use computers to network with colleagues all over the world.

 Networking

Computer networking is not new to health care. Since the late 1950s, when health care institutions began using mainframes connected to terminals in various offices for financial processing, networking has progressed to the point where institutions are connected to a worldwide network known as the Internet. Computer networks exist whenever two computers share the same data. A network can range in size from a connection between a palmtop and a PC, to the worldwide, multi-user computer connection—the Internet.

The variation in network size is often seen in the name used to denote the network, such as a local area network (LAN) or wide area network (WAN). A LAN is a network in which the connected computers are physically close to one another, such as in the same department or building. A WAN is a network in which the

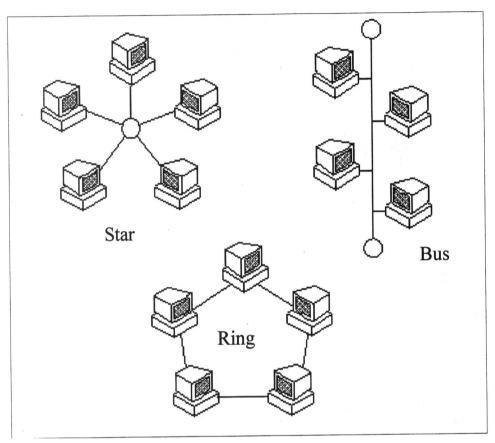

Star

Bus

Ring

Figure 12-1 • Network topologies. (Printed with permission of Mecklermedia & Sandy Bay Software Company. PCWebopaedia network.)

connections are further apart. Often a WAN is an internetwork of LANs. WANs are sometimes referred to as enterprise networks, because they connect all of the computer networks throughout the entire organization or enterprise.

Networks are connected physically with a variety of materials, such as twisted-wire cables, phone lines, fiber optic lines, and even radio waves. How the connections are designed is referred to as the *topology* of the network. Basically, there are three types of topologies—a star, a ring, and a bus (Fig. 12-1). Under the bus topology, each computer is connected to one cable called the backbone, or bus. In the star topology, all computers are connected to a central hub, whereas in a ring, they are all connected to each other.[1] These topologies vary in cost as well as in advantages and disadvantages. Computers connected to a network are referred to as nodes.

[1]The physical topology of a network does not necessarily dictate the logical topology or how it is connected. For instance, a Token-Ring network is logically defined as a ring network. However, the physical layout may be in a star configuration, in which every computer has a physical wire back to the central hub (star topology). The hub takes care of maintaining the logical ring network (Quiggle, 1998).

Like a computer, networks also require an operating system. Although the Macintosh operating system has built-in networking functions, the term network operating system generally refers to special software. Some examples are Artisoft's LANtastic™, Microsoft's Windows NT™, and Novell's Netware™. Most networks found in health care institutions have a computer that functions as a file server. A file server is a high-performance computer with a large hard drive that is reserved as a central location for data that will be accessed by all. Networks without a dedicated file server, called peer-to-peer networks, are also possible.

▼Telephony

Telephony refers to computer software and hardware that can perform functions usually associated with a telephone. It is this technology that forms the basis for voice mail. However, it is not limited to voice mail. It is possible for individuals to use telephony to communicate with a computer. With the purchase of a sound card, speakers, microphone, and the appropriate software, a computer can be set up to function as a telephone (IW Labs, 1996). The computer should have a chip equivalent to at least a Pentium, and the sound card needs to be capable of full-duplex communication, that is, it can both transmit and receive at the same time.

Because as this text is written there are no standards for telephony transmissions, both parties involved in communication need to be using the same software (IW Labs, 1996). Additionally, if both parties are not online with the telephony software open, no connection will be made.[2] To overcome this situation, most phone packages are designed to be used with a host server. The host server accepts an incoming connection, lets the user know who is connected, and notifies the other users that another person is now online. From the list provided by the host server, the user selects a caller and establishes a direct connection. The sound settings of microphones and speakers might have to be checked before achieving understandable conversations. When all of this is worked out, expect latency, or a half-second to 1-second delay in hearing what is said. Like all new technologies, the bugs in telephony are yet to be worked out.

▼The Internet

The Internet is a worldwide, amorphous network of interconnected computers (Fig. 12-2). What makes the Internet workable is that each computer connected to the Internet uses specific rules in communicating called protocols. These protocols make it possible for a person using a Macintosh to send a message to a person using a PC or any other type of computer.

THE BEGINNINGS OF THE INTERNET

The Internet was devised as a means of communication that would survive a nuclear war and provide the most economical use from scarce computer resources (Medenis,

---

[2]This is not completely true; if the called party has what is called a static IP address, some programs will still make the connection. Static, or unchangeable, IP addresses are used mainly by those who connect to the internet without benefit of a network or ISP.

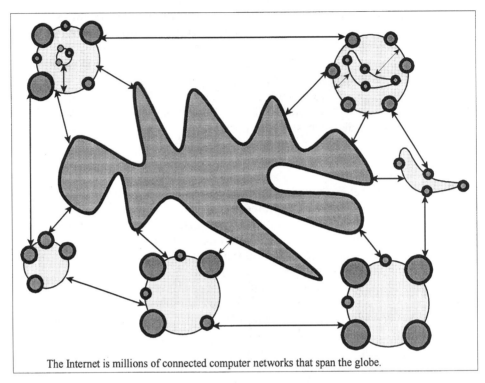

The Internet is millions of connected computer networks that span the globe.

Figure 12-2 • The Internet.

1997). It Internet began in 1969 as a single network known as Advanced Research Projects Agency NETwork (ARPANET), which was built to connect four nodes, the University of California Los Angles, Stanford Research Institute, University of California Santa Barbara, and the University of Utah. It did not remain four nodes for long. By 1971, there were 15 locations connected to ARPANET, and the next year, the first international connections linking the University College of London (UK) and the Royal Radar Establishment (Norway) were established.

At the same time, other networks were being developed, all of which used different methods for intercomputer communication (Medenis, 1997). To overcome this problem, it was necessary to develop common communication protocols that would be used by networks that wished to communicate with each other. These protocols, the Transmission Control Protocol (TCP) and Internet Protocol (IP) were introduced in 1974 and are still in use.

The term *Internet* was first used in 1983 to describe the interconnected networks developed by the NSF (National Science Foundation), which were known as the NSFNET (National Science Foundation Network). By 1983 the term denoted connectivity to the NSFNET (Rickard, 1997). A noncommercial governmental enterprise, the NSFNET found itself in competition with private companies. The result was a solicitation for bids in 1993 to replace the NSFNET service. On April 30, 1995, NFSNET was shut down and replaced by a worldwide commercial backbone, today's Internet.

NATIONAL INFORMATION INFRASTRUCTURE

As a means of making network technologies useful to the public, business, libraries, and other nongovernmental entities, the U.S. federal government is now in the process of creating the National Information Infrastructure (NII), sometimes called the Information Superhighway (The National Information Infrastructure, 1996). Information available through this entity will be in many different formats, including video, databases, images, and audio. To make this network a reality, software that allows users to access and manipulate the information, and network standards that ensure privacy for individuals and security for information also need to be developed.

INTERNET WORKINGS

Before mass transmission of the items that the NII envisions becomes a reality, improvements need to be made in the speeds that data can be transmitted (the infrastructure of the Internet). The speed of transmission depends on several factors: the device that is directly connected to a computer that performs the physical act of sending and receiving the data (modem), the transmission lines that connect the user to the Internet, and the ability of the Internet to handle increased transmissions.

CONNECTIONS TO THE INTERNET

A computer can be connected to the Internet by being directly wired to a network that is connected to the Internet, by using a modem, or even by wireless transmission. When institutional networked computers are connected to the Internet, the connection is generally provided at the network level. Stand-alone computers, unless they are connected to the Internet with a cable modem or special line, require a device that translates computer output (digital format) to electronic impulses that can be transmitted over telephone lines (analog format). These devices then translate the data received through telephone lines back into the digital format that the computer can understand. Known as modems, these devices can be internal (card inside the computer) or external (a box that is outside the computer and connected to the computer). Whether internal or external, the modem is connected to a telephone jack with the same type of line that is used to connect a telephone.

Telephone Modems

A telephone modem is one that uses a regular telephone line as its first step in connecting to the Internet. They vary in the speed with which they transmit data, a characteristic measured in kilobits (1024 bits) per second (Kbps). Do not confuse kilobit with Kilobytes (a bit is 1/8th of a byte). Most users today have modems theoretically capable of transmitting data at 28.8 or 33.6 Kbps. This does not mean that the data is always transmitted that fast. Besides a modem capable of these speeds, the phone lines must be clear of noise, or interference. The more noise in the line, the slower the connection. Generally, older lines have more noise.

Impaired phone lines have a great effect on the 56.6 Kbps modems that are available for regular telephone lines. Depending on the phone line, a 56.6 modem may or may not give users an increase in data transmission speed (Bay Networks, 1997; Snyder, 1997). The use of technology that enables the transmission of a digital signal over a line without converting it to analog is what permits a 56.6 Kbps modems to achieve this speed (Quiggle, 1998). This speed, however, is attainable only downstream, from your Internet Service Provider (ISP) to you. Even faster connections can be achieved with an asymmetrical digital subscriber line (ADSL) modem. These modems permit speeds of about 6 Mbps (megabits per second) receiving data, and from 16 to 640 Kbps when sending (Asymmetric Digital Subscriber Lines, Undated).[3] All of these modems use regular telephone lines, known as plain old telephone service (POTS), which are not terribly robust. Undue noise on the line can break a connection. Picking up a phone extension while the line is being used for a computer connection and call waiting can also interrupt a POTS phone connection.

Cable Modems

Those who have surfed the net or have had information transmitted to their computer from various Internet connected computers have discovered that there can be a long lag time between asking for information and receiving it. In reality, the time lag is not generally that long, but anything exceeding 3 seconds is seen as too long by most computer users conditioned to instant response. The slow response times are often a result of the slowness of the modem in transmitting data. Cable modems, which use the transmission devices of the cable television network, can attain transmission speeds up of 10 megabits per second (Mbps) (National Cable Television Association, 1997). Like the 56 Kbps modems, however, this speed is available only for data that is transmitted to a computer. Additionally, the data transmission speed is not consistent. It is affected by a number of factors, including oddities in the cable networks, the number of other people in the neighborhood who are online at the same time, and traffic on the Internet.

Bandwidth

Increasing the speed of a modem alone will not increase the speed with which Internet information is received. It is also necessary that the bandwidths of the various connections between the user and the source of anything to be retrieved are able to transmit quickly all current data traffic. Bandwidth is a measure of the speed at which a line (wire) transmits data. The higher the bandwidth, the higher the speed (Table 12-1). Bandwidth varies throughout the Internet. The line used to reach the Internet usually has the lowest bandwidth. The line that an ISP uses to connect to the Internet is greater, whereas the highest bandwidth is found in the Internet backbone. Bandwidth becomes very important when large files are transmitted. Although plain text files can be transmitted at very slow bandwidths, graphical files, sound files, and especially moving picture segments are very large files whose speed of transmission is greatly affected by bandwidth.

---

[3]One megabit is 1000 times faster than a kilobit.

TABLE 12-1 ● *Bandwidths (Speeds) of Various Network Connectors*		
Connection	**Common use**	**Speed**
POTS (**P**lain **O**ld **T**elephone **S**ervice)	Connects home computers using telephone modems to their Internet Service Provider	Theoretically capable of sending up to 33.6 Kbps. Will be lower if the line is old and there is noise on the line. May be able to receive 56.6 Kbps. Only guaranteed to 14,400 Kbps.
ISDN (**I**ntegrated **S**ervices **D**igital **N**etwork)	May be used by home users or by an ISP to connect to the Internet	64 Kbps to 128 Kbps
Wireless	May be used by home users, more often is used in WANs	400 Kbps
T1 line	ISPs to connect to the Internet backbone	Simultaneously carries 24 separate data transmissions at 64 Kbps with resulting speed of 1.5 Mbps.
T3 line		Simultaneously carries 672 separate data transmissions at 64 Kbps with resulting speed of 43 Mbps.
Fiber optic cable	Internet backbone	With today's technology, actual speed is 2 gigabytes per second, but fiberoptic cable is theoretically capable of 250 gigabytes per second.

Wireless Transmission

This type of transmission for Internet traffic is still in its infancy. One disadvantage to wireless Internet services is the limited broadcast spectrum that is available. Wireless options must compete for a share of the unallocated broadcast spectrum, whereas there is no limit to the amount of cable that can be installed.

Wireless transmission within health care institutions is used successfully today. These transmissions are limited in distance; thus, they do not have to compete with other radio traffic.[4] When a wireless system is installed, receivers are placed at strategic locations throughout the institution, locations that are determined by a thorough building assessment. These receivers pick up the signals sent by a user and transmit them to the central server; then they transmit signals back to the user's computer.

HOW DATA ARE TRANSMITTED

The TCP/IP protocol agreed on at the birth of the Internet is actually two protocols, the TCP and the IP. The IP protocol allows computers to find each other on the In-

---

[4]Unfortunately, some health care institutions have been using some of the broadcast spectrum illegally for wireless transmissions within their institution. When a legal entity, such as a television station, starts to use this frequency, problems result.

ternet (Quiggle, 1998). Before a message is sent, the TCP protocol breaks it into smaller manageable pieces called packets, numbers them, and assigns a control feature called a *checksum*. These packets range in size from 1 to 1500 bytes. When the packet is received at the destination computer, the computer looks at the checksum to verify that the packet is identical to the one that was sent. If the checksums do not agree, the destination computer requests that the packet be resent. When the checksums for the received packets agree, the destination computer looks at the packet numbers assigned by the sending computer, and reassembles the message based on those numbers. If the computer finds that there is a missing packet, it will request the missing packet from the sending computer. The TCP protocol is what permits reliable transmission of a message.

The IP protocol on a computer sends each packet to a router. In turn, the router scans the routes available to the final destination, and selects what looks the shortest (least number of hops) and least congested route, and sends the packet on to another router (Quiggle, 1998). The next router repeats this process until the packets finally end up at the destination computer. These protocols are what allow for a guaranteed transmission of your message (Fig. 12-3).

Each packet that is sent out carries with it a Time To Live (TTL) variable. At each step of the way, the router decrements the TTL (Quiggle, 1998). Once the TTL reaches zero, the router that decremented it to zero, sends an internet control mes-

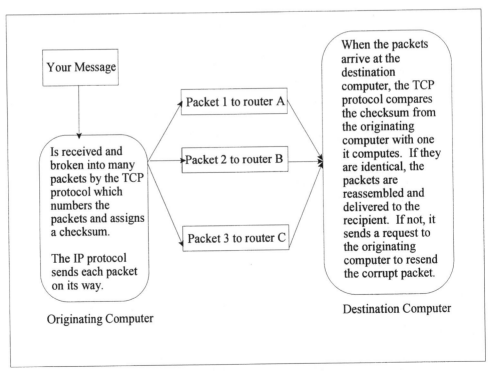

Figure 12-3 ● Transmission Control Protocol (TCP) and Internet Protocol (IP) for sending information.

saging protocol message to the originating computer, stating that the packet expired. This keeps undeliverable packets from floating around the Internet and creates an error message for the sender stating that there have been too many hops. When a user receives this error message, the message must be resent because it was not delivered.

INTERNET SERVICE PROVIDERS

There are four things that are necessary to surf the net. A computer, a modem or network connection, a communication package, and a link to the Internet. Most computers purchased today as stand-alone units come with a modem. Additionally, modern operating systems contain communications packages. Thus, when you purchase a computer, the only thing lacking is an internet service provider (ISP) (Fig. 12-4).

Finding an Internet Service Provider

There are two types of ISPs: online services and basic ISPs. Online services such as America Online™, Microsoft Network™, and Prodigy™ offer not only a connection to the Internet but proprietary content and features that are not available on the general Internet. Basic ISPs, however, may provide fewer busy signals and more readily accessible technical help. Many ISPs provide a flat rate monthly service. To find an ISP, talk with several acquaintances who are Internet users, and get their recommendations (Display 12-1).

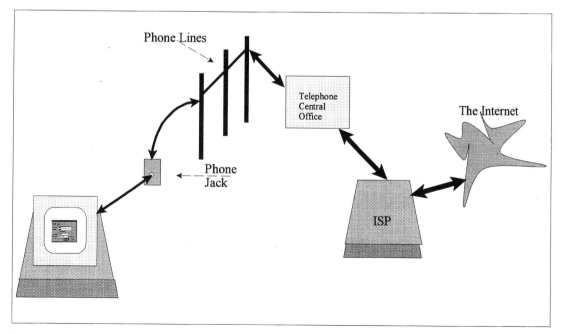

Figure 12-4 ● Connecting to the Internet through an internet service provider (ISP).

●▼●▲●▼●▲●▼●▲●▼●▲●▼●▲●▼●▲●▼●▲●▼●▲●▼●▲●▼●▲●▼

Display 12-1 • CONSIDERATIONS IN SELECTING AN INTERNET SERVICE PROVIDER (ISP)

Should I use an online service or an ISP? The big commercial ISPs like America Online and Prodigy have easy to use interfaces and a very easy set up; additionally, they provide many resources not generally found on ISPs. You may, however, encounter more busy signals than with a local or regional provider, as well as other user limitations.

How much will I be using the Internet? All ISPs have different plans. Many ISPs provide unlimited hours for around $10 to $20 a month. If there are time limitations, they are often in the 600-hour range. Choose the most economical plan for yourself. Keep in mind that Internet use tends to increase as one discovers the myriad of items to be found there.

Is the number my computer dials to access the ISP a local phone call? Long distance phone charges will add greatly to the cost of an ISP. Find a provider that offers local service or an 800 number. Anyone who needs Internet service while traveling will want to know if there are methods of connecting to their ISP from other locations.

What software do I need to get connected? Most ISPs provide diskettes or allow you to download the necessary software. The downloading can be done using the built-in communication packages provided with your operating system. A good service provider will give you detailed instructions for both downloading and installing the software.

How often are the phone lines to the ISP busy? A cheap ISP for which the phone lines are always busy is probably not a bargain. To evaluate how often the line is busy, try calling the number you would use to connect at the times when you would be connecting. If you repeatedly get a busy signal you may wish to look elsewhere. If you get a high-pitched whining sound, the number you called is available for your computer to use.

Do the hours for technical support coincide with the hours that you will be using the Internet? You may also want to determine how helpful the ISP is when you have a difficulty. Are the personnel patient? Unless you are a computer guru you can expect to occasionally have some questions about your service. A helpful, readily available human being is very welcome.

What bandwidth does the ISP use to connect to the Internet? The higher the bandwidth to the Internet, the faster your data will be transmitted. Use the information in Table 12-1 to make comparisons.

EMAIL

Email, or electronic mail sent and received on the computer, is one of the primary uses of the Internet. It has been estimated that there are 25 million email users sending 15 billion messages per year, a figure that increases annually (PCWebopaedia, 1997). Before 1995, users could send email only to those who shared the same network connection. Those using Compuserve™, for instance, could only email others who also used Compuserve. Today, with most computer networks part of the Internet, the exchange of email is possible with anyone on the globe who has an Internet email address. Email, however, does not always have to involve the Internet. Many companies network their computers and provide in-house email without connecting to the Internet.

Email offers many advantages to nurses and other health care professionals. It is a way to avoid "phone tag" and to create a written message that the receiver can read several times, if needed. Most mail packages keep a copy of all messages that are sent, so the sender can check to be sure that a given message was transmitted. Additionally, all email packages provide some way to preserve incoming mail and organize it into folders for future reference. Email is the perfect vehicle for communicating over time zones, not only because the sender and receiver can respond in times that are most convenient but because it saves postage and telephone expenses. Although plain email is ASCII, files created by word processors, spreadsheets, or other programs can be added to an email message as an attachment.

Internet Email Addresses

Like all mail, email requires an address. At first, email addresses look forbidding, but as you become more familiar with them, patterns are seen, which makes them easier to use (Fig. 12-5). All Internet email addresses have two parts, which are separated by the @ sign. The first part, or the letters before the @ sign, is called a *login name* or a *userId*. These login names are assigned to individuals. The part after the @ is the name of the computer used to access the Internet or the Internet address of the ISP one is using. No two ISPs can have the same address. The characters after the @ sign are identical for all those using the same ISP. The login or userId part of an email address varies with the ISP. Many use first and last names separated by a dot; others use a combination of first, last, and middle names; whereas some randomly assign userIds. Regardless of the method used, every individual has a unique email address.

Nonalphanumeric characters, such as an underscore (_) or a hyphen, may be found within an email address. One always seen is the dot (.). Email addresses never have a space.

When entering email addresses, it is imperative that they be accurate. To make this job easier, most email software provides an option that allows the user to create an address book for email addresses, or as they are sometimes called, nicknames. To create such a file, follow the directions for the email package and enter the email address and name of any individual to whom email is frequently sent. The next time this individual is sent a message, access this file, find his or her name, and click on it. Or, in some communication packages, just enter the intended recipient's name. This process places the email address and name in the appropriate place in your message. Besides saving time, using this feature prevents errors in typing the email address, a situation that results in messages that are returned for an improper address.

The characters after the last dot in an email address indicate the *domain* or main subdivision of the Internet to which the computer belongs. They provide a clue as to the type of organization that the sender is using as an ISP. Outside of the United States, and even for some addresses within the United States, the country of origin can be determined by the last part of an email address. A complete list of countries

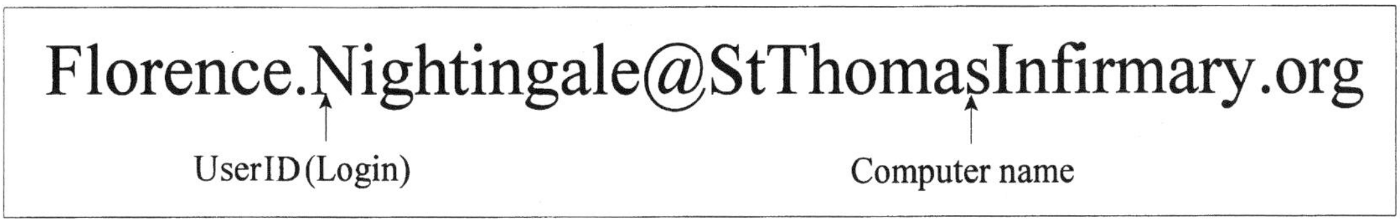

Florence.Nightingale@StThomasInfirmary.org

UserID(Login)   Computer name

Figure 12-5 • Email address.

and the letters used to indicate that country can be found at ftp://rs.internic.net/netinfo/iso3166-countrycodes.

Email Etiquette

Email is a special form of communication that is not as interactive as the telephone but is more interactive than written communication. Because it often seems very personal and quick, there is a tendency to regard it as a verbal conversation and to forget that the recipient may been involved in many complicated matters since she or he last sent you a message. For this reason, mailers provide an option to include the prior message with the original when you reply. To prevent messages that rapidly become too large and uncommunicative, edit this message so that only the parts pertinent to your reply are included. To edit the message, an email package provides word processing functions such as select and delete.

Emoticons and Acronyms

Email is devoid of the nonverbal commands of face-to-face communication. To meet this need, icons called *emoticons* (emotional icons) were devised by telecommunicators with a sense of humor and knowledge of the difficulties that lack of body language in communication can cause. These figures are created entirely with characters that can be entered from the keyboard. :-) is one that is seen frequently. When tilting one's head to the left, which is the position for viewing all emoticons, a smiling face can be seen. Emoticons are useful only if the recipient understands their meaning (Display 12-2). Use them sparingly, if at all, in business situations.

With the informality of much email and the limited typing skills of many who send messages, it is only natural that common acronyms will develop. Like emoticons, they are valuable only when the recipients understand them, too (Table 12-2).

Signature

Considerate emailers always include their signature and email address on a message. Assuming that the recipient knows who sent the message can cause miscommunication. Most email software has a feature that allows you to design a signature that is

TABLE 12-2 ● Common Email Acronyms	
Acronym	**Meaning**
BTW	By the way
FAQs	Frequently asked questions
f2f	Face to face
FWIW	For what it's worth
\<g\>	Grin
IMO or IMHO	In my opinion or in my humble opinion
OTOH	On the other hand
\<s\>	Smile
TIA	Thanks in advance
TTFN	Ta ta for now

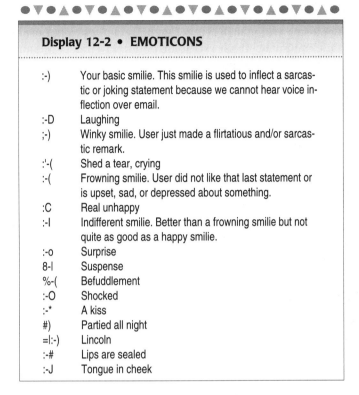

Display 12-2 • EMOTICONS

:-)	Your basic smilie. This smilie is used to inflect a sarcastic or joking statement because we cannot hear voice inflection over email.
:-D	Laughing
;-)	Winky smilie. User just made a flirtatious and/or sarcastic remark.
:'-(	Shed a tear, crying
:-(	Frowning smilie. User did not like that last statement or is upset, sad, or depressed about something.
:C	Real unhappy
:-I	Indifferent smilie. Better than a frowning smilie but not quite as good as a happy smilie.
:-o	Surprise
8-I	Suspense
%-(	Befuddlement
:-O	Shocked
:-*	A kiss
#)	Partied all night
=I:-)	Lincoln
:-#	Lips are sealed
:-J	Tongue in cheek

automatically affixed to all your outgoing mail. Check the help files for the word "signature" for further instruction.

Subject

Although one is sometimes at a loss as to what to state as the subject, when this is omitted, it may cause the reader to assume that your note is junk mail and delete it unread. When sending a message to a group, including a subject is doubly important.

Spamming

Spam is the electronic equivalent of junk mail, except that it shifts the costs of advertising to the receiver. It also fills the Internet with unwanted messages. The best way to fight back against this practice is to never buy anything from an organization that advertises in this manner.

TELNET

Although it is an old feature, telnet is still popular. It allows a user to log into a distant computer and use its features. Telnet is often used by people who are traveling and want to access their email on a distant computer. Some features are available only by using telnet, but slowly they are being converted to web features.

FILE TRANSFER PROTOCOL

File transfer protocol (FTP) is the method by which a user can retrieve files from a distant computer, much as she or he might request a book from a library. In most cases, today it is not necessary to learn the commands associated with FTP because most computers with files that others may want provide automatic FTP retrieval through the World Wide Web.

To speed the transmission, most files retrieved in this manner are compressed. More specifically, algorithms have been used to make them smaller for storage and transmission.[5] If the file is not self-extracting (when you execute or install it, it extracts the files needed to use it), a special decompression program will need to be used.[6] Most operating systems today come with such programs; others can be downloaded from the Internet.

FTP may be used by individuals who telecommute—who work physically separated from the institution that employs them—to transfer files to and from a central location. These individuals usually install special FTP software that can be configured to make using FTP as simple as copying a file from one folder or disk to another.

CLIENT-SERVER TECHNOLOGY

Much networking and many of the tools on the Internet, such as telnet and FTP, are based on client-server technology. In this scheme, a connected computer can be either a client, a server, or both. A client computer has software that allows it to request and receive files from the server. The server has software that can accept these requests, find the appropriate file, and transmit it back to the client (Fig. 12-6). The software for both the client and server are designed for the type of transmission for which they are used. For example, client-server networking software is designed to facilitate the workings of the network; client-server software for FTP is designed to work with FTP protocols; and telnet client-server software is designed for telnetting protocols.

When users on a client computer want a file from the server, they request it using the client side of the software. The server uses its special software to accept and implement the request. The client side then receives the transmission and interprets it. Beyond making the initial request, rarely is any of this process visible to the user, just as when one makes a long distance telephone call, the process of making the connection is invisible to a caller.

▼ Summary

Computer networks are a natural outgrowth of the use of computers to manage information. Very few computers exist today that are not somehow tied into a network, either as part of a LAN or by access to the Internet. From its earliest beginning, the In-

---

[5]This book could be compressed by assigning a symbol to stand for frequently used words. "&" might mean "computer" and "#" the "Internet."

[6]Be sure to check the file with a virus checker before decompressing or installing it.

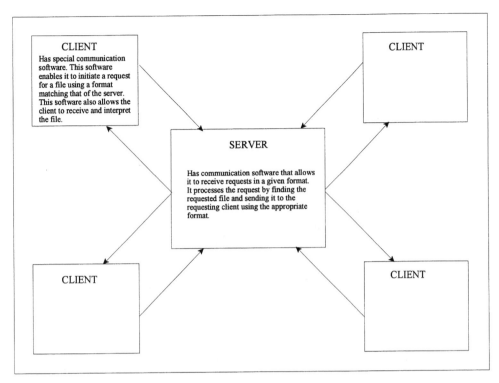

Figure 12-6 • Client-server architecture.

ternet has had a part in distributing data, information, and knowledge. Given that distributing these phenomena plays an important part in creating more information and knowledge, the Internet is an important link in the general increase in knowledge. In a relatively short time, the Internet has changed the way we communicate between individuals, communities, and countries.

The Internet is like having a library in your computer, but today retrieving this information is slower than we would wish. This speed is affected by the modem or device that connects the computer to the Internet, the bandwidth of all the connections to the computer that has the information, and the number of other individuals also seeking information at that moment. A feature of the Internet, email, is now such an accepted part of daily life that many people include their email address on business cards.

Many tools have been developed to enable users to retrieve information from distant locations. Special client-server software, working behind the scenes, has removed much of the work and memorizing of commands formerly needed to use these features. As more people become connected, the Internet produces an environment that will shrink the globe and provide us all with a library on demand. It is impossible to predict the changes that will be created by these developments.

EXERCISES

1. How is rapid communication and availability of knowledge via the Internet affecting society in general? Health care?

2. List some things that you might want to ask if you were considering using an ISP.

3. What advantages are there to communicating with email?

4. Relate the use of email etiquette to other types of communication.

5. What are some ways computer communication is being used by health care professionals in
   a. Clinical practice?
   b. Administration?
   c. Education?
   d. Research?
   e. Entrepreneurial work?

REFERENCES

Assymetric Digital Subscriber Lines. (Undated). Available: http://www-inst.eecs.berkeley.edu/~domviola/project/adsl.html.

Bay Networks. (1997). *White paper.* Available: http://www.baynetworks.com/Products/Papers/2745.html#mak.

Halfhill, T. R. (1996, September). Break the bandwidth barrier. *Byte.* Also Available: http://www.byte.com/art/9609/sec6/sec6.htm.

IW Labs. (1996, June). Internet phones: The future is calling. *Internet World, 40,* 42–46;48–52.

Medenis, M. M. (1997). *Internet backbone networks and the NII.* Available: http://web.ece.arizona.edu/~medenis/hw1/assign1.htm#docindex.

National Cable Television Association. (1997). *Surfing the Internet at lightening speed: The high speed cable modem.* Available: http://www.ncta.com/modem.html.

PCWebopaedia email. Available: http://pcwebopaedia.com/e_mail.htm.

PCWebopaedia network. Available: http://pcwebopaedia.com/network.htm.

Quiggle, A. L. (1998). Personal correspondence.

Rickard, J. (1997). *Internet architecture.* Available: http://www.boardwatch.com/isp/archit.htm.

Snyder, J. (1997, December). Want speed? Go digital. *Internet World, 34,* 38.

The National Information Infrastructure: Agenda For Action Executive Summary. (1994). Available: http://sunsite.unc.edu/nii/NII-Executive-Summary.html.

CHAPTER 13

The Internet:
A Generative Environment

Objectives:

After studying this chapter you should be able to:

1 Compare and contrast the various non-WWW Internet communication tools

2 Discuss the different types of search services

3 Evaluate information found on the net

4 Discuss plug-ins

5 Identify some of the newer technologies found on the WWW

With many people in different environments sharing their knowledge and skills, the Internet has proven to be a fertile ground for innovation. These innovations have revolutionized the way knowledge is shared and managed. Given the desire of people to communicate in real time (synchronously), many of the next innovations will improve these capabilities. Although the World Wide Web (WWW) has captured people's imagination, there are still computer communications that are independent of the WWW.

Non-World Wide Web Communications

BULLETIN BOARDS

Bulletin boards were one of the first attempts to use computers to provide up-to-date information and a place for people with similar interests to exchange ideas. Known colloquially as bulletin board systems (BBSs), they are one of the last remaining computer communication devices that do not require one to use the Internet for access, although some are now also available through the Internet. Those who operate a bulletin board are called *sysops*. Setting up a bulletin board is relatively inexpensive. All that is needed is a computer that is constantly on, a modem, an available telephone line, and bulletin board software. Many organizations, both nonprofit and profit had bulletin boards for their constituents. The features that a bulletin board offers are determined by the sysop. Some are read only; others allow posting.

To contact a bulletin board, besides a computer, one only needs a modem, communication software, and the telephone number used for a connection. Bulletin boards may duplicate many features found on the WWW, such as email, real-time interactions, database applications, and file libraries (Crowe, 1996). Because they are text only, bulletin boards can be used with older computers. Some bulletin boards provide Internet access, although the interface will be text only. Because BBSs are contacted by regular telephone lines, unless the BBS has an 800 number, few users are found outside a local calling area.

NEWS GROUPS

News groups are an electronic discussion forum. First established in 1979 as Usenet News at the University of North Carolina to provide a forum for the discussion of politics, religion, and other subjects, users from all over the world soon joined (Timeline, 1997). Although the term news is used for these groups, the news refers to messages sent by *any* individual who chooses to do so and replies to those messages. For the most part, these messages are *not* refereed. As originally conceived and distributed under Usenet News, these groups were organized in hierarchical levels under seven different headings. As more groups developed, some did not fit into the seven original categories and an Alt category was created to house them (Oliver, 1996).

A loose network of computers developed that agreed to carry the messages and replies that had been posted to these groups and make them available to the public. The number of groups grew to cover many different topics, including health-related and nursing-related topics. By 1995, there were more than 12,000 such groups generating 300 megabytes of information a day (Fleishman, 1995). There are two for nursing—alt.npractioner and sci.med.nursing. Today, many local groups exist that are available only locally and are intended for communication about area issues.

To access news groups requires a special news reader. Most browsers include this software, but more extensive news readers are also available. A good reader keeps track of the messages you have read and allows you to subscribe to a particular group. A subscription, which is free, just means that you can easily access the group without going through the hierarchy to locate it. The reader also provides ways to post messages to the group.

MAILING LISTS

A mailing list group is a different form of network news. Like network news, there are many groups, each of which focuses on specific topics. But instead of using a special reader to read the messages, they are sent to your email address. Like Usenet news groups, subscriptions are free. Once a user subscribes to a group (Display 13-1), copies of any message posted to the group are sent to the subscriber's mailbox (Fig. 13-1). The user can reply to any of the messages or send an entirely new message to the group. The tasks of keeping track of subscribers and sending copies of messages is accomplished by a software program. The original program was called *ListServ*™, which is why mailing lists are often called listservs.

•▼•▲•▼•▲•▼•▲•▼•▲•▼•▲•▼•▲•▼•▲•▼•▲•▼•▲•▼•▲•▼

Display 13-1 • HOW TO SUBSCRIBE TO A MAILING LIST

To subscribe to a list, you send a message to the mailing list software at the list address. The message varies with the type of software used to manage the list. For most of the software packages, the message is Subscribe [listname] [first name] [last name].[1] For example, if Florence Nightingale were to subscribe to NurseRes, she would send a message to:

listserv@listserv.kent.edu

Her message would be:

subscribe nurseres Florence Nightingale

You do not need to include a subject or any other information in the message. In fact, extraneous information can confuse the software that manages the list. Within a short time after sending this message (some-times within one or two minutes), you will probably receive a message telling you that you must confirm your subscription within 48 hours. Unfortunately, the information about how to respond is not always clear, but the proper response is to use the reply function and to type OK as your message. This confirmation protects the list from false subscriptions to nonexistent addresses by nefarious souls who have time on their hands, a behavior that creates much extra work for the list owner—who in most cases is an unpaid volunteer.

A few minutes after your confirmation is received, you will receive a welcome message giving you information about the list. **Save this message!** It contains information about how to post a message to the group, and about other functions that you can use to tailor the messages you receive to your needs.

[1]The word *join* instead of *subscribe* is used by the mailing list software Mailbase; most others use the word *subscribe*.

Mailing list software offers many options for subscribers beyond just sending messages (Table 13-1). For this reason, there are two addresses for each group. One address is used to subscribe or evoke any of the many functions, such as temporarily suspending your mail or unsubscribing, and another address is used only when one posts a message to the group.

Lists can be either unmoderated, moderated, or moderated with editing. On unmoderated lists, all messages posted to the group's address are automatically sent to the group. On a moderated group, messages first pass to the list's *owner*, or the individual who takes responsibility for the list. This individual may or may not post a message, depending on the criteria of the group. In a moderated with editing group, the messages not only go to the owner but this individual may edit a message before posting. There are advantages and disadvantages to all formats. On an unmoderated list, you get all messages including obvious errors or requests mistakenly sent to the group. The messages, however, are posted immediately. On lists that are moderated, the owner does not post obvious mistakes and can keep items off the list that do not meet the list criteria. Also, there is usually a delay between when a message is sent and when it is posted to the group itself.

Mailing lists can also be private or read only. A private mailing list is one set up by a group that wishes to exchange information among its members, such as a class, or organization. It can serve both as a communication tool and a forum for discussion of issues pertaining to that group. A read only mailing list is intended only for the distribution of information to a fixed group. Subscribers cannot post messages to a read only list (Table 13-2).

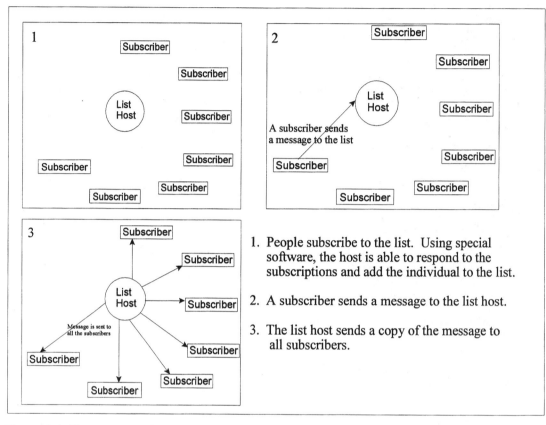

Figure 13-1 • Listserv topography.

1. People subscribe to the list. Using special software, the host is able to respond to the subscriptions and add the individual to the list.

2. A subscriber sends a message to the list host.

3. The list host sends a copy of the message to all subscribers.

Listserv Etiquette

Although most mailing lists that you join are open to the public, membership is a privilege. The number of members varies. Some, especially private ones, have only 10 or 15 members. Others have a membership that numbers in the thousands. If a list is to meet the needs of this many subscribers, members should not only follow normal email protocol but recognize that many people, most of whom a member does not know, will read any message that is posted to the group. Although all groups welcome *lurkers,* or members who never post to the group but read all messages, lists are only as helpful as those who contribute to the group.

A user will feel more comfortable posting to a mailing list when he or she understands some of the unwritten conventions that enable groups to be convivial. Most groups welcome new members, especially those who contribute postings, but the best idea is to lurk for a few days to a week before posting to the group. This enables you to get a feel for the types of message that are posted. In most cases, they will be loosely focused around the topic of the list. When you do post, always include a sub-

TABLE 13-1 • Mailing List Options

The following table gives some options that most mailing list software makes available to subscribers. The message may differ somewhat depending on the software that is used to manage the list. Some of the more popular mailing list packages are Listserv™, Mailbase™, and Listproc™. All mailing list software sends new subscribers a set of instructions that detail how to invoke the options. Keep this original message and refer to it when you need help.

Option	Purpose	Message (should all be on one line)	Example
Subscribe	Place yourself on the mailing list so you will receive all messages sent to the group	sub group name First Name Last Name	sub nurseres Florence Nightingale
Unsubscribe	Remove yourself from the mailing list	unsub group name	unsub nurseres Florence Nightingale
Digest	Places all messages for a day into one message which is sent to you as a single message with a list of subject headings at the top. You then select only the messages you wish to read by number	set group name digest	set nurseres digest
NoMail	Allows you to temporarily suspend mail from the group	set group name nomail	set nurseres nomail
Mail	This option resumes messages from the group	set group name mail	set nurseres mail
Review	Retrieves information about the group and a list of subscribers organized alphabetically by email address	rev group name	rev nurseres
By name	Retrieves information about the group and a list of subscribers organized alphabetically by email address	rev group name by name	rev nurseres by name
By country	Retrieves information about the group and a list of subscribers organized by country	rev group name by country	rev nurseres by country

TABLE 13-2 ● *Posting and Replying to Mailing Lists*		
To	**Send to**	**Example**
Post a message to the group	The name of the group and address	nurseres@listserv.kent.edu
Set a function, e.g., unsubscribe, nomail	The name of the mailing list software that manages the list	listserv@listserv.kent.edu
Your objective	**How to post**	**Explanation**
Reply to a message to the group	Use the reply function	Generally, if you use the reply function
Initiate a new topic of discussion	Initiate a new message: specify the new subject on the subject line	when replying to a mailing group message, the message will be posted back
Reply individually to a poster	Initiate a new message and use the email address of the individual who posted the message	to the entire group as a message on the same topic.

ject and sign your name and email address. Sometimes members will wish to contact you privately instead of replying to the list.

When replying to a message, include enough of the original so readers will grasp the full meaning. Members may have read the message a day or more ago and be completely in the dark about the original message. To avoid messages that can grow to astronomical lengths, in including the message to which you are replying, edit out text that is not pertinent. Putting the word "snip" where text was removed and retaining the signature of the original poster are also helpful methods. If initiating a new topic of discussion, be sure to send a new message with a new subject line. This approach not only helps readers but some mailing lists have their messages indexed by subject and archived for retrieval on the WWW. It is disconcerting to find a posting about one topic grouped with another topic.

Most mailing lists are global in scope. Unless the focus is a specialty, they include members from many different walks of life. This factor can cause a lack of understanding when acronyms are used. It is not unusual to see a message posted that has as its main topic an acronym that is unfamiliar to people with different backgrounds. When using an acronym, be sure it is defined in every message the first time it is used, even when replying to a message that has used it within the last few days.

List members use many types of Internet connections for email. Although some mailers are capable of sending messages in other formats, they will not be readable by many members. Always send plain ASCII text messages when posting to a mailing list. Subscribers may also be irritated when members set their email to deliver an automatic reply stating they will be unavailable until a certain date. Using this setting generates an unwanted reply to the group for every message, which can be avoided if a member sets the NoMail option (see Table 13-1).

Someone has to mind the list. This involves taking care of *error messages,* or messages to members that are returned, often because a member did not unsubscribe from the list but terminated his or her account. Error messages are also created by members who go on vacation, but do not temporarily suspend their list mail, and fill up their mailboxes. Looking at all of these error messages and disposing of them appropriately takes time on the part of the owner, time that is unpaid. Considerate mailing list members know to what lists they are subscribed, use "nomail" appropriately, and unsubscribe before they terminate an account. Instructions for performing these functions are included in the welcome message that is sent to new subscribers.

FORUMS

Forums are similar to news groups, but they are sponsored by individual organizations and are usually web based. To visit a forum, visit the web site of the sponsoring organization. From there, follow the instructions for entering a forum of choice. Depending on the organization, there may be one or more forums, but the topic of discussion for each will be related to the mission of the organization. Often, newcomers are asked to register by name and password. Use this password each time you return to the forum.

SIMILARITIES AND DISSIMILARITIES

The biggest similarity among all of these groups is that they are a means of asynchronous communication (Table 13-3). All of the various mailing lists and news groups generally all follow the same procedures for their type of group, whereas the format for bulletin boards and forums varies from group to group.

THREADED MESSAGES

When messages are threaded, they are organized by the topic of the message. The first message for that topic starts the thread, with other messages about this topic following. Often the number of other messages on this topic are in parentheses after the

---

TABLE 13-3 ● *Organized Computer Asynchronous Communication*

Group	How to receive messages	How to post messages
UseNet News—a bulletin board where individuals post messages about a common interest; organized by areas	Access the news reader. Varies from ISP to ISP	Depending on the news reader, most are similar to sending email
Mailing List—group of individuals who share a common interest and communicate on all facets of this topic	Subscribe by sending a message to the ListServ at the group's address; all messages then are sent to your mailbox	Send them to the name of the group at the host address
Forums—Discussion groups available at some web sites	Visit the web site, enter the forum; you may need to have a login name and a password	Differs for each forum; follow the instructions
Bulletin Board—computer communication organized by a sysop to provide information and other services	Connect by using communication software to dial the local phone number	Follow the established protocol; it is NOT necessary to be connected to the Internet to use most bulletin boards

topic of the group. News groups and most forums have threaded messages. Bulletin boards may have them, whereas mailing lists do not, although some are archived in threads. The threading concept works only when posters use the reply function or use the exact wording for the original subject for messages on a given topic. Threading breaks down when posters use the reply function to start a new topic.

READING MESSAGES

To read messages for all of the groups except mailing lists, it is necessary either to access a reader or to visit a site. In these groups, topics can be selected by the user. Mailing lists, however, deliver all messages to your email box, whether they are of interest or not. For this reason, mailing lists sometimes feel more personal but can also overwhelm a person with the volume of mail.

FLAME WARS

A flame is derogatory mail sent by a poster who takes umbrage at another's message. A message of this sort can easily deteriorate into a flame war when others take up one or the other position. In most groups, this ends on a conciliatory note when cooler heads prevail. Flame wars can happen in any group but tend to be more common in groups that discuss volatile topics.

Worldwide discussion groups have opened a new chapter in inter-personal relations, one in which we are still learning to see our communications from many different points of view. Rereading all messages before posting and trying to imagine how they will look to others who do not share our view or background goes a long way toward preventing flame wars. It also opens the door to a real understanding.

SYNCHRONOUS COMMUNICATION

Synchronous communication is available through the use of chat. Originally, synchronous conversation was limited to two people, but in the late 1980s, internet relay chat (IRC) was developed, making it possible for multiple users to engage in live discussions (IRC, 1997). Although responses are immediate, they are text based. IRC requires special software on your computer and regular connection to the Internet. IRC is plain text, but graphical interfaces are now available for web chats.

Some ISPs build in the needed software and provide chat rooms as one of their features. Generally, unless it is prearranged, in most chat rooms, users talk with whomever is online at that time. Consequently, most of the use that has been made of chat has been for socializing. However, with the graphical features of the WWW, it holds great promise for health care and educational uses, especially when it is combined with the features of a multi-object-oriented system (MOOS).

Going beyond chat rooms, purposeful conferencing is also available. Although available for many years, the introduction of a graphical environment with the WWW has increased the number of functions available. Versions of most web browsers created since early 1997 include software that permits users to conduct a conference with other users. Attendees at these conferences can share files, view a common whiteboard,[1] and work collaboratively. Live audio is also available with a microphone through a user's sound card. Connections for these conferences can be as simple as entering the email address of the individual or individuals with whom a user wishes to connect.

Gophers

Although they are mostly a part of Internet history, gophers were the first tool that eased the chore of finding information on the Internet. There had been previous tools for finding files that could be retrieved using File Transfer Protocol (FTP), such as Archie and Wide-Area Information Server (WAIS), but using them involved knowing some commands and accessing very busy sites. Like many of the Internet tools, Gophers were built on the client server model. They presented users with menus that were often hierarchical, that is, making one selection led to another menu. Using a Gopher, a user could browse through the Internet's resources and make selections from menus.

Everything on a gopher is text based, but unlike FTP, users could read a document before deciding if they wish to download it. It was also possible to add a bookmark for selections to which one wished to return. There was even a tool, Veronica (very easy rodent-oriented netwide index to computerized archives), that was updated at least every 2 weeks, which provided searching ability. Gophers have declined in use with the rise of the WWW. Most documents that are available on Gophers have now been converted to web documents.

World Wide Web

The WWW can be regarded as a huge, worldwide library. By using it, a user can find very valuable information, such as the latest in cancer treatments, the full wording of bills pending before Congress, and any information that someone who has a point to push and access to a web site wants to publish. Starting in 1989, the original purpose of the WWW was to enable the sharing of research materials and collaboration between physicists at many different locations. The WWW is based on providing links to other files in the form of hypertext. Hypertext is a type of cross-referencing in which text that is linked to another file is specially marked (Fig. 13-2). In a web document, this marking is usually blue and underlined. Placing the mouse pointer on that word and clicking on it retrieves the document linked to that word. Linking, however, is not limited to text. Objects also can have links.

BROWSERS

After its inception, WWW tools were made available to other interested users. These tools include browsers that request and read the files; documents that are specially formatted using a language called Hypertext Markup Language (HTML); and the use of a transmission protocol called Hypertext Transmission Protocol (HTTP). Using client-server conventions, the browser is the client software. The server also has specialized software that permits it to receive and respond to requests.

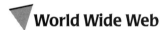 [1]A whiteboard is a display in which multiple users can write or draw while others watch.

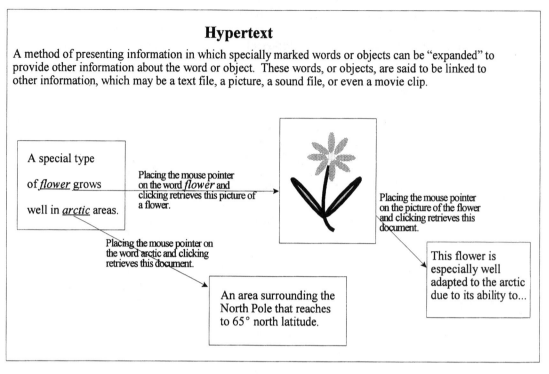

Figure 13-2 • Hypertext.

Although there are text web browsers, the development of a graphical browser, Mosaic, along with the arrival of graphical user interface (GUI) operating systems that could use a graphical browser, enabled the WWW to take off in popularity. The two most popular browsers today are Microsoft Internet Explorer™ and Netscape™. Browsers work by using the HTTP protocol to request a HTML-formatted document from a web server (Fig. 13-3). This formatting tells the browser how to display the document on the user's screen. These instructions may include links to other web pages, provide for the color and position of the text, and set locations for various images that the document contains.

USING THE WORLD WIDE WEB

To use the WWW, besides the usual computer communication hardware and software, a connection to the Internet is needed, preferably one that permits a graphical interface and a web browser. To use a browser, open the browser and then connect to the Internet through an ISP. If one is connecting through a networked computer, it is possible that the connection is always open, and that as soon as the browser is open,

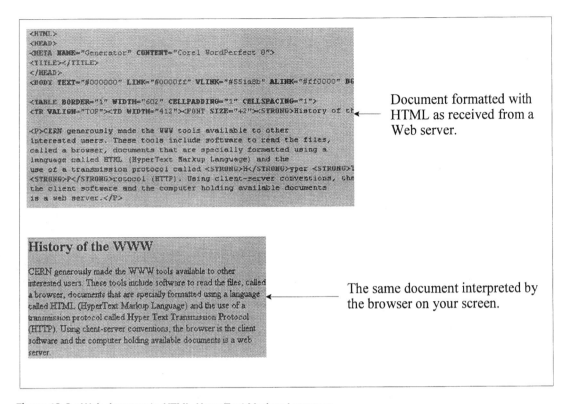

Document formatted with HTML as received from a Web server.

The same document interpreted by the browser on your screen.

Figure 13-3 • Web documents. HTML, HyperText Markup Language.

the WWW can be accessed. Whichever browser in use, the top of the screen will look somewhat like the one in Figure 13-4.

There will be a location line that lists the Universal Resource Locator (URL), or address of the computer that hosts the document that is on your screen. There will also be a way to go to the previous screen and to any already accessed. However both options may be grayed out when the browser is first opened because only one docu-

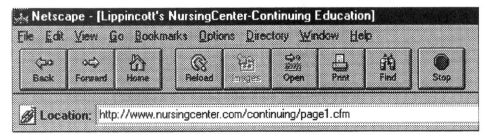

Figure 13-4 • Browser interface.

ment is viewed during this session. A button that will allow the user to print the document, find a word or phrase, and request a new document will also be available. There are several ways to access a URL. The quickest is to type it (or paste from the clipboard using Ctrl-V) on the location line. All browsers also provide either an open button, or a choice on the file menu that presents the user with a dialog box into which the URL can be entered. Small objects in an icon in the right hand corner of the screen will then start moving to indicate the request is being filled. These objects will continue to move until the document requested has been completely downloaded. Very seldom will the return be instantaneous. Be prepared to wait a minute or two, depending on the document requested as well as the traffic on the Internet.

Occasionally, instead of the requested file, an error message will be received. In general, there are three types of error messages. One type tells the user that the computer whose name was entered in the URL does not exist. Another informs the user that the computer in the URL is not responding. The third relays that the file requested does not exist. See Figure 13-5 for the error messages and Table 13-4 for thoughts on remedying these errors. Occasionally, either a site is too busy, or Internet traffic is too great and a site will *time out:* that is, the calling computer will be unable to make contact with the called computer.

If the user discovers a mistake after a request is made, clicking on the stop button cancels the command. There are other times when a transfer seems to get interrupted

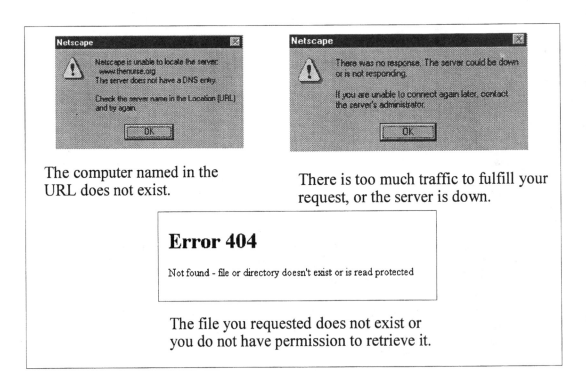

Figure 13-5 • Error messages. URL, Universal Resource Locator.

TABLE 13-4 ● *Possible Responses to Error Messages*	
Error	**Thoughts on correcting**
	Click on "OK" and then:
The computer does not exist. (The server does not have a DNS entry.)	Check the URL you entered, it may be incorrect. Correct and try again. This error can usually be avoided when you can copy and paste the URL.
There is too much traffic at the site or the server is down. (There was no response.)	Try again later.
The file does not exist or you do not have access to it. (Error 404)	1. Check the name of the file. 2. Go up one level in the address and see if you can find the file from there. Do this by deleting the part of the URL to the right of the last forward slash.
File request has timed out.	Try once more, usually best course is to try again at a different time.

or only part of the requested file appears on the screen. This problem can sometimes be remedied by clicking on the reload button, or if the status line says that the document is done, clicking the back button and then the forward button.

Navigation of a web document is identical to that used for a word processing document, including the use of the arrow keys, page down and up, and vertical and horizontal scroll bars. There are a few properties, owing to the hypertext abilities, that are not part of word processing navigation. Clicking on any area where the mouse pointer changes to a hand will retrieve the document or object to which that item is linked. If the so-called hot area is a text word, it will be underlined and probably colored blue. If the hot area is a graphic, moving the mouse pointer over it and seeing it become a hand, instead of an arrow, will tell the user that clicking on that graphic will retrieve another file. Like turning to another page in a book that is cross-referenced, a reader sometimes wishes to return to the original document. This can be done by clicking on the back button on the tool bar, or clicking the right mouse button, which will provide a menu of options, one of which will be back.

Once you start using the hypertext feature in a document, it is possible to get so far away from the original document that returning to it becomes a lengthy procedure. A feature of browsers, called either History, or Go, keeps a record of the last nine or more documents that you have retrieved (Fig. 13-6). To return a document to the screen, click on this button and click on the name of the document on the drop down menu.

URLS

All documents on the WWW have an address, or URL. These addresses are seen in advertisements on television or in print sources. Although it may not always be stated, all URLS start with http, the acronym for hypertext transfer protocol; a colon,

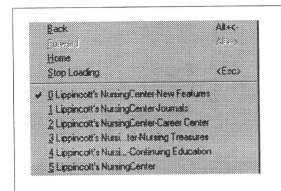

The history of documents retrieved during this WWW session. The check mark indicates the document that is currently on the screen.

Figure 13-6 • Web document history. WWW, World Wide Web.

and two forward slashes. Many then follow with www.[2] The rest of the address varies. Like email addresses, URLs may look like a conglomeration of characters when they are first seen, but there is a pattern to them just as there is to email addresses (Fig. 13-7). The name of the computer that hosts the document follows either the double forward slash (//) or the dot after www. It ends with the next forward slash (/). The letters after the name of the computer are directories (folders) on the host computer. These directories are organized in a hierarchy identical to the files on the hard drive. A forward slash (/) separates each folder from the one above it and from a file name if there is one in the URL. The URL may end with a folder or a file name.

Nonletter characters may be seen in a URL, such as an underscore (_), hyphen (-), or a tilde (~). These elements are all integral parts of an address and should not be omitted. When a tilde is in an address, it denotes a personal web page versus an institutional one. One thing that all web addresses (like email addresses) have in common, is that there are no spaces. Note that the slashes in a URL are forward slashes.

WHAT IS ON THE WORLD WIDE WEB?

What is available on the WWW can be summed up in one word: information. Health care information for professionals and laypersons can be found in abundance. Many organizations such as the American Nurses Association and Sigma Theta Tau have

---

[2]Newer versions of browsers do not require you to enter the http://www as part of the address.

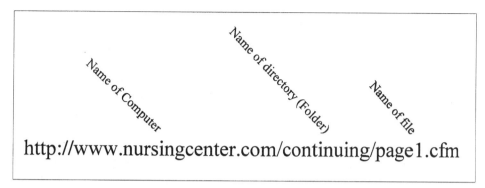

Figure 13-7 • Universal Resource Locator (URL) dissected.

web pages, as do health care institutions, governments, and individuals. There are even online journals with full-text articles, several of which pertain to nursing. The full text of many books can also be found. Besides bibliographical databases, there are other databases, some from the government, others from private institutions. Advertisements and catalogs also proliferate.

Most items on the WWW are free, but this feature could change. Although there are no printing costs with web pages, there is a cost involved in preparing the information to be placed on the WWW and maintaining the site. At present, many sites try to support themselves with advertising. It remains to be seen how effective this will be.

FINDING INFORMATION ON THE INTERNET

Cataloging items on the Internet and indexing them in a manner in which they can be delivered to those who need them is a monumental task. It is not surprising that finding what you need on the Internet can be time consuming. One of the best sources of information is word of mouth. Members of mailing lists, forums, or news groups often post web sites that they have found to be helpful. URLS for helpful information can also be learned from print sources and on television. Many useful sites are also discovered by following links in a document. When all else fails, there are search services.

There are basically three different types of search services—directories, or web guides; search engines; and meta searchers. There are also specialized searchers that allow the user to look for specific items, such as a mailing list, an address, a company, or an email address, and search engines that search in specific categories such as law or health. Additionally, there are sites that help choose the search engine best suited to specific needs.

Web Guides

Directories, or web guides, are search services that attempt to cut down irrelevant hits by including only items that they approve. McKinley's Magellan Internet Directory™, Yahoo™, and Lycos™ are web guides. When these services are accessed, the user is presented with a list of subject categories. Each category links to several layers of subcategories. At the bottom level is a listing of links. At each level, it is also possible to search for a term either from the category currently on the screen or the entire search service. Some web guides use symbols to indicate how they have rated a site, but getting information on how the ratings are calculated is difficult.

Search Engines

Search services, categorized as search engines, have software called *spiders,* which perpetually roam the Internet looking for a new site or one that has changed. The information a spider collects from a site varies depending on the dictates of the search site (Sparks & Rizzolo, 1998). Some spiders are programmed to capture every site, whereas others attempt to rate sites based on how often they are accessed and how frequently they change (Maskin, 1997). The indexes created may contain the words in a document as well as other information about a site. Because there may be thousands of sites containing words that match a given query, most search engines rate the sites. For example, some use the number of times the word appears in the document as a rating guide.

When using a search engine, what is searched is the index that the search engine has built. From this index, the search engine returns a list organized by the ratings that the proprietors have assigned, with the site with the highest rating at the top. This list often has a brief description of the site, which is sometimes the first few lines of the document.

Mega Searchers

Mega searchers search a given set of search engines, eliminate duplicates, and report the list back to the user. When there is a great deal of information available on a topic, the mega searchers can often focus on the most pertinent sites. Although they do not find as many sites for a given topic, any that they miss can often be located with links. No matter what search engine is used, the results will be different with each search engine due to the different ways they search and archive.

Image Searching

It is also possible to search just for images. If a user prefixes a search on Alta Vista with the word *image,* a list of URLS for images, instead of documents, will be received. Yahoo has a category devoted to images, and there are search engines that specialize in finding them. If one is downloading an image, be sure to comply with copyright laws.

Hints for Better Searching

Selecting a search tool should be based on the information that is needed. If the topic is very broad, such as diabetes, select a web guide. If the topic is very narrow, or if the user doubts there is much information available, start with a mega searcher. If the search is unsuccessful, try one of the search engines. Take the time to become familiar with help, hints, or frequently asked questions (FAQs) option that each search service provides.

WEB COOKIES

Web cookies are a piece of data that is sent to a computer by some web sites. The browser stores the information in a cookie file, which is an ASCII text file. When the site is visited again, the server asks the browser to return any information it might have about the user's visits to the site (AnimEigo, 1997). When a site places a cookie in a cookie file, this information tells how long the cookie is valid. It also uses a keyword so it can identify the cookie and any information about the user's visit to the site that it wants to be able to access. Cookies do not capture any information from the user's computer. Essentially, cookies are a way for a server to better meet user needs. In some sites in which the user needs to register, the password and login name is stored in a cookie that is retrieved when the site is visited. This means the user does not have to reenter this information each time the site is visited. It is possible to set your browser to ask each time a site wants to send a cookie and for the user to refuse.

REPEATED VISITING OF HELPFUL SITES

When a site is found that a user wishes to visit frequently, click on bookmarks (or favorites), a word on the second screen line of most browsers. Then click on the phrase add bookmark (or favorite). This process adds the URL for this site to a list of items that will drop down when this button is clicked. When accessing this site again, click on bookmark (favorites), and click on the name of the entry in the list. Assuming you are online, this procedure will request the named document. Once a sizeable number of these URLS are gathered, organize them into folders. A description for each item can be included. It is also possible to search the list in case the placement of a specific document is forgotten. Use the help function to learn to do this. This file is a separate file, just like a word processing file. The difference is that it is in HTML code and is an ASCII, or text file.

EVALUATING INFORMATION ON THE INTERNET

This freedom of publication on the Internet allows an airing of ideas, many which are not in the main stream. The authenticity that we count on in the print world with the reputations of various newspapers and journals is not yet available on the WWW. Evaluation is a subjective endeavor. In conducting an evaluation of a resource, whether on the WWW or elsewhere, the first step is to have the need for the resource clearly in mind. There are a series of criteria that are often helpful in evaluating a resource, which include accuracy, authority, objectivity, currency or timeliness, coverage, and usability.

Accuracy

When referring to a source for information, it is often difficult to evaluate its accuracy. There are, however, some items that should be considered in making a judgment. Sometimes you will find excerpts from print material. In these cases, the entire source might have to be looked at to evaluate the piece. If terms like prove are used, be suspicious. Research results never prove anything, they either lend support to a hypothesis, have no effect on it, or show a lack of support.

Authority

With print text, authority is often judged by source. If an article is published in *Nursing Research,* we are reasonably certain that it has had an extensive review by others with knowledge of the subject. If it is published on the Internet, it will fall on a continuum from a reviewed article to someone's highly opinionated soapbox.

There are criteria that can be considered in deciding if the source is reliable. The most important is the source of the document. What is the reputation of the organization at whose site you found the document? If the document does not reveal this information, the URL can be used to gain this information. If you see a tilde (~) in the URL, you are looking at a personal page. By looking at the part of the URL directly following the www, one can tell what type of organization, and sometimes the name of the organization that hosts the server and perhaps sponsors the site. You can also use the domain name to tell the type of organization. If the domain name is org, for instance, it is a nonprofit organization.

If an author is listed, what is the reputation of the author? Any initials after the name can give information about credentials. Some authors are linked to their home page, which may list some of their accomplishments. Another avenue is to determine whether the name can be found in a bibliographical database appropriate to the field, for example, CINAHL or the International Nursing Index, in nursing.

Not finding any of these things does not automatically mean the document is faulty, it just means other criteria need to be used when making a decision. Is the information in the document verifiable? Are thought-provoking statements supported by references to other sources that are reliable? If so, is the reference stated fully enough so that it can be found? Are there outside evaluations of the site? By whom? Do any of the web guides include it? Inclusion in these guides lends some reliability to the document. Is the site or document peer reviewed or edited? If so, by whom?

Objectivity

Information is rarely neutral. Because data are used in selective ways to form information, they generally represent a point of view. When evaluating information found on the Internet, it is important to think about any biases that may be present in the document. The popularity of the Internet makes it the perfect venue for commercial and sociopolitical publishing. These areas, in particular, are open to highly subjective uses of data.

Is the page intended for entertainment, business or marketing, reference or information, news, or a personal page? Does this purpose lead you to expect that the author has an agenda such as to inform, explain, or persuade? If so, what point of view would you expect? If you find biases, what are they and do they render this piece unusable for your purpose or can you still use it? Finding biases is not necessarily bad. Most of us have opinions on many things. This does not make our writings or speech unacceptable.

Currency or Timeliness

Like print information, data on the Internet can become dated. Well-designed pieces carry the date when they were last updated. If the document is undated, look at View/Document Information to see the date that it was last updated. Another way to determine the date is to test the links. Many nonfunctional links are a sign that the information may be old.

Coverage

Criteria in this category are very specific to your purpose. If you are searching for a professional description of a disease condition, an article for a lay audience will probably be inadequate. On the other hand, if you are looking for information for a client, a professional article may contain too much depth.

Usability

There are many criteria that determine the overall usefulness of a site or document. What they are is determined by the purpose of the site. Sound, for example, when used for effect, can be nuisance, but if a user wishes to hear breath sounds, it is a necessary accompaniment to the site. Color can contribute to functionality or be a distraction. Graphics that take a long time to download and that are necessary for understanding can limit a site's usefulness. Whether or not it is easy to navigate the site also determines usability.

Overall Rating

It is tempting to want to make a checklist for evaluation. This endeavor is based on the assumption that all pieces on the Internet are alike. It is hoped that the criteria that are discussed will be used as considerations when evaluating items from the WWW, not as an end in themselves. The WWW is a new medium. To deal with it effectively requires critical thinking abilities, not checklists. The usefulness of a resource depends on the reason the information is used and criteria, which vary with the type of resource.

PLUG-INS

A plug-in is a helper program for a browser. Browsers are capable only of interpreting certain types of files, such as those in the html format, gif or jpeg images, or au or wav audio files. The Internet, however, is capable of transmitting other types of files, such as those created by multimedia authoring languages. Before a user can use these files, his or her computer must have a program that can interpret the file and show it in the browser. Plug-ins fill this function.

One of the most common plug-ins is Adobe Acrobat Reader, which is used to read files that are printer definition format (PDF) files. These files are designed to print a specific way, unlike regular web pages that print according to the dictates of the printer used to print them. Adobe Acrobat Reader, like most plug-ins, can be downloaded for free.

JAVA

It is very hard to be on the Internet for any length of time and not be aware that there is something, besides an island in Indonesia or coffee, called Java. Java is a programming language that was originally developed for small consumer electronic devices.

What makes Java important is that programs written in this language can be run on computers using any operating system, such as Macintosh™, Windows™, or Unix™. This means that instead of producing a different version of a program for different operating systems, the same Java program can be used on any Java-enabled operating system. The spirit of Java generally accepted in the programming community is to avoid modifications to enhance one operating system at the expense of others. Java programs that are available from the Internet are called applets. Java can also be used to write full programs such as a word processor or a spreadsheet (Quiggle, 1998).

STREAMING

Streaming is a technique for transferring data that allows the user to start seeing the file before the entire file has downloaded. This technique is becoming important because of the increase in the number of large files, such as multimedia applications, that users want to download. Its ability to work depends on the receiving computer's ability to collect the data and deliver it in a steady stream, even when the data is received faster than is necessary. Audio files and movie clips are sometimes sent in this manner.

Display 13-2 • INEXPENSIVE VIDEOCONFERENCING

Relatively inexpensive desktop conferencing is available with a golfball-sized camera for $100 or more, and free software from Cornell University known as CU-SeeMe. An expanded version of this software is also available for a fee. Both versions of this software permit both point-to-point and multipoint conferencing. Although the equipment is easily installed, video is a very demanding application and requires a computer with at least a Pentium 133 and 16 megs of memory and at least a 28.8 Kbps modem.

Once the software is installed, you can connect point to point with another individual in one of two ways. You can connect to what is called a reflector site, which is analogous to an audio chat room. Essentially it is a server that allows people to log in to their site for the purpose of videoconferencing.

Or, if you prefer more privacy, you and another individual can connect by using internet protocol (IP) addresses. An IP address is a number assigned to everyone who is connected to the Internet. Because there are a limited number of these addresses available, instead of assigning a permanent one to each client, ISPs assign what is called a dynamic IP address. That is, each time you connect to your ISP, you are assigned a different IP number. If you are using Windows 95™ you can discover what your IP address is by clicking on Start/Run and entering winipcfg. (See *http://www.langara.bc.ca/vnc/ipaddress.htm* for instructions on how to do this with a Mac.)

This type of conferencing is not broadcast-quality. Limitations imposed by modems, telephone lines, and Internet connections make only small images possible, plus movement is somewhat disjointed due to the number of frames per second that are able to be transmitted. With a very good connection, you may be able to transmit 15 frames per second as opposed to the 30 that are necessary to have movie-like movement. More often, the transmission is at 4 to 10 frames per second. Audio is also sometimes a problem. Although this type of application is still in its infancy, expect to see major improvements as connections to the Internet and data transmissions on the Internet itself become faster. At present, like telephony, expect to spend time playing with the settings to achieve a satisfactory connection.

PUSH

Push is a technology that allows data to be sent without a user request. Email is the oldest example of push. With push technology, a site sends the user information that the web master believes will be of interest to that individual instead of waiting for the user to visit the site and obtain the information. It can be used to keep people up to date on topics of their choosing.

VIDEOCONFERENCING

Videoconferencing is a conference between participants at different locations, during which the participants can see each other (Display 13-2). The conference may involve only two people (point to point) or more (multipoint). In addition to a computer, a sound card, camera, speakers, and specialized software are needed. The quality of videoconferencing depends on the quality of the items mentioned and the speed of data transmission. There are two types of videoconferencing systems—desktop and room. The desktop systems are less expensive, whereas the room systems offer higher quality.

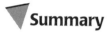

Summary

The culture of sharing resources on the Internet has led to many tools that today are taken for granted. Bulletin boards and email were the earliest of these tools. Email spawned news groups and mailing lists.

The arrival of the WWW has greatly increased the use and popularity of the Internet. Finding information on the Internet is made easier by the use of special search engines. Not only are there different types of search services but search engines within the same group vary in how they index and present items to a user.

Evaluating web sites must be done with an eye to the type of site, the purpose of the site, and the reason for which the site will be used. Criteria that should be considered when evaluating a web site include accuracy, authority, objectivity, timeliness, depth of coverage, and usability. Some files available on the WWW require a plug-in, or helper program, to be used. Plug-ins are generally freeware and available for downloading from the Internet. As the WWW and Internet infrastructure matures, expect to see many more developments that affect how the world communicates.

EXERCISES

1. Find two documents on the WWW, and document them as if they were being used as a resource for a paper or a report.
2. Find four documents on a given nursing topic and evaluate them for:
   a. Professional use
   b. Layperson use
3. What are some ways Internet tools are being used by health care professionals in
   a. Clinical practice?
   b. Administration?

c. Education?

d. Research?

e. Entrepreneurial work?

REFERENCES

AnimEigo. (1997). *What is a cookie?* Available: http://www.animeigo.com/Resources/FAQs/ COOKIES.html.

Crowe, E. (1996, Feb 27). *Internet basics: BBS: Not gone, not forgotten.* Available: http://www. currents.net/magazine/national/1405/intb1405.html.

Fleishman, G. (1995). Looking for the right Internet connection. *Info World, 17*(5), 51–52.

IRC. (1997). Available: http://pcwebopaedia.com/IRC.htm.

Maskin, D. (1997, December). Power search. *Internet World,* 79-80, 82-84, 86, 88, 90, 92.

Oliver, D. (1996). *Netscape 3 unleashed.* Indianapolis, IN: Sams Net.

Quiggle, J. H. (1998). Personal conversation.

Sparks, S. M., & Rizzolo, M. M. (1998). World Wide Web search tools. *Image, 30*(2), 167–171.

Timeline: PBS life on the internet. (1997). Available: http://www2.pbs.org/internet/timeline/ index.html.

The Internet:
The Other Health Care Revolution

 The Internet

One change the Internet has already made in health care is that patients come to health care professionals with knowledge about their medical condition. Using search tools on the World Wide Web (WWW), clients find it easy to locate information about a disease. Sites providing current information for various conditions, such as arthritis, cover a broad range of topics, including research, exercise, medication, surgery, and complementary therapies. It is easier to work with patients in planning care when they have a more thorough understanding of their condition. Patients may also want to take more responsibility in making decisions about their care—determinations that used to be made solely by health care professionals.

As cable modems become more common and easier to use, thus making Internet access more universal, clients will be referred to various web sites to reinforce teaching. This will involve health care professionals in a thorough evaluation of these sites. Health care professionals, such as nurses, may also be designing information to be placed on a web site for patient viewing. Knowing how to present information in a hypertext environment and how to design information that stands alone are skills that health care professionals will find useful.

Like anything, there is another side to easily available information. Nurses will also need to work with patients who have gained misinformation from the Internet. This creates a situation in which nurses have to decide whether something is misinformation or a fact that is unknown. Nurses must be open minded and be ready to investigate all sources that patients use for information. This may be particularly difficult with news groups, listservs, and forums, which are not referred. Becoming familiar with some alternative news groups, such as alt.folklore. herbs or alt.support.arthritis, and support listservs and forums, may be necessary in order to be prepared for ideas that clients bring to consultation rooms.

INTERACTIVE MEDICAL ADVICE

It will become more common for patients to check with online sources before seeking medical advice. There is at least one site that offers a so-called expert system to assist a user to diagnose the status of a symptom. At this site, before starting the consultation, the user clicks on a agreement not to hold the site responsible for any complications from the information that may be obtained. The user then selects whether the problem pertains to men, women, children, or is general, then makes another selection from a list of possible problems. Next, the user supplies information about his or her gender and age, and then answers a number of questions. At the end, the program may state that it is impossible to make a diagnosis, or it may present a list of possible diagnoses with a recommendation about whether the condition requires immediate medical attention. Information about each possible diagnosis is also presented.

DATABASES

Increasingly, governments are placing databases of information on the WWW. The U.S. government has made available many national health care databases. A user can obtain the average length of stay (LOS), average total charge, and co-morbidities for all of the diagnosis-related groups (DRGs) at http://www.ahcpr.gov/data/index.html. If the file is downloaded, it may open in a spreadsheet or database (Display 14-1) and be used in queries.

●▼●▲●▼●▲●▼●▲●▼●▲●▼●▲●▼●▲●

Display 14-1 • WORKING WITH DOWNLOADED DATA FILES

When the data is in an HTML table format, once it is downloaded, you may be able to open it directly into a database.

When the data is in columns, it can often be opened into a spreadsheet. Then select the rows that you need and copy them to another sheet in the notebook. At this point you will probably need to clean up the labels. Text that takes two cells but belongs to the same record will need to be placed together. When you have cleaned the data, it can be exported to a database or a statistical package.

FREE-NETS OR COMMUNITY NETWORKS

Another source of health information may be found in community networks, sometimes referred to as *free-nets*. A free-net is a free public computer network that provides information and Internet access to citizens of that community. It can be seen as an electronic community center, local hang-out, and public library rolled into one (Stallings, 1996). As a community center, free-nets may offer access to service agencies and local office holders. The function as a local hang-out is fulfilled through forums in which citizens can discuss civic issues through conferences and email. In a library role, free-nets provide online information resources. Many also offer citizens the ability to ask questions of nurses, doctors, and other health care professionals. In an effort to reach citizens who do not have their own computers, these groups attempt to place as many terminals in public places as their funding allows.

The first free-net was an outgrowth of a bulletin board system (Schuler, 1995). Users could leave questions for nurses, doctors, dentists, or other health care professionals that were answered within 24 hours. Access to governmental entities as well as hundreds of community organizations who agreed to maintain their own information was added. These organizations included many with a health promotion focus such as Alcoholics Anonymous, the Handicap Center, Center for International Health, and the Pediatric Information Resource Center.

The growth of community networks was furthered by the U.S. National Telecommunications and Information Administration in 1994, when they announced federal support for people and organizations to use telecommunications in their communities (Stallings, 1996). Community networks, such as the Rural Information Networks (RINs), which were created to deliver market-, agriculture-, and health-related information to rural areas, were one result of these grants.

SUPPORT GROUPS

Support groups for various conditions have been part of the health care scene for several decades. In traditional support groups, face-to-face contact is required. For many individuals who lack the time to travel to a meeting or who are separated by a large distance from meetings, the Internet provides this service. Support groups, such as Computerlink, can be organized that not only provide networking between caregivers of patients with Alzheimer's disease but also allow questions to be left for a nurse (Brennan, 1994). Another example of this type of network is the bulletin board system AIDSNET, which is sponsored by the Decker School of Nursing at SUNY Binghamton. AIDSNET offers rural patients an opportunity for consultation with nurses, the ability to send and receive messages, and the ability to download information that has been gathered from the national AIDS-related network (Atav, 1998; Parietti & Atav, 1994).

Support groups can also operate independently of health care personnel. A good search engine will locate many such groups, some for relatively rare conditions. Additionally, there are many news groups, forums, and mailing lists that act as support groups.

PSYCHOLOGY

A web site called Shrink Talk is an online forum for the *San Diego Magazine* (Gold, 1998). This site allows users to learn about concerns related to psychology. A few of the topics that have been discussed are addictive behaviors, adult learning principles, anxiety, changes in the workplace, and family. A recent email study found that psychiatric nurses on the Internet who are part of an international community of psychiatric nurses found that it helps ". . . to reduce the sense of isolation that many psychiatric nurses may feel as a result of being geographically isolated from peers or working in hostile environments" (Lakeman, 1997, p. 86).

EDUCATION

The educational opportunities available on the Internet are not limited to classes or individuals pursing information. The Internet is a rich source of images, which along with textual information found on the Internet, can be used by educators to create multimedia presentations for use in the classroom, a waiting room, or in one-on-one teaching. The Visible Human, which can be found at http://www.crd.ge.com/esl/cgsp/projects/vm, has many images that can be downloaded for use in a presentation. The Visible Embryo at http://visembryo.ucsf.edu/ is another site with images.

QUALITY OF INFORMATION AVAILABLE

The felt need to evaluate health-related items found on the Internet is universal in the health care community. An organization entitled The Health on the Net Foundation,[1] was originally founded to advance the development and application of new information technologies in health and medicine. This group responded to concerns regarding the varying quality of medical and health information available on the WWW by developing six criteria for medical and health web sites. The criteria include the provision that only appropriately trained medical professionals give advice, that the advice be scientifically supportable, and that the site not interfere with any physician or patient relationship (Health on the Net Foundation, 1997). Sites that agree to abide by these criteria are entitled to display the organization logo (Fig. 14-1). Compliance is voluntary, and a site that displays the organization logo must provide a link to the Health on the Net Foundation page, where the criteria are visible. The decision about whether this logo is warranted is left to site visitors, who are responsible for reporting to the foundation any deviance from the criteria.

Expect to see more attempts to evaluate sites that contain health care information. There are, however, many difficulties associated with regulating web sites. First, the WWW is truly world wide, and acceptable health care information in one country may not be acceptable in another. Even within political boundaries there are differences in opinions about health-related information. Additionally, it is very easy to

---

[1]The Health on the Net Foundation is an International nonprofit foundation supported by donations. The web page can be found at http://www.hon.ch/.

Figure 14-1 • Health On the Net Foundation logo. (Printed with permission of Health On the Net Foundation, a non-profit international foundation, which can be found at http://www.hon.ch/)

We subscribe to the HONcode principles of the Health On the Net Foundation

change a web page after it has been approved. In fact, it is necessary to make changes to stay current.

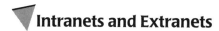 ## Intranets and Extranets

The concept of hypertext in web browsers has also been appropriated for use in private Internets, or networks that are not available to the general public. There are two types—an *intranet* and an *extranet*.

INTRANET

Intranets are networks that are accessed using a web browser but are only available to users within a specific organization. They are useful in making information that is needed by those within an organization freely available. Anyone in an organization who has either struggled to find the latest version of a procedure or to see that all who need updated information have it in their possession can appreciate an intranet. Intranets can be very useful for storing documents that need frequent updating, such as procedures, policies, and drug information. Because there is only one official copy of these items, all that is required to have current information accessible is to update the one document on the intranet.

An intranet may or may not be connected to the Internet. If it is connected, the contents of the intranet will be protected by a *firewall* or encryption. Those within the institution, therefore, can access both the intranet and the Internet, but outsiders cannot access the information on the intranet. Intranets can also provide some of the features provided on the Internet, such as email, mailing lists, or news groups, although unless they are connected to the Internet, these features will be limited only to the intranet.

Information on an intranet is not limited to text. Graphics and multimedia files can also be transmitted this way. This makes the intranet an ideal way to offer inservice and continuing education programs. Preparing these document is not difficult if one uses one of the many programs available. Additionally, all the major application programs (word processors, databases, spreadsheets, and presentation programs) convert documents to web documents with a few mouse clicks. When preparing material for the intranet, thought should be given to adapting the material to take full advantage of browser capabilities.

EXTRANETS

An extranet is an extension of an intranet. It provides accessibility to the intranet to a specific group of outsiders. To access the extranet, a valid user name and password is needed. Besides offering the same services as an intranet, an extranet can be used by health care providers to access patient care information from outside of the institution. They are also used to provide access to current patient data from patient monitors for authorized health care professionals who are not physically present in the hospital (Nenov & Klopp, 1996).

▼ Nightingale Tracker

An innovative use of computer communication technology is the Nightingale Tracker, developed by FITNE, Inc. (formerly the Fuld Institute for Technology). The tracker system uses a client-server architecture, consisting of field clients that are personal digital assistants (PDAs) and a central server. Students or nurses in the field can, therefore, receive their assignments electronically. They can also develop a plan of care and electronically transmit this data back to the agency. In the field, the user can have real-time communication with an instructor or supervisor by using the tracker's built-in telephone connection. Clinical data relative to the encounter can be processed and the user can perform point-of-care documentation. The PDA also provides the user with communication features such as e-mail, faxes, and access to the WWW. In addition, information collected by the server can serve as a long-term clinical data repository (Elfrink, 1998).

▼ Research

Researchers can take advantage of the Internet to gain study participants from many countries. Electronic mailing lists, news groups, and forums provide a venue for asking for subjects to participate in a study, either by responding to a message or by visiting a web site where a questionnaire is posted. Although most Internet studies to date have involved questionnaires, some researchers have engaged in qualitative studies. To date, several studies in nursing have been conducted on the Internet, including a cancer survivors survey questionnaire, a case study of usage of the NURSE Gopher, a qualitative analysis of mailing lists, and a survey to establish nursing priorities for nursing research (Fawcett, 1995; Murray, 1995).

Most of the disadvantages to using the Internet for data gathering revolve around sample. Researchers using this method of data collection need to consider not just the usual convenience sampling difficulties but also those involved with access to the Internet. Although access to the Internet is available in many libraries and for many college students, those who are inclined to participate may not reflect the general population. There are, however, advantages to using the Internet for data collection. When the research is about a topic of great interest to many people, it is easy to find subjects. Not only can using the Internet increase the breadth of a study when subjects are included from other countries but it can reduce the cost of administering a questionnaire from hundreds of dollars to nothing (Lakeman, 1997). Cost and time savings are also seen in preparing data for analysis. Questionnaires posted on the WWW can be designed so that the data collected is in a structured format that is ready for analyzing. Data collected by email in a qualitative study, moreover, do not require transcription.

Telehealth and Telemedicine

The terms telehealth and telemedicine are sometimes used interchangeably, but each has a separate meaning. Telehealth is defined as using communication networks to transmit health data and education that focuses on health promotion and disease prevention. Telemedicine is a part of telehealth and is exemplified by a physician in one location using electronic technologies for the diagnosis or treatment, or both, of a patient in another location (Cyberoptions, 1997).

Some of the things that telehealth makes possible include a cardiologist listening in real time to a patient's heart sounds from 8000 miles away, a distant radiologist reviewing a magnetic resonance image (MRI) immediately after it is taken, a pathologist reviewing a slide from a lab in another country, and nursing and medical students learning from an expert nurse or doctor many miles away (Bonace, 1997). Although telehealth technology has experienced great growth with the advent of the Internet, telemedicine was reported in the literature 40 years ago, when teleradiology data was transmitted over standard telephone lines. Closed-circuit television also has a history of use in telemedicine and telehealth. Telenursing (note: in Europe this term has another meaning), which is another form of telehealth, is more commonly used with the telephone, rather than the computer. Telenursing is used both for triage and consultation. Telenursing involves nurses interacting via telecommunications technology with clients at a remote site (National Council of State Boards of Nursing, 1998). Health care institutions in rural areas were the first adopters of telehealth. At the end of 1996, approximately 30% of the nation's rural hospitals were equipped with telehealth capabilities (Siwicki, 1996).

Although a full-fledged telehealth-dedicated network can run $100,000 for an installation, there are other effective lower cost alternatives. In a process known as *store and forward,* photos, patient records, and images are digitized and transmitted from one location to another. Store and forward provides the ability for patients to be seen at a time convenient to them, and for the consultant to view or listen to the information when time is available. It has been estimated that about 60% of telemedicine is store and forward (Barrett, 1997).

ISSUES IN TELEHEALTH

As with all new methods, the introduction of telehealth brings new issues. The benefits of this technology will permit people in any area with access to the Internet to have the benefit of health care consultation from experts. It also allows health care professionals anywhere to learn first hand from experts. As the technology of wireless computer communication becomes more generally available, almost any place on earth can become a possible consultation room or classroom. Before this vision becomes a reality, issues beyond technology must be addressed.

Regulatory Issues

At present, professional health care licenses are issued by states, yet telehealth allows a nurse in Maine to provide consultation for a client in Montana. The nursing profession is working to resolve such an issue. A proposal has been approved by delegates to the National Council of State Boards of Nursing, in which nurses will be licensed in the state of residency but will be able to practice in any state, provided that he or she adheres to the laws and regulations of the state in which practice is to take place (National Council of State Boards of Nursing, 1998). Surprisingly, international regulation does not seem to be an issue. Regulatory barriers in Europe are generally lower than those in the United States, creating a so-called prime telemedicine market (Barrett, 1997).

Other regulatory issues involve reimbursement. In some cases, medicare has restricted reimbursement for remote health care delivery. In 1997, California dropped these restrictions with the passage of the California Telemedicine Act (Barrett, 1997). Other states are considering this type of legislation as well. States with at least partial medicaid coverage for telemedicine, include Arkansas, Georgia, Kansas, Montana, North Dakota, Oklahoma, South Dakota, Virginia, and West Virginia.

Security

Anytime patient data is transmitted electronically, there is a security issue. In addressing this problem, the American Nurses Association (ANA) argues for the development of policies, standards, and regulations in this area. The belief is that patients should be informed of any security limitations and benefits to be gained in telehealth. The ANA contends that patients should be able to determine who has access to their data. They also believe that patients themselves should be able to view any information that is generated in the process. The ANA further stipulates that enforceable penalties must be applied to anyone who violates established security policies (ANA, 1996).

Supplement or Replacement

The issues surrounding how telehealth will be used will also come under scrutiny. Some fear that in the rush to reduce health care expenses, the technology will be used in place of face-to-face consultation. The ANA has taken the position that telehealth should augment, not replace, traditional health care (ANA, 1996). The ANA sees a potential for misuse of the technology by replacing professionals in patient care in homes, schools, and other settings with computers.

▼ Summary

Health care is changing due, in part, to an increasing knowledge base and communication enabled by the Internet. Health care professionals must increasingly work with patients who have knowledge about their conditions and those who have misinformation. Web technology is used in private networks by health care organizations, both internally to provide up-to-date information for various departments and externally to accord access to data for a given group of individuals. This technology creates a need for new skills in those who develop informational and educational material if it is to be used to its fullest advantage.

Telehealth, in all its forms, is changing the face of medicine. It enables people in remote locations to have access to specialists without traveling great distances. With a larger market, telehealth may also permit practitioners to specialize in narrower areas, which could either fracture or enhance health care. Other questions that telehealth raises include whether it will ultimately be used as a supplement or in place of regular care. Provision for security of health care data is also an important issue.

EXERCISES

1. A need arises for teaching diabetic patients via the WWW. How might a nurse go about doing this task? Some thoughts: using information from another web source, teaming up with other institutions to create a virtual patient care site, or designing your own information.

2. Visit and evaluate the Global Medic site, the expert patient consultant (http://www.globalmedic.com/).

3. Examine the pros and cons of an online expert patient consultation service. Come to a conclusion, and support it with rationale.

4. What are some recommendations for resolving the presence of questionable health care misinformation on the Internet? Consider all of the ramifications of any suggestions; no solution is without pros and cons.

5. What uses might be proposed for an intranet and an extranet?

6. What are some ways telehealth is being used by health care professionals in
   a. Clinical practice?
   b. Administration?
   c. Education?
   d. Research?
   e. Entrepreneurial work?

REFERENCES

ANA. (1996). *Telehealth—issues for nursing.* Available: http://www.ana.org/readroom/tele2.htm.

Atav, S. (1998). Personal communication, February 13, 1998.

Barrett, R. (1997, May). Telemedicine on the rise on the Internet. *Interactive Week, May 12.* Available: http://www4.zdnet.com/intweek/print/970512/inwk0024.html.

Bonace, A. (1997). Telemedicine. *Tri-State Nursing Computer Network Newsletter, 8*(1), 8–10.

Brennan, P. F. (1994). Computerlink: An innovation in home care nursing. In S. Grobe & E. S. P. Pluyter-Wenting (Eds.), *Nursing informatics: An international overview for nursing in a technological era: Proceedings of the Fifth IMIA International Conference on Nursing Use of Computers and Information Science* (p. 407). San Antonio, TX, June 1994. Amsterdam: Elsevier.

Cyberoptions. (1997). *Definition of telemedicine.* Available: http://www.cyberoptions.com/def.html.

Elfrink, V. (1998). *The Nightingale Tracker: 1998 Update.* Available: http://www.ev.net/fitne/tracker/default.htm.

Fawcett, J. (1995). Using the Internet for data collection: An innovative electronic strategy. *Computers in Nursing, 13*(6), 273–279.

Gold, J. (1998). Mental health and the Internet. *Computers in Nursing, 16*(2), 85–86, 89.

Health On the Net Foundation, a non-profit international foundation. (1997). *HONcode principles.* Available: http://www.hon.ch/HONcode/Conduct.html.

Lakeman, R. (1997). Using the Internet for data collection. *Computers in Nursing, 15*(5), 269–275.

Murray, P. (1995), Using the Internet for gathering data and conducting research: Faster than the mail, cheaper than the phone. *Computers in Nursing, 13*(6), 206, 208–209.

National Council of State Boards of Nursing. (1998). Personal correspondence.

Nenov, V. & Klopp, J. R. (1996). Remote access to neurosurgical ICU physiological data using the World Wide Web. In S. J. Weghorst, H. B. Sieburg, & K. Morgan (Eds.), *Studies in health technology and informatics* (pp. 242–249). Amsterdam: IOS Press in conjuction with Ohmsha, Ltd.

Parietti, E. S., & Atav, A. S. (1994). AIDSNET: An innovative strategy of nursing outreach. In S. Grobe & E. S. P. Pluyter-Wenting (Eds.), *Nursing informatics: An international overview for nursing in a technological era: Proceedings of the Fifth IMIA International Conference on Nursing Use of Computers and Information Science* (p. 816). San Antonio, TX, June 1994. Amsterdam: Elsevier.

Schuler, D. (1995, December). Public space in cyberspace. *Internet World,* 89–95.

Siwicki, B. (1996). Telemedicine projects beginning to multiply. *Health Data Management, 4*(3), 18.

Stallings, B. (1996). *A critical study of three free-net community networks.* Available: http://ofcn.org/whois/ben/Free-Nets/.

UNIT FOUR

Computers as Patient Care Tools

CONTEMPORARY health care requires that health care institutions have information systems. Using a hospital information system as an example of such a system, Chapter 15 addresses the many facets involved in these systems, including what they incorporate, how they are implemented, and benefits that they provide. Hospital information systems will benefit nursing most when we can unambiguously document what we add to health care. In Chapter 16, the efforts that are being put forth to build classification structures that will permit this are discussed. Computerization of health care records can lead to a the production of a computerized patient record that will follow an individual from birth to death. In Chapter 17 some of the pros and cons of this approach to comprehensive health care are presented. The last chapter of the book briefly introduces the emerging field of nursing informatics.

CHAPTER 15

Information Systems
Margaret Hassett, MS, RN,C[1]

*D*elivering quality nursing care requires that practitioners be aware of, and contribute to, a vast pool of data and information. Clinicians regularly gather and document assessments, problem lists, treatment plans, outcome goals, patients' progress, and interventions. Information reported by other practitioners, lab and radiology results, interventions, policy and procedure documents, reference data, and various schedules are constantly being used. Information systems enable a speed, integration, and accuracy of information sharing that is shaping clinical practice. As active health care providers, nurses must be aware of and use the information technology now found in every clinical practice area, from stand-alone clinics to bustling acute care settings.

 Hospital Information Systems

A hospital information system (HIS) is a collection of applications and information systems linked or interfaced together to support information exchange in hospital organizations (Spurr & Hassett, 1996). The assembly of systems and the structure by which they support each other is individual for each organization. Health care organizations have always had some type of HIS in place, although for much of the time it has been a manual paper system (Ball, 1995). Today, however, the development of computerized HISs is necessary to permit the ef-

[1]Senior Consultant, First Consulting Group, Inc., Long Beach, California.

ficient communication of information vital to the existence of organizations in today's world of health care. Computerized systems have expanded from fiscal systems with manual form supports to multi-application systems that are interfaced to share data and networked to support several institutions in one health care organization.

Organizational strategic goals and business plans determine the composition of an HIS. The type of data and information that can be collected or reported in an efficient manner is determined by the composition of the HIS. Available information empowers departments and organizations to make informed decisions that enhance the development and direction of services to be provided.

The development and integration of the various components of an HIS enable a single piece of data (such as a patient's ID number) to be used many times by a variety of practitioners in a multitude of locations without constantly reentering it. The aim of any system is to improve patient care, and the HIS is no exception. The development and planning of an HIS depends on:

▼ Strategic goals of the institution
▼ Practice needs of the care providers
▼ Business needs of the organization

▼ Information Systems Configurations

An information system is a collection of computer technologies that takes data keyed in by a user or transferred from other systems (input) and processes them to provide reports in the form of printouts or screen displays (output). There are many ways an information system can be constructed or configured to maximize the collection and communication of data and information between users. The configuration depends on the organizations' existing information systems, applications, and needs.

The mainframe configuration is typically designed to meet the primary or entire computing needs of a large organization. Information is input from video-character terminals and sent to the mainframe computer, where it is stored, sorted, and reported from the mainframe to printers or back to the video-character terminals on the care units. All applications and data are obtained by accessing the mainframe as opposed to residing on individual PCs.

In another type of configuration, microcomputers or PCs are *networked*, or linked to other PCs in organizations by using client-server architecture. Data and files can then be shared throughout an organization as determined by security and access policies. This configuration allows an institution to share applications such as word processing or databases in what is called a networked application. This configuration is becoming the most popular in clinical environments but can present important security issues.

PCs can also be configured to function not only as a separate processor but as workstations. This configuration refers to a personal computer that communicates with a file server or a central computer through a network. The benefits to this configuration are that the system shares applications and data from a central site. Standardization of the system is supported, and exchange of data can be enhanced.

Some systems use point-of-care devices or computers located where information is either generated or accessed (McDermott, 1994). For example, a handheld computer may be used by a clinician at the bedside to record pertinent data at the time it is obtained, or laptops or PCs may be placed in a clinically strategic location. This practice saves time and prevents data errors. The clinician can record patient information immediately at its final destination instead of writing it down and then later transferring the information to the chart, hoping that she or he has remembered which piece of paper belongs to which patient.

The use of radio frequency in HISs is becoming more and more common. This technology allows clinicians to work with input devices that are mobile. They are usually portable computers or personal digital assistants (PDAs) that link to the hospital networks via radio waves. A drawback to radio frequency is the cost involved in preparing older buildings. Also, the technology may provide users with more portability, but the processing of information and data may be slower than when computers are hard wired to the hospital network.

▼ Types of Computer Applications

There are many different types of computer applications that are used by patient care facilities to support and communicate the variety of information that is necessary to maintain good patient care. The individual application is usually clear to the user of an HIS. It is important, however, for users to be aware that several different applications comprise an HIS, and that the display of complete information depends on each of the applications functioning properly and integrating with the others.

In a well-designed system, there is an interface, or an exchange of information between systems to support the sharing of data so it does not have to be reentered. An order entry system, for instance, would combine the order with patient demographic information from the admission, discharge, and transfer system, send the information to the department responsible for discharging the order, and in turn, send the information to the fiscal system, where a cost would be attached and a bill created.

ADMISSION, DISCHARGE, AND TRANSFER

The Admission, Discharge, and Transfer (ADT) application is the backbone of the clinical portion of most hospital systems. This application provides and tracks patient details, such as demographic and insurance information, medical record number, care provider, next of kin, and so on. All patient interactions are tracked or linked to this basic information. Laboratory results will find their way to the appropriate provider or care area based on the information contained in this portion of the HIS. It is important, therefore, that this information be updated and verified on a regular basis.

FINANCIAL SYSTEMS

Financial systems are another distinct application in the HIS. They are considered by some as the second backbone of the HIS, because they track financial interactions and provide the fiscal reporting necessary to manage an institution. Fiscal reporting includes patient and services billing, accounts receivable (AR), and general ledger (GL).

ORDER ENTRY

Order entry applications, which are in place in many health care institutions, are usually the second application with which clinicians must regularly interact, the first being the ADT system. A number of ancillary departments can be represented in an order entry system. An order entry system provides the ability for a clinician to place an order by simply selecting a patient and the needed service from a computer screen. When the selection is made, the order is immediately sent to the appropriate department. This replaces the manual writing and waiting for the order to be transported to the department responsible for the service. It also prevents transcription errors. Additionally, order entry systems allow financial information to be captured easily. An order entry system may include results.

ANCILLARY SYSTEMS

Ancillary applications—such as those for physical therapy, laboratory, or radiology—that integrate or share information with the other systems provide for some of the specific informational needs of these ancillary services. Ancillary applications may provide quality control, testing in a laboratory, assessment write up, and equipment billing in a physical therapy department, or film tracking in a radiology system. The use of these systems can also improve reporting and documentation efforts.

DOCUMENTATION APPLICATIONS

Documentation applications are available in a variety of formats. A good documentation system is part of the clinical workflow and provides communication of real-time information. These systems avoid the need to go find the chart and allow all who must use the chart to access it when needed. For example, at the change of the shift, several practitioners can use the patient record at the same time. When properly designed, the data collection supports clinical workflow as opposed to distracting from it.

Screens can be designed to support assessment documentation by listing systems, or practitioners can be cued by the system with a pop-up box to complete or verify vital information, such as allergies. In a well-planned documentation system, there is little need for free text entry, although the ability to do should be there for the occasional outlier. When these systems work well, it is because the nurses working on the clinical unit where the system is used were involved in the system's design.

SCHEDULING

Scheduling applications are another type of application that can be found in the HIS network. Scheduling applications support the scheduling of patients, procedures, supplies, and staff. They can schedule patients, staff, or services with a department such as radiology or the operating room. Staff scheduling systems can share information with hospital personnel and the fiscal system. Patient scheduling systems are enhanced when they share information with materials management for supplies related to the scheduled procedure, the ADT system for patient demographics, and the financial system for cost accounting purposes.

ACUITY APPLICATIONS

Acuity applications, which have been in use in some form for two decades, provide for the classification of patients or services in an attempt to predict and provide the appropriate resources. Given the unpredictable nature of health care, they are not always satisfactory. In a cost-conscious health care system, however, they are necessary. An acuity system may be integrated with other systems such as ADT, staffing, and documentation, in an effort to create more accurate predictions.

SPECIALTY SYSTEMS

Specialty systems are continually being developed to meet the specific needs of groups. In these systems, patient information consisting of elements specific to the practice are collected. Selected test results are recorded and placed in a report designed to meet specific practice needs. For example, in a system developed to meet the needs of a gastrointestinal practitioner, specific patient history information related to gastrointestinal symptoms is collected. When a procedure such as an endoscopy is performed, the images from the test are automatically attached to a report generated from the accumulated information.

One of the biggest challenges associated with most of the specialty systems is the integration of information between systems. Ideally, patient information should be provided automatically from the ADT system. Data should be provided to the practitioners through the results reporting system, and the bills should be generated by the financial system. Many specialty systems are unable to provide for that exchange of information. The specialty system, therefore, must generate reports and billing information in an alternate form, such as a hard copy report. This information is then distributed to the appropriate places and, in many cases, reentered into a system—a method that is prone to errors.

DECISION SUPPORT SYSTEM

Decision support systems provide information that undergirds a variety of decisions that are based on data and information that is either contained in the HIS or accessible by the HIS. The information could be fiscal, clinical, bibliographical, statistical, or a combination of these forms. Logical and relationship statements can be incorporated into the systems in order to generate integrated documentation and order entry systems.

COMMUNICATION SYSTEMS

Communication systems, such as email and Internet connections, facilitate the exchange of information needed by the various health care disciplines. Although these systems are not usually integrated with the above-mentioned systems, they enhance the information flow in an organization and are already demonstrating an impact on practice.

Benefits of HIS

Information systems permit health care providers to collect and communicate patient data in a more effective and efficient manner. Information can be easily shared between involved disciplines to facilitate quality patient care. Information systems also provide access to the patient chart regardless of the location of the patient. For instance, a patient may be scheduled for a radiograph the following day. Without leaving the department, personnel from the radiology department can view patient demographics for the patient's health history and insurance information. Meanwhile, the physician can be notified that an NPO and prep orders are needed. Once they are given, they can be automatically communicated to the dietary, pharmacy, and nursing staff.

REAL-TIME INFORMATION

Another benefit of an HIS is the ability to have real-time information. Information systems promote effective and efficient communication of information. An example is the patient who is referred to a facility for an outpatient test, such as an MRI. The referring office, if it is connected to a referring facility information system, would be able to view available appointments and schedule the patient for the MRI before the patient leaves the office. On completion of the tests, results can then be communicated directly back to the referring doctor in a timely fashion. Treatment plans are enhanced with this type of rapid information exchange, which supports efficient and informed practitioner decision making.

EASILY OBTAINED AGGREGATE DATA

The collection of information relative to the effectiveness of patient care and the treatment of identified outcomes is another advantage to automated patient and treatment documentation. Documentation systems can be structured behind the screens to aggregate data input for specific reports. One is able to easily extract information that previously had been obtained only through exhaustive chart reviews.

Critical Pathways

HISs also allow for the construction of critical pathways. Critical pathways provide a foundation for multidisciplinary documentation that focuses on the attainment of a specific outcome within a given length of time. The pathway identifies the patient and desired outcomes. The outcomes and time required for their achievement are predetermined by representatives of the multidisciplinary groups involved in the care of patients with that diagnosis. The structure of the path allows for documentation of assessment elements, interventions, patient response to interventions, and coordination of documentation by all disciplines.

In an HIS, all disciplines document on the same tool, which is focused on the desired outcome. In the case of a total knee replacement, the desired outcome is discharge to home in 3 days. Specific criteria include pain control, range of motion, ambulation, and medication knowledge met by a stated time. The respective practitioners note the element of care that is their responsibility. For example, physical therapy would document progress in range of motion and ambulation, nursing would record the results of pain control and the client's medication knowledge, and the physician would document related medication changes.

This form of documentation permits more cost-efficient care through better communication. Each discipline participating in the patient's treatment plan can see the whole picture and know the patient's current status. Care provider documentation is used to compare the patients' progress by noting results or patient responses in a progressive and interrelated format. This type of record-keeping also allows for comparison of clinical data regarding interventions, outcomes, and multidisciplinary approaches.

▼ System Implementation

The systems development life cycle of an information system consists of specific activities. These activities provide for an informed system selection and design process, followed by effective implementation and efficient utilization. Nursing can and should participate in as many of the activities as possible to ensure that systems address their practice and information needs.

There are many similarities between the system development life cycle and the nursing process used every day in the planning and delivery of patient care (Table 15-1). Nurses are well suited by their professional practice to assume responsibilities related to working with information systems. Assessment and analysis complemented with problem solving and priority setting skills are important attributes in working with end users and information system support personnel.

OBSERVATION AND REQUIREMENTS DEFINED

Requirements definition is very similar to the observation phase of the nursing process. The nurse analyst gathers information pertaining to users' expectation of the information system, cost and benefits of implementing the system, and the impact on workflow. This process can be accomplished in a variety of ways:

TABLE 15-1 ● *Comparison of Nursing Process and System Life Cycle*	
Nursing process	**System life cycle**
Observe	Requirements defined
Assess/diagnose	Analysis
Plan	Design/preliminary testing
Implement	Training/implement
Evaluate	Testing/evaluate

Adapted from: Douglas, M. (1995). Butterflies, bonsai, and buonarroti: Images for the nurse analyst. In M. J. Ball, K. J. Hannah, S. Newbold, & J. V. Douglas, (Eds.), *Nursing and informatics: Where caring and technology meet* (2nd ed.) (pp. 84–94). New York: Springer-Verlag.

▼ Interviews with end users of the system
▼ Site visits
▼ Establishment of workgroups
▼ Surveys
▼ Workflow and environment observations

The gathering of these observations and user input is a very important phase of this process and will determine its future success or failure. The relative cost of fixing an error in the project increases exponentially as the development and implementation progress. The cost of fixing an error that is not found until the system is operational can be as much as 40 to 1000 times what it would cost to fix it in the analysis phase (Douglas, 1995).

ASSESS AND DIAGNOSIS VERSUS ANALYSIS

Once the initial expectations and current workflow impact are determined, efforts in the analysis phase challenge the analyst to be creative and open to new ways of doing the work. This phase requires an effective melding between an appreciation for the users' needs and the required workflow.

An understanding of the impact of change on nursing and other health care workers' roles is essential (Zielstorff, 1994). In addition, the analyst must communicate and demonstrate an understanding of technological solutions that are attainable. An appreciation and awareness of the organization's strategic and business goals, coupled with the development status of an Information Systems Department and their service objectives, is another crucial component.

Questions such as the following need to be answered:

▼ What is to be accomplished or provided by the information system?
▼ How does the implementation of a system impact on current workflow?
▼ What are the costs and benefits of the system?
▼ Can the system be supported and maintained with current organization structures and personnel?

PLAN VERSUS DEVELOPMENT, DESIGN, AND TESTING

The development and design phase provides the nurse analyst with opportunities to influence the ability of a system to meet the defined needs of nursing practice. Without adequate input and participation from nursing users, vendor and information systems staff responsible for a system implementation may overlook crucial design features such as

▼ Screen design: displaying data elements in a manner that facilitates the entering and use of data
▼ Information access: creating an intuitive, yet secure way to access information
▼ Data sharing: optimizing the system so it supports multidisciplinary communication and information sharing

Adherence to standards in the system design and data collection enhances data sharing and aggregation between other systems, practices, and organizations, greatly expanding the ability to create data reports. Standardizing collection and reporting of data allows for increased benchmarking across institutional structures. Such standards may be technical such as HL-7 (the communication standard for exchanging health care data), or practice languages such as Nursing Intervention Classifications (NICs) (Zielstorff, 1994).

Initial testing of the system design not only allows so-called bugs to be worked out but also allows end users to gain experience in working with the system. The use of end users in initial testing provides the design team with valuable developmental information. Users can verify that the system is functioning appropriately for inclusion in a workflow. Training needs are highlighted in the testing phase by observing users. Many times, something that is considered intuitive by the design team may prove confusing for the targeted user.

TRAINING FOR IMPLEMENTATION

Adequate and appropriate training is essential for the successful implementation and use of a system. When practitioners take responsibility for learning to use a system, ask questions, and provide feedback on functionality, the system better serves their needs. Some institutions use clinical workgroups that meet on a regular basis or identified super users during an implementation process and on an ongoing basis.

Training activities should be viewed as multipurpose activities. The trainer does not only teach intended users how to use a system but determines specific system support required by the users, as well as system design or function issues missed in earlier steps. It is during the training sessions that security and data integrity must be addressed. By discussing the issues in the context of system use, the user responsibilities related to security are more meaningful. It is necessary for users to understand and practice security and confidentiality, and to employ the steps necessary to ensure data integrity.

METHODS OF IMPLEMENTATION

Several methods are used to support the implementation of a system, or to go live.

One method is called the *big-bang approach*, or direct or crash conversion, in which the entire institution implements at the same time. This method can be the most disruptive to an environment. This method is used most frequently when there is no initial system, the system in use is old, or there is a requirement for implementation on a specific date, such as a beginning of new fiscal year.

Pilot conversion enables the testing of a system on a smaller defined scale. For instance, a new documentation system or point-of-care device may be implemented on one care unit for a period of time. This type of conversion requires that specific evaluation criteria be established and that the pilot testing be completed within a defined period of time. Usually a pilot implementation is used in order to determine operational or training needs for a future implementation of the system.

Phased conversion requires the operation and support of the new and the old system for a period of time. The implementation plan will normally address the specific operational needs and define the timing of the implementation. This approach can be used in the case of an order entry or documentation system. Specific departments or care units may be targeted with specific dates for switch over to the new system. This approach allows an organization to allocate resources in a more efficient manner.

Regardless of the method of implementation, adequate system and user support is crucial for the success of the implementation of the system. Initially, 24-hour, on-site support may be required, with later phasing directed from a help desk. Vendor support is important in the initial stages of implementation to trouble shoot unforeseen issues that need to be resolved quickly, especially if the method used is the big-bang approach.

EVALUATE

Implementation of any system highlights issues regarding system use, supports, and needs. End users make recommendations for system redesign, which must be captured and then followed with a response. These recommendations can be gathered from end user input as they are voiced to help desk personnel, shared through workgroup participation, or observed during information services rounds. Established teams and analysts must continually evaluate any system. They need to develop plans to deal with identified issues and upgrades.

▼Need for Security

General access to an HIS depends on hospital security and access policies. Although information is available through computers, access may be limited depending on user sign-on or departmental definition. HISs differ in who has access to what information or programs, but ultimately, users are responsible for system security. Users need to regard their privileges professionally, just as they would with a written record. Passwords must be viewed as what they are—a private entry into a system. If they are shared, the system is compromised, and the owner of the password becomes responsible for whatever is done on the system when that password is used. HISs are built with tracking mechanisms, so that what an individual has looked at in a system is a matter of record.

▼Summary

Computers and the integration of existing clinical technology are beginning to assist nurses in the capture, documentation, and reporting of clinical data. As practitioners become more accustomed to the presence of information systems in practice areas, they will become more adept at applying and using the data to support clinical decision making.

The time is now for clinician involvement in the development of information systems. Practitioners must take the time to express to system developers what is needed and expected from a system to support practice. Practitioner participation can be accomplished within a hospital or network through user workgroups that integrate clinicians and information system analysts. Another effective method is with vendor user groups that actively solicit user input in the redesign of the vendor's product and information systems.

Information and data are vital portions of any clinical practice, and a cooperative effort is required between clinicians and information specialists. Care providers in practice areas can express what information is valid in the care scenario and how it should be displayed, while information specialists provide current technology facts and advice to meet the clinicians' information needs. New and exciting roles and relationships are being forged to accomplish clinical information systems development.

EXERCISES

1. Identify the types of systems that are in place in a clinical area in which you are practicing. Ask those who are using them what they like about them and what they would change if they could.

2. Select one decision point in a practice field, such as administering a medication or scheduling a procedure. List the various pieces of information needed to make the decision or perform the activity. Then identify where you have to get the information. Is it all in one place or several?

3. Patient information is to be kept confidential. Take a critical look around your care area and identify the different ways to obtain and view patient information, such as the phone, computer screen, chart, reports, and so on. Evaluate the means employed to keep that information confidential.

4. What are some ways that health care information systems are being used by health care professionals in
   a. Clinical practice?
   b. Administration?
   c. Education?
   d. Research?
   e. Entrepreneurial work?

REFERENCES

Ball, M. J., Simborg, D. Albright, J. W., & Douglas, J. V. (Eds.). (1995). *Healthcare information management system* (2nd ed.). New York: Springer-Verlag.

Dick, R. S. & Steen, E. B. (1991). *The computer-based record, an essential technology for health care.* Washington, D.C.: National Academy Press.

Douglas, M. (1995). Butterflies, bonsai, and buonarroti: Images for the nurse analyst. In M. J. Ball, K. J. Hannah, S. Newbold, & J. V. Douglas (Eds.), *Nursing and informatics: Where caring and technology meet* (pp. 84–94) (2nd ed.). New York: Springer-Verlag.

McDermott, S. (1994). Interfacing and linking nursing information systems to optimize patient care. In S. J. Grobe & E. S. P. Pluyter-Wenting (Eds.), *Nursing informatics: An international overview for nursing in a technological era* (pp. 197–201). New York: Elsevier.

Spurr, C. & Hassett, M. (1996). *Guide to nursing informatics.* Chicago, IL: Healthcare Information and Management Systems Society.

Zielstorff, R. D., Hudgings, C. I., & Grobe, S. J. (1994). *Next-generation nursing information systems.* Washington, D.C.: American Nurses Publishing.

Nursing Classification Systems

A major problem that nurses encounter today is the seeming invisibility of their profession (American Medical Association, 1990). Occupational therapists, pharmacists, physical therapists, dieticians, and respiratory therapists can define their tasks. Not only do nurses have difficulty describing what they do, but on evenings and weekends nurses are often responsible for the tasks of other departments. Although the hospital may charge the patient for these non-nursing tasks performed by nurses, the money rarely is credited to the nursing department. Instead, it flows to either the hospital at large or to the department responsible for the treatment during regular working hours.

Although nurses conscientiuosly document care, nursing notes are often viewed as simply a means of communication between physicians and nurses, hence they are of little use to either administration for billing or medicine for research (Bowker, 1996). Nursing information is never included in patient discharge abstracts that are prepared by hospital medical records departments (Hannah, Ball, & Edwards, 1994). These abstracts, used by different agencies for a variety of funding and statistical purposes, have no indication that nursing care is part of hospital care.

It is difficult to plan for nursing resources if those in the profession are unable to communicate the nature of nursing and nursing care in a manner that allows it to be classified with other health care professions (McCloskey & Bulechek, 1996). Documentation, therefore, must make clear what nurses do beyond procedures and following orders, and it must be done in a manner so that

249

it becomes a part of permanent records used by others. To accomplish this aim, it is necessary for nurses to examine what is documented and how it is done. To this end, effort must be focused on building classification structures that can be used to computerize nursing documentation in a database.

▼ Nursing Minimum Data Set

One of nursing's first attempts to standardize and make nursing data visible was the Nursing Minimum Data Set (NMDS). The NMDS was modeled on the Uniform Minium Health Data Set (UMHDS), which was developed as the minimum set of health data necessary to assist in decision making about health care. To make these standards viable, several criteria were defined:

▼ The data must be useful to most potential users, for example, legislators, health care professionals, administrators, and regulatory bodies.
▼ The items in the set must be readily collectable with reasonable accuracy.
▼ The items should not duplicate other available data.
▼ Confidentiality must not be violated.

Using these standards, three patient-focused UMHDSs were constructed—one in the area of long-term care, another in ambulatory care, and the third for hospital discharge (Werley, Ryan, & Zorn, 1995). The minimum data set developed for discharge, the Uniform Hospital Discharge Data Set (UHDDS), was mandated in 1972 to be collected on all hospitalized medicaid patients. In 1987, the U.S. Congress ruled that a nationwide system for the collection of long-term care be established. None of these data sets, however, contained information pertaining to nursing.

Recognizing this lack, attendees at the 1977 Nursing Information Systems Conference originated the idea for the NMDS (Werley, Ryan, & Zorn, 1995). In 1985, the NMDS was formalized at a conference attended by 64 national experts who used a process similar to that used to develop the UHDDS. The participants included nurses with expertise in clinical practice, administration, research, and education, as well as a health policy spokesman and those with specialties in information systems, health records, and the development of the UMHDS.

The purposes of the NMDS are to

▼ Make it possible to compare data from different clinical settings, populations, and geographical areas
▼ Describe nursing care in a variety of settings, including institutional and noninstitutional settings
▼ Show or project trends regarding nursing care and resources needed for clients with various nursing diagnoses
▼ Stimulate nursing research by providing links to data
▼ Provide nursing data to influence clinical, administrative, and health policy decision making

The elements in the NMDS consist of three broad categories: nursing care, demographics, and service elements. As can be seen in Table 16-1, all but six of these items are already collected as part of the UHDDS. With the exception of intensity of nurs-

TABLE 16-1 ● *Elements of the Nursing Minimum Data Set (NMDS)*		
Nursing care elements	**Patient or client demographic elements**	**Service elements**
1. Nursing Diagnosis*	5. Personal identification	10. Unique facility or service agency number
2. Nursing Interventions*	6. Data of Birth	11. Unique health record number of patient or client*
3. Nursing Outcomes*	7. Sex	12. Unique number of principal registered nurse provider*
4. Intensity of Nursing Care*	8. Race and ethnicity	13. Episode admission or encounter date
	9. Residence	14. Discharge or termination date
		15. Disposition of patient or client
		16. Expected payor for most of this bill (anticipated financial guarantee for services)

*These six items are NOT comparable to items in the UHDDS.
Adapted from Leske, J. S., & Werley, H. H. (1992). Use of the nursing minimum data set. *Computers in Nursing, 10*(6), 259–263.

ing care, the general meaning of the elements are clear to the casual observer, but all have a written description. Intensity of nursing care is not a synonym for patient acuity (Werley, Devine, & Zorn, 1988). Instead, it is an element determined by the total hours of nursing care and the ratio of the types of nursing personnel involved in the care. As if to demonstrate the need to make nursing more visible, when the NMDS was pilot tested, of those institutions taking part in the study, only 31% could easily retrieve the nursing care elements (Leske & Werley, 1992).

The NMDS is not meant to provide all of the information needs of the nursing profession. Rather, it is intended as the basic set of items needed to describe nursing practice in all settings, including the hospital, home, industry, schools, or any location in which professional nurses provide client care (Werley, Ryan, & Zorn, 1995). Emergency room nurses have demonstrated the ability to modify the NMDS to meet the needs of their specialty with the development of the Emergency Nursing Uniform Data Set (ENUDS). The American Organization of Nurse Executives, along with researchers from the University of Iowa, have built on the NMDS and established a Nursing Management Minimum Data Set (NMMDS), that focuses on nursing environment, nurse resources, and finances (Simpson, 1997).

▼ Nursing Language

A nursing minimum data set, or any nursing data set, demands standard definitions. If different terms are used, data from one institution cannot be compared with data from another institution. This situation leaves nurses unable to determine which interventions are the most effective. It also leaves those in the profession unable to communicate what nurses do to facilitate the well-being of clients. This lack of communication also affects patient care. When one person defines a skin problem as raw, red skin whereas another describes it as a stage one pressure sore, the type of care given may vary with the hospital and the individual giving care (Shuttleworth, 1993). Thus, patient comfort, quality of care, and cost effectiveness are compromised because treatment may be withheld when the description does not match the requirement for care. The wide variations in vocabulary used to describe the same characteristic also make it difficult to make meaningful comparisons.

LINKING TO OTHER SOURCES OF INFORMATION

The use of standardized language will also enable nursing to link their data to the literature. Work on a medical standardized language began in 1986, when the National Library of Medicine (NLM) commenced a long-term research and development project to build the Unified Medical Language System (UMLS®) (Lindberg & Humphreys, 1995). The objective is to develop a link between clinical records, factual databases, knowledge databases, and the literature. Nursing through the American Nurses Association (ANA) has developed a Unified Nursing Language System (UNLS) that has been incorporated into the UMLS (McCormick, 1995). The metathesaurus of the UMLS provides a bridge between the nursing and other terms by providing the linkages between nursing and non-nursing terms.

There are many advantages to be gained from a UNLS. Integrating patient records with scientific data would allow those in the profession to use key words to search nursing records, just as is done in searching bibliographical records (McCormick & Zielstorff, 1995). It will also provide the practicing nurse the ability to easily link patient problems to research findings in the literature, thus narrowing the gap between research and practice and providing immediate continuing education.

In constructing both the UMLS and the UNLS, there are many issues that need to be decided (Table 16-2). The difficulties involved in this project stem from the many different ways the same concept can be expressed and the problem of locating the appropriate database to provide the needed information.

TABLE 16-2 ● *Creating a Unified Nursing Language System (UNLS)*

Defining formats to add and delete content
Determining public access
Establishing rules for ownership
Defining use of proprietary content
Determining a maintenance schedule
Establishing timeliness of content
Ensuring an update schedule
Identifying who is responsible for updates
Ensuring resources to develop new content and maintain content
Establishing procedures to delete content
Instituting educational strategies to teach about the UNLS

From: McCormick, K. A., & Zielstorff, R. (1995). Building a unified nursing language system (UNLS). In American Nurses Association (Eds.), *An Emerging Framework: Data System Advances for Clinical Nursing Practice* (p. 146). Washington, D.C.: American Nurses Association.

THE EUROPEAN SCENE

The United States is not alone in working to promote standardized terminology for health data. Concerned with the growth of telecommunications and its effect on health care, in 1976, the nations in the European Community started work on a medically oriented European Minimum Data Set (EMDS) (Clark, 1994). In 1989, the International Council of Nurses launched a concerted action to develop an International Classification for Nursing Practice (ICNP). Its worldwide purpose is to enable the description and comparison of nursing data for clinical populations, to support nursing care, and to provide the knowledge needed for cost-effective nursing care (Lang & Murphy, 1995). This work stems from the belief that throughout the world, nursing is central to patient encounters with the health care system. It is important, therefore, that health care data reflect not only medical data but the reasons for nursing care.

In 1991, European nurses started work on forming a network of nurses interested in identifying and classifying nursing elements (Hannah & Anderson, 1995). It became clear that those in the profession from all over Europe were interested (Goossen, 1998). In 1995, many in this group started to develop an international classification and forge a link with the International Council of Nurses' ICNP project.

Some of the goals of the ICNP are to name the actions that nurses engage in to produce outcomes related to human needs, and to explain what nurses do to assist people in achieving and maintaining good health (Clark & Lang, 1992). Other aims include the discovery of problems or situations that concern nursing; nursing contributions to preventing, alleviating, or solving these problems; and the outcomes that nursing activity achieves.

In 1996, the International Council of Nurses Foundation received a second 3-year grant to continue the work of developing the ICNP (News from ICN, 1996). In this phase, the council will work at describing nursing activities and practice for community-based health and primary care. Nurses worldwide whose work is in primary health care will be involved in these efforts to develop an international nursing language. At the same time, a European consortium is promoting the use of the emerging ICNP, along with a clinical nursing minimum data set in electronic patient care records (Telenurse, 1997). Using field test sites in Europe, an alpha version of the ICNP has been tested to determine its usefulness for European health care institutions. Efforts have been focused on analyzing the ability of the NMDS (European) to summarize and compare nursing activity between various units, hospitals, and countries. Nurses in Australia are also working on language standardization and unified language projects.

THE NURSING INTERVENTION LEXICON AND TAXONOMY

Susan Grobe is developing a standardized language named the Nursing Intervention Lexicon and Taxonomy (NILT). Grobe (1996) is approaching this task from the perspective of preserving the holistic nature of nursing. Believing that the traditional methods of classification—in which membership in categories is determined by common properties—is inadequate for describing nursing care, her team is developing a system that uses a cognitive view of classification. Using this view, items are classified by meaning. This approach allows abstract entities, or free text entries, to be classified based on the language used to express them.

NILT is based on capturing and analyzing the natural language that nurses use to describe interventions instead of forcing the nurse to choose from a given set of alternatives (Grobe, 1996). In analyzing the language that nurses use to describe interventions, these researchers have found that there are about 115 verbs continually used by nurses in their intervention statements. Using these verbs and other commonalities, statements are subjected to a computer algorithm that classifies them into one of seven categories (Table 16-3). The central concept for all of the categories is care, a concept that undergirds all nursing interventions. Using this system, the natural language of nurses can be computerized and used to quantify care, examine the care pattern for the course of care, and compare care across various dimensions. This system also permits asking questions about whether intensity, focus, and comprehensiveness are related to outcomes.

PATIENT CARE DATA SET

Nurses at Wright State University-Miami Valley College of Nursing and Health teamed with the Blue Chip Computer Company of Dayton, Ohio, to develop a longitudinal patient health record and medical history (Renner & Swart, 1997). Called the Patient Care Data Set (PCDS), it is consistent with HL7 criteria. The idea behind the development of the system was to provide data that could be available for each health care encounter. Ideally, the data set would be used to update a patient record by health care practitioners or used in a regional data depository, or both.

▼ Data Set Classifications

A data set is a collection of related items. A collection of nursing memorabilia could be seen as a data set. Once the collection grew beyond a size that could be managed by intuition, a way of organizing the collection would become necessary. The form

---

TABLE 16-3 ● *Nursing Intervention Lexicon and Taxonomy (NILT) Categories and Meanings*

Category name	Meaning	Primary concept
CND*	Care need determination	Determining need for care
CV***	Care vigilance	Monitoring physical status
TCG***	Therapeutic care–psychosocial	Performing therapeutic procedures
TCP***	Therapeutic care–cognitive understanding and control	Providing emotional support
TCCU&C**	Care environment management	Encouraging control and self-care
CEM**	Care environment management	Managing the care environment
CIP***	Care information provision	Informing and teaching

***>90% **>80% *>70%
Adjusted average means for agreement between computer categorization of interventions and human categorization
Adapted from Grobe, S. J. (1996). The Nursing Intervention Lexicon and Taxonomy: Implications for representing nursing care data in automated patient records. *Holistic Nurse Practitioner, 11*, 48–63.

that this organization takes would be decided by those responsible for the collection. This classification would be based on the purpose to which the collection would be put. Decisions would need to be made about the various categories, definitions written to define the categories, and rules for cataloging or coding the items developed. This same procedure is used in developing nursing data sets. A nursing data set has to provide the data routinely needed by decision makers about a given dimension of the health care system (Johnson & Maas, 1997a). It also must provide standard measurements, definitions, and ways to organize the data.

CLASSIFICATION SYSTEMS

Classification is a method of organizing or structuring information in a manner that facilitates using it. How data are classified depends on how they are used.

TAXONOMIES

Various classification systems are known as taxonomies. A taxonomy is a method of organizing items that follows a given perspective. Filing cabinets can be an example of a taxonomy. Different drawers, for instance, may be selected to contain items that belong to a given category, such as letters and financial information. Inside the letter drawer, letters may be organized by a suborganizing concept, such as the project to which they are related, then organized at an even lower level by the individual to whom they were written. Another drawer may hold financial information, which is also organized into subcategories inside the drawer. The objective is to facilitate finding needed information. Thus, the categories used in a filing system involve decisions about the categories to be used in the classification as well as the overriding concept for the organization.

Taxonomies are a way of collapsing items into mutually agreed-on concepts. These larger categories make working with the individual pieces of data easier and facilitate finding data that belong to a category. Once it is known, for instance, that a given piece of data is in the x category, one knows where to look to find it. Developers base their classification on an overriding concept, then develop rules to guide the development of the classification system and taxonomy. The resulting data set is then field tested, with revisions made based on these tests. The work of refining a system is continuous. New situations are constantly developing that require additions, deletions, and modifications to a system.

▼ Some Current Nursing Data Sets

The ANA has been very active in promoting the development of nursing data sets for use in computerization of nursing documentation. They have also adopted a set of policies for data set development, among them the stipulation that databases will be classified by assessment, diagnosis, interventions, and outcomes, and that the data sets will be evolutionary and subject to regular review by the profession. For a full list of these policies, see the position statement at http://www.nursingworld.org/ readroom/position/practice/prdatabs.htm. At present, the ANA has recognized the NANDA's Taxonomy I, the Omaha System, the HHCC, the NIC, the NOC, and the Patient Care Data Set.

Each of these classifications represent concerted research efforts and consideration of many philosophical and practical issues on the part of the developers. This discussion of these classification schemes, however, focuses mainly on how they would be used to code nursing efforts for use in a database. The goal is to present a brief overview of each system and to promote a beginning understanding of the efforts to define and record nursing interventions.

NORTH AMERICAN NURSING DIAGNOSIS ASSOCIATION

The NANDA data set had its origins in the early 1970s, when two nurses participated in a demonstration project requiring that patient data be computerized (Warren & Hoskins, 1995). The frustration of these nurses when they realized that they were not able to do this resulted in the first meeting of the National Conference Group for the Classification of Nursing Diagnoses in 1973. Thus began the formal work of identifying, developing, and classifying nursing diagnoses. Nursing diagnoses are statements that identify patient care problems that nurses are licensed to treat independently. The objective of nursing diagnoses is to emphasize the unique role of the nurse.

Difficulties arose, however, when this group attempted to classify the diagnoses. Their first attempt was an alphabetic listing (Carpenito, 1983). At the third conference, a group of nurse theorists began to work on developing a better classification system. It was not until the fifth conference, however, that this group presented the nine patterns that were to form the organizing framework for the NANDA taxonomy. It was also at this conference that NANDA was officially organized. Since then, NANDA has assumed responsibility for maintaining and developing the nursing diagnoses taxonomy (Warren & Hoskins, 1995).

One pattern used to classify nursing diagnoses was Gordon's 11 functional health patterns (Carpenito, 1983). This pattern, however, was intended only for assessment. The taxonomy developed for computerization uses nine patterns for the top level of the taxonomy: exchanging, communicating, relating, valuing, choosing, moving, perceiving, knowing, and feeling. Each pattern has sublevels, with each level being more specific in its description. NANDA's Taxonomy I uses a coding pattern in which the code starts with the number assigned to the top domain and continues with numbers from levels below (Table 16-4).

OMAHA SYSTEM

The Omaha System developed through the efforts of community health nurses in Omaha, Nebraska, and agencies in seven other geographical areas. The objective of this system is to provide a consistent vocabulary for collecting, sorting, classifying, documenting and analyzing data pertaining to individuals, families, or communities. The Omaha System has three components: problems, interventions, and outcomes.

The Problem Classification Scheme is a taxonomy of client problems that was developed using actual client data with extensive research and testing (Martin & Scheet, 1992). From these studies evolved a four-level scheme consisting of four domains (Table 16-5), 40 problems, two sets of modifiers, and signs and symptoms. The nurse assesses the four domains and identifies any problems in each. Each prob-

TABLE 16-4 ● *One Branch of Nursing Diagnosis Taxonomy*	
Code number	**Description**
1.	**Exchanging**
1.6.2	Altered protection
1.6.2.1	Altered oral mucous membrane
1.6.2.1.2.1	Impaired skin integrity
1.6.2.1.2.2	Risk for impaired skin integrity

Adapted from Warren, J. J., & Hoskins, L. M. (1995). NANDA's nursing diagnosis taxonomy: A nursing database. In American Nurses Association (Eds.), *An emerging framework: Data system advances for clinical nursing practice* (pp. 49–59). Washington, D.C.: American Nurses Association.

lem is then referenced as health promotion, a potential or actual impairment, and as to whether it applies to the family or the individual. If a problem is identified as an actual problem, using the assessment data, the nurse further describes the problem using a cluster of problem-specific signs and symptoms. See Table 16-6 for an example of the problems in the environmental domain and a sample problem statement.

The Intervention Scheme consists of four categories: health teaching, guidance and counseling, treatments and procedures, case management, and surveillance. One or more of the categories can be used to document or plan care for a given problem. The user selects a general category for the intervention that describes the nurse's primary function, then the nurse selects a target from a list of 62 options (Martin & Scheet, 1995) (Table 16-7). A target is an object of a nursing intervention or activity. Examples of targets are bonding, cardiac care, and cast care. To describe an intervention in which the nurse identified a problem with exits from the residence and discussed this with the client, she or he would document category I, health teaching, guidance and counseling, and then select the related activity (target) of safety (see Tables 16-6 and 16-7). The problem would be coded as residence, which would then be modified as actual and applying to the family. The description of the problem from the nurses' observation would be stated as inadequate or obstructed exits.

TABLE 16-5 ● *Problem Domains in the Omaha System*			
I. Environmental	**II. Psychosocial**	**III. Physiological**	**IV. Health related**
Material resources and physical surroundings	Patterns of behavior, communications, relationships and development	Processes that maintain life	Activities that maintain or promote wellness, recovery, or maximize rehabilitation

Adapted from FITNE. (1997). The use of a standardized language with the Nightingale Tracker. Available: *http://www.ev.net/fitne/tracker/omaha.htm.*

TABLE 16-6 • Items in the Environmental Domain in the Omaha System

Domain	Environmental				
Problem	*01 Income*	*02 Sanitation*	*03 Residence*	*04 Neighborhood*	*05 Other*
Signs and symptoms associated with actual impairment	01 Low/no income 02 Uninsured medical expenses 03 Inadequate money management 04 Able to buy only necessities 05 Difficulty buying necessities 06 Other	01 Soiled living area 02 Inadequate food/storage/disposal 03 Insects/rodents 04 Foul odor 05 Inadequate water supply 06 Inadequate sewage disposal 07 Inadequate laundry facilities 08 Allergens 09 Infectious/contaminating agents 10 Other	01 Structurally unsound 02 Inadequate heating/cooling 03 Steep stairs 04 Inadequate/obstructed exits 05 Cluttered living space 06 Unsafe storage of dangerous objects/substances 07 Unsafe mats/throw rugs 08 Inadequate safety devices 09 Presence lead based paint 10 Unsafe gas/electrical appliances 11 Inadequate/crowded living space 12 Homeless 13 Other	01 High crime rate 02 High pollution level 03 Uncontrolled animals 04 Physical hazards 05 Unsafe play area 06 Other	Other

Situation | House has only two exits, back door is from an enclosed porch. Porch is used as storage area which makes it impossible to negotiate a path to the door without moving many heavy objects

Problem | Problem 03 Residence

	Choices to further describe the problem	*Example (when problem is actual)*
Modifier 1	Health promotion, potential, or actual impairment	Actual
Modifier 2	Family or individual	Family
Signs/symptoms	The statement of an actual problem is further described by the use of a cluster of problem-specific signs and symptoms	04 Inadequate or obstructed exits

Adapted from FITNE. (1997). *The use of a standardized language with the Nightingale Tracker. Available: http://www.ev.net/fitne/tracker/omaha.htm.*

TABLE 16-7 • *Matching of Interventions with Targets*				
Intervention category	I Health teaching	II Treatments and procedures	III Case management	IV Surveillance
Target	Select from a list of 62 Problem 03 Residence 46 Safety (instructed on importance of free exits)			

Adapted from FITNE. (1997). *The use of a standardized language with the Nightingale Tracker.* Available: *http://www.ev.net/fitne/ tracker/omaha.htm.*

The Problem Rating Scale for outcomes is a five-point Likert scale, which is used to measure an individual's or family's progress throughout the period of care. Using the scale, each problem is rated in three major areas: knowledge (that a client has), the behavior or client activities that the client is using to work toward alleviating the problem, and the status (psychological or physiological) of the problem. Outcomes are assessed at the time of admission, at periodic and stated intervals, and at discharge (Table 16-8).

TABLE 16-8 • *Evaluation of Outcomes*					
Each problem is rated on each of the three concepts at time of admission, at periodic intervals, and at discharge.					
Concept	1	2	3	4	5
Knowledge	No knowledge	Minimal	Basic	Adequate	Superior
Behavior	Not appropriate	Rarely appropriate	Inconsistently appropriate	Usually appropriate	Consistently appropriate
Status	Extreme	Severe	Moderate	Minimal	No signs and symptoms
Problem	03 Residence				
	Category	Coding		For this situation	
	Knowledge	3 (Moderate)		States that the back porch exit would be difficult to use and that it should be cleared of "junk"	
	Behavior	2 (Rarely appropriate)		Talks about clearing away clutter from exits but has not done so, says is "too busy"	
	Status	3 (Moderate)		Moderate amount of clutter, some but not all exits obstructed	

Adapted from FITNE. (1997). *The use of a standardized language with the Nightingale Tracker.* Available: *http://www.ev.net/fitne/ tracker/omaha.htm.*

The Omaha System has been in use many years and has been found to be useful both nationally and internationally in many areas including home care, public health, school health, clinics, ambulatory care, and with faculty and students. To see the complete problem list, visit the site http://www.ev.net/fitne/tracker/omaha.htm.

HOME HEALTH CARE CLASSIFICATION

HCCC was developed at Georgetown University by Saba and colleagues. Their goal was to develop a method to assess and classify medicare home care patients in order to determine the resources required to provide home health services and the expected outcomes of care (Saba, 1995). They used data on 8961 newly discharged medicare patients from 646 randomly stratified home health agencies. They studied the nursing diagnoses and problems related to the reason for the home care, and the outcome of each at discharge, along with all the nursing activities provided during each home visit.

From this study, a classification scheme was developed for nursing diagnoses, nursing interventions, and outcomes. Under this scheme, there are 20 nursing components that are the unifying feature of this system and provide the first level of coding. Nursing diagnoses are classified in 50 major categories and 95 subcategories, which form the second and third levels of coding. The final code is for the outcome, which is classified as either improved, stabilized, or deteriorated. To code a nursing problem, one selects a nursing component (Table 16-9), then one of the listed nursing diagnoses and a subcategory, if applicable. At discharge, the code is modified further by adding a 1 if the status is improved, 2 if it is stable, and 3 if the problem is worse (Table 16-10).

In studying the nursing interventions, it was found that there were two facets to nursing interventions: the intervention itself, and a modifying action. The nursing or modifying actions are assessment, direct care, teaching, and management of nursing services. The first two levels of coding for an intervention are identical to those for a problem, the third lists the intervention, and the last the modifying or nursing actions (Table 16-11). For a full list of the components of the HHCC, visit http://www.dml.georgetown.edu/research/hhcc.

TABLE 16-9 ● *Nursing Components in the Home Health Care Classification*			
A. Activity	F. Fluid Volume	K. Physical Regulation	P. Self-Concept
B. Bowel Elimination	G. Health Behavior	L. Respiratory	Q. Sensory
C. Cardiac	H. Medication	M. Role Relationship	R. Skin Integrity
D. Cognitive	I. Metabolic	N. Safety	S. Tissue Perfusion
E. Coping	J. Nutritional	O. Self-Care	T. Urinary Elimination

Adapted from Saba, V. K. (1995). Home health care classifications (HCCCs); Nursing diagnoses and nursing interventions. In American Nurses Association (Eds.), *An emerging framework: Data system advances for clinical nursing practice* (pp. 61–103). Washington, D.C.: American Nurses Association.

TABLE 16-10 ● Problem and Outcome Coding in HHCC				
Nursing component	**Nursing diagnosis**		**Discharge status**	**Coding**
	Major category	*Subcategory*		
D. Cognitive	**08** Knowledge Deficit	**.5** Medication Regimen	**1** Improved	**D.08.51**
J. Nutritional	**24** Nutrition Alteration	**.3** Body Nutrition Excess	**2** Stabilized	**J.24.32**
The bold characters indicate the code for each item.				

Adapted from Saba, V. K. (1995). Home health care classifications (HCCCs); Nursing diagnoses and nursing interventions. In American Nurses Association (Eds.), *An emerging framework: Data system advances for clinical nursing practice* (pp. 61–103). Washington, D.C.: American Nurses Association.

NURSING INTERVENTIONS CLASSIFICATION

NIC is an approach to standardizing the language for nursing interventions. It was developed beginning in 1987 at the University of Iowa by a large and diverse research team. To guide their work, this group first developed a set of principles to ensure consistent wording, then used references such as nursing textbooks, care planning guides, and nursing information systems to construct a list of nursing interventions (Table 16-12) (Bulechek & McCloskey, 1996; Donahue, 1995). Results were then validated through a systematic process involving surveys, focus groups, and testing in various clinical settings.

Like NANDA, the first classification set for NIC was alphabetical, but after the process of validation, a taxonomy consisting of three levels was created to provide for easy location of related interventions (McCloskey & Bulechek, 1996). The first level consists of the six domains—physiological: basic, physiological: complex, behavioral,

TABLE 16-11 ● Coding Scheme for Interventions in Home Health Care Classification (HHCC)					
Service	**Nursing component**	**Intervention**		**Nursing action**	**Code**
		Major category	*Subcategory*		
Evaluate for hyper/hypo-glycemia	**H.** Medication	**24.** Medication Administration	**3** Side Effects	**1.** Assess	**H.24.31**
Give insulin injection	**I.** Metabolic	**27.** Diabetic Care	**0**	**2.** Direct Care	**I.27.02**
Need to eat regularly	**J.** Nutritional	**24.** Nutrition Alteration	**1** Body Nutrition Deficit	**3.** Teach	**J.24.13**
Arrange for meals on wheels	**J.** Nutritional	**24.** Nutrition Alteration	**1** Body Nutrition Deficit	**4.** Manage	**J.24.14**

Adapted from Saba, V. K. (1995). Home health care classifications (HCCCs); Nursing diagnoses and nursing interventions. In American Nurses Association (Eds.), *An emerging framework: Data system advances for clinical nursing practice* (pp. 61–103). Washington, D.C.: American Nurses Association.

TABLE 16-12 ● Examples From Top Two Levels From the Nursing Interventions Classification (NIC)					
Level 1 **Domains**	Physiological: Basic	Physiological: Complex	Behavioral	Safety	Family	Health System
Level 2 **Classes**	**A.** Activity & Exercise Management	**G.** Electrolyte and Acid-Base Balance	**O.** Behavior Therapy	**U.** Crisis Management	**W.** Childbearing Care	**Y.** Health System Mediation
	B. Elimination Management	**H.** Drug Management	**P.** Cognitive Therapy	**V.** Risk Management	**X.** Lifespan Care	**a.** Health System Management
Level 3 **Interventions**	See Table 16–13					

Adapted from Iowa Intervention Project. (1995). Validation and coding of the NIC Taxonomy Structure. *Image: Journal of Nursing Scholarship, 27*(1), 43–49.

safety, family, and health systems. These are coded by a number. The second level consists of 27 classes, each of which belongs to one of the six domains. These are represented by a letter. The class codes are upper case with the exception of two, which, although they might not be billable costs, the developers believed are important to the patient. At present, they have identified more than 400 interventions, each of which is assigned a four-digit number (Table 16-13). To code an intervention, one starts with the number of the domain, adds the letter of the class and the number assigned to the intervention. The coding is further modified by adding a code for the specific activity performed for the intervention, which is placed to the right of a decimal point.

NURSING OUTCOMES CLASSIFICATION

The NOC is a classification system for outcomes. It is intended to be used with NANDA and the NIC classifications as one large system. NOC defines outcomes as measurable, variable patient states or behaviors, including patient perceptions, that

TABLE 16-13 ● Example of Coding for Nursing Intervention Classification (NIC)		
1. Domain	**4.** Safety	**Coding**
2. Class	**U.** Crisis Management	
3. Intervention	**6140** Code Management	**4U-6140.**
	6200 Emergency Care	**4U-6200.**

Each intervention has a list of activities with a code for each. These numbers are added after the decimal point.

Adapted from Iowa Intervention Project. (1995). Validation and coding of the NIC Taxonomy Structure. *Image: Journal of Nursing Scholarship, 27*(1), 43–49.

result from nursing interventions (Johnson & Mass, 1992; 1997b). Although the outcomes may be stated as goals, they are not intended as such. Outcomes are selected based on the judgment of the nurse as to their appropriateness, and they are not tied to a specific nursing diagnosis or intervention.

There are four levels in the outcomes taxonomy: domains, classes, indicators, and the empirical measurement scale. See Table 16-14 for the six domains and some examples of the classes in each domain. Outcomes are rated on a scale of 1 to 5, using one of 16 measurement scales, each of which is matched to an outcome in a manner that gives a definition to the outcome. See Table 16-15 for examples of three of the 16 measurement scales. For more information see the site at http://www.nursing.uiowa.edu/noc/QUESTION.HTM.

PATIENT CARE DATA SET

Since 1992, the Patient Care Data Set has been under development. The objective has been to develop a data dictionary for clinical terms used in acute care settings by nurses and other nonphysician health care disciplines that can be used to record patient problems, patient care actions, and expected patient outcomes (Ozbolt, 1997). It has been designed to be compliant with Health Level 7 (HL7) standards for patient care data (a protocol for exchanging data among health care applications).

The definitions recognize that problems, interventions, and goals are multidimensional. For example, problems are characterized by persistence and severity. Interventions are implemented at various times and have a duration, and goals entail evaluations and dates for review. Using this system, problems can be described based on their potency (are they potential, active, or resolved?), their severity (are they potential, mild, moderate, severe, or life-threatening?), and their status (are they currently addressed or not?) (Ozbolt, 1997).

Patient care orders may be identified as protocols, pathways, or specific items of care. Details for these actions specify the responsible discipline, the frequency with which each order is to be performed, and times for initiating and stopping the action. Goals describe patient conditions or behaviors that are expected to be achieved as a result of care. Outcomes (intermediate or ultimate) are viewed as goal achievement status. They are rated as achieved, progressing ahead of schedule, progressing on schedule, delayed, regressing, or failing to achieve. Because the terms of the Patient Care Data Set were compiled from those actually used by nurses and others to record information in patient records, they are expressed in language familiar to caregivers, at the level of detail used to plan and document care.

ISSUES IN EFFORTS TO STANDARDIZE THE LANGUAGE

Each of these data sets is intended to provide a standardized language for inclusion in a computerized patient record (Table 16-16). In order to fulfill the needs of a computerized record, three components must be present: problem statements, interventions, and outcomes. NANDA, NIC, and NOC each address only one of these components, but the developers of NIC and NOC state that all three are to be used together

TABLE 16-14 • Nursing Outcomes Classification (NOC) Domains, and Two Classes for Each Domain

Level 1 Domains	1 Functional Health	2 Physiological Health	3 Psychosocial Health	4 Health Knowledge & Behavior	5 Perceived Health	6 Family Health
Level 2 Classes and designated code letter	**A** Energy Maintenance **B** Growth Development	**E** Cardiopulmonary **F** Elimination	**M** Psychological Well-Being **P** Social Interaction	**Q** Health Behavior **R** Health Beliefs	**U** Health & Life Quality **V** Symptom Status	**W** Family Caregiver Status **X** Maltreatment Resolution

Adapted from Iowa Outcomes Classification (NOC). (1997). *Taxonomy of nursing outcomes.* Iowa City: IA College of Nursing, The University of Iowa.

Rating Scale	1	2	3	4	5	Two outcomes with which this scale is associated
B	Extreme deviation from expected range	Substantial deviation from expected range	Moderate deviation from expected range	Mild deviation from expected range	No deviation from expected range	Growth, Physical Aging Satisfactory
E	Not at all	To a slight extent	To a moderate extent	To a great extent	To a very great extent	Joint Movement Active, Joint Movement Passive
M	Never demonstrated	Rarely demonstrated	Sometimes demonstrated	Often demonstrated	Consistently demonstrated	Decision Making, Parent–Infant Attachment

There are 16 different measurement scales, each of which is appropriate for a given outcome. They are coded with the letters A–P.

Adapted from Johnson, M., & Maas, M. (Eds.) (1997). *Iowa Outcomes Project: Nursing Outcomes Classification (NOC)*. St. Louis: Mosby.

TABLE 16-16 ● *Summary of Some Nursing Classification and Language Systems*

Purpose	System	Problem	Intervention	Outcome
Develop a set of data to make nursing data comparable to assist health care decision makers	NMDS			
Adaptation of the NMDS for use by nurses in the emergency room	ENUDS			
Adaptation of the NMDS for nurses in management	NMMDS			
Map to disparate clinical terms used by the various classification systems to facilitate finding information	UNLS			
Develop a method to computerize the natural language that nurses use to describe interventions	NILT		X	
Develop a data dictionary for clinical terms in acute care settings for recording patient problems, patient care actions, and expected patient outcomes	Patient Care Data Set	X	X	X
Provide a long-term patient history and health record for use in health care encounters and regional data repositories. (Patient Care Data Set)	PCDS	X	X	X
Provide a description and comparison of nursing data for clinical populations around the world	ICNP			
Provide consistent language for collecting, sorting, classifying, documenting, and analyzing data pertaining to a family's situation for home health care	Omaha	X	X	X
Assess and classify Medicare home care patients in order to determine the resources required to provide home health services as well as the expected outcomes of care	HHCC	X	X	X
Identify, develop, and classify nursing diagnosis	NANDA	X		
Provide a comprehensive, standardized language for nursing interventions	NIC		X	
Provide a comprehensive classification of nursing-sensitive patient outcomes with a standardized measure of nursing intensity	NOC			X

as a set. In all of the classifications, the highest level of the taxonomy is the most abstract, and the lowest level is the most concrete. Each data set also has a specific definition for each item to guide the practitioner in selection of the appropriate label. The ultimate aim of computerization of nursing data is to provide data for analyses. Data collected using these data sets could provide much information about the nature of nursing and the value nursing adds to health care.

The different systems that are discussed earlier are not presented as perfection but as approaches to a standardized language. Each evolved from a different need. The different needs indicate the breadth of practice in which nurses are involved. What is encouraging is the that various data sets have all been mapped to each other, thus providing comparability and visibility without disrupting managements' prerogative of selecting the system they deem most workable.[1] Each system has its advantages and disadvantages. The challenge is not to try and select the perfect system but to select the one that best suits the needs of the institution. There are serious concerns about all of the standardized languages. Cody (1995) voiced the opinion that NIC was reductionistic, reflected only an objectivist view of nursing, and was linked to the technical task-based approach to nursing. Others are worried that a standardized language will be inflexible, will not be clinically useful, or is cookbook nursing (McCloskey & Bulechek, 1994). Any of these concerns may be true. The approach used by the person administering the nursing care may well be the determinant. For instance, Cody states that none of NIC reflects mutual nurse–client decision making. Using NIC, however, or any of the standardized languages, does not preclude it. Like standardized care plans, the system used in classification can produce cookbook nursing, but it may also enable the nurse to document any individualized care that she or he gives to the patient. The determining factor in the type of nursing care a patient receives is the approach of the individual nurse, and the culture of both the unit in the health care institution and the institution itself. Standardized data will allow the comparison of nursing care among institutions and may demonstrate that institutions with an individualized approach to nursing or who engage in mutual nurse–client decision making have better outcomes with the same interventions than those with a more functional task,oriented approach.

There is a push for health care institutions to develop an electronic or computerized patient record. If nursing data is to be included in the collected data, hence visible to the world beyond nursing, it will be necessary to use some form of language standardization. Computerization always involves difficult decisions that invariably exclude or provide less emphasis for some items and more for others. What nursing needs to decide is if the need to provide visible nursing data, so nursing care can be recognized for the value it adds to health care, outweighs the concerns mentioned earlier. It is unlikely, given the richness of nursing and the breadth of practice areas, that a perfect standardization will ever be developed. All of the systems, however, are constantly being evaluated and updated to meet new concerns that develop as the health care environment changes.

▼ Other Health Care Classification Systems

The use by the government and other payors in the 1980s of DRGs for billing, catapulted health care into modern health care classifications. Much of the emphasis to this point has been in the development of classification systems for billing purposes, although development of the UMLS and Systemized Nomenclature of Human and Veterinary Medicine (SNOMED) demonstrate the efforts of clinicians to have access to information needed for practice. See Table 16-17 for a summary of some of the billing classification systems and some other health-related nomenclatures.

---

[1]To map the terms means to match a term in one language with one in another language that has the same meaning.

TABLE 16-17 ● Some Other Coding Systems

Acronym	Definition	Purpose/Use
UMLS	Unified Medical Language System	Developed by the National Library of Medicine as a standardized medical language to facilitate linking clinical records, factual databases, knowledge databases, and the literature.
UNLS	Unified Nursing Language System	A standardized nursing language being developed for the purpose of facilitating the searching of nursing records and making research findings available at the bedside.
ICD-9	International Classification of Disease–9th version	Released by WHO in 1975, provided a classification system for surgical, diagnostic, and therapeutic procedures. Consists of a tabular list containing a numerical list of the disease, and alphabetical index to the disease entries.
DRG	Diagnosis Related Group	A classification of patient's hospital stay in terms of what was wrong with and what was done for a patient. The DRG classification is based on diagnoses and procedures coded in ICD9-CM, and on patient age, sex, length of stay, and other factors. The DRG frequently determines the amount of money that will be reimbursed, independently of the charges that the hospital may have incurred.
ICD9-CM	International Classification of Disease–9th edition with Clinical Modifications	Based on the official version of the World Health Organization's 9th Revision, International Classification of Diseases and modified for use in the United States by the National Center for Health Statistics. It classifies morbidity and mortality information for statistical purposes, for the indexing of hospital records by disease and operations and for data storage and retrieval. Diagnoses and procedures coded in ICD9-CM determine the DRG that controls reimbursement.
ICD10	International Classification of Disease, 10th edition	An enlarged version of ICD9. Has added information for ambulatory and managed care encounters, expanded injury codes; combined the diagnosis/symptoms codes to reduce the number of codes needed to fully describe a condition. Although widely used in Europe, is not yet accepted in the United States because ICD9-CM is an integral part of hospital billing systems. The National Center for Health Statistics has developed the goal of having ICD10-CM in use for morbidity diagnoses in the year 2001.
DSM-IV	Diagnostic and Statistical Manual of Mental Disorders, 4th Edition	System of codes for psychiatric care maintained by the American Psychiatric Association. The DSM-IV diagnostic codes are also valid ICD9-CM codes.
CPT-4	Current Procedural Terminology, 4th Edition	Published annually by the American Medical Association. Contains a listing of descriptive terms and identifying codes for reporting medical services and procedures performed by physicians. Required by most payors and HCFA for physician billing.
SNOMED	Systemized Nomenclature of Human and Veterinary Medicine	Designed as a system for representing clinical information by the College of American Pathologists. It's designed to permit the full integration of all medical information into an electronic medical record. The classification includes signs and symptoms, diagnoses, and procedures.
UMLS	Unified Medical Language System	A long-term research project begun in 1986 by the National Library of Medicine to facilitate the development of systems that integrate electronic biomedical information. The system will allow users to retrieve all data on a given topic whether the data is in electronic patient records, bibliographical databases, factual databases, or expert systems.

(continued)

TABLE 16-17 • *Some Other Coding Systems (continued)*		
Acronym	**Definition**	**Purpose/Use**
Read	Read Codes	Developed in Great Britain, the Read Codes are a comprehensive list of terms intended for use by all health care professionals to describe the care and treatment of their patients. They include topics such as occupations, signs and symptoms, investigations, diagnoses, treatments and therapies, and drugs and appliances.
NCVHS	National Committee on Vital & Health Statistics	Although not a coding system, this organization, which is responsible for the collection, analysis, and dissemination of health and health-related information, has as one of its goals to accelerate the evolution of public and private health information systems toward more uniform, shared data standards.

Adapted from *Links to Coding System.* (1996). Available: http://www.mcis.duke.edu/standards/termcode/codehome.htm.

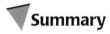 ## Summary

The need to use a computer to manage the data generated in health care is part of today's reality. Like items in a filing cabinet, data in a computer are useless unless they are organized in a manner such that they can be retrieved. What the data are and how they are structured determine what facts a theoretically objective computer will produce. Although computerizing efforts are now under way to facilitate the retrieval of clinical information, most of the effort in the past has been on developing billing systems.

To this point, nursing has been mostly a sideline player in these efforts, not through discrimination but due to lack of a way to document contributions in a manner amenable to computerization. To stand up and be counted, nurses need to adopt a standardized way of recording and presenting the data that documents what nursing adds to health care. The classification systems are an indication that nurses are making progress in this area (Fig. 16-1).

Beyond economic realities, a systematic way of recording practice provides a way to think about skills and improve them, both individually and as a profession. In one pilot study of nursing classification systems, both nurses and students reported that it enhanced their practice (Lunney, 1997). The profession will benefit when we can look at data for many patients and determine which interventions offer the most benefit and at what time in a patient's condition. Nurses also gain an advantage when databases such as the SNOMED and the UMLS permit the integration of health care literature into their information structure.

Like all things, standardized languages and data sets can be misused. They can be employed to regulate nursing or produce cookbook-style nursing. On the other hand, they can be used to improve patient care greatly and influence the public's perception of nursing as a crucial and professional field.

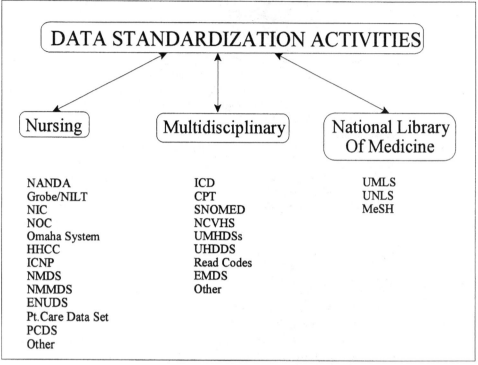

Figure 16-1 ● Some of the current data standardization activities. (Structure of this figure credited to Simpson, R. [1998]. *Nursing informatics: Nursing's newest specialty.* Presentation at February 1998 *Caring* Meeting, Washington, D.C., who credits conversations with Kathy Milholland as basis for figure.)

EXERCISES

1. What issues can you foresee in efforts to make the NMDS a part of a discharge record?
2. Given data from any of the data sets or languages presented earlier, demographic data about a patient, length of stay, and primary and concurrent medical diagnoses, what information could you derive?
3. Make a case for or against standardized documentation.
4. What are some ways standardized data might be used by health care professionals in
   a. Clinical practice?
   b. Administration?
   c. Education?
   d. Research?
   e. Entrepreneurial work?

REFERENCES

American Medical Association. (1990). Troubled past of "invisible" profession. *Journal of American Medical Association, 264*(22), 2851–2857.

ANA. (1997). *Position statement: A national nursing database to support clinical nursing practice.* Available: http://www.nursingworld.org/readroom/position/practice/prdatabs.htm.

Bowker, G. C. (1996). *Lest we remember: organizational forgetting and the production of knowledge.* Available: http://alexia.lis.uiuc.edu/~bowker/forget.html.

Bulechek, G. M. & McCloskey, J. C. (1996). *Nursing interventions classifications (NIC)* (2nd ed.). St. Louis: Mosby–Year Book.

Carpenito, L. J. (1983). *Nursing diagnosis: Application in clinical practice.* Philadelphia: J. B. Lippincott Company.

Clark, J. (1994). The international classification of nursing. In J. McCloskey & H. K. Grace (Eds.), *Current issues in nursing* (4th ed.; pp. 143–147). St Louis: C. V. Mosby.

Cody, W. K. (1995). Letter to the editor. *Nursing Outlook, 43*(2), 93.

Donahue, W. J. (1995). Nursing interventions classification (NIC): A language to describe nursing treatments. In N. M. Lang (Ed.), *Nursing data systems: The emerging framework.* (pp. 115–131). Washington, D.C.: American Nurses Association.

Duke University. (1996). *Links to coding system.* Available: http://www.mcis.duke.edu/standards/termcode/codehome.htm.

Grobe, S. J. (1996). The Nursing Intervention Lexicon and Taxonomy: Implications for representing nursing care data in automated patient records. *Holistic Nurse Practitioner, 11,* 48–63.

Goossen, W. T. F. (1998, March 24), Personal Communication.

Hannah, K. J. & Anderson, B. J. (1995). Determining nursing data elements essential for the management of nursing information. In M. J. Ball, K. J. Hannah, S. K. Newbold & J. V. Douglas (Eds.), *Nursing informatics: Where caring & technology meet* (2nd ed.; pp. 130–143). New York: Springer-Verlag.

Hoskins, L. M. (1995). NANDA's nursing diagnosis taxonomy: A nursing database. In N. M. Lang (Ed.), *Nursing data systems: The emerging framework.* (pp. 49–59). Washington, D.C.: American Nurses Association.

Johnson, M. & Maas, M. (1997a). *Nursing outcomes classification (NOC).* St. Louis: Mosby–Year Book.

Johnson, M. & Maas, M. (1997b). *Nursing-sensitive outcomes classification (NOC): An overview.* Available: http://www.nursing.uiowa.edu/noc/overview.htm.

Johnson, M. & Mass, M (Eds.). (1992). *Nursing outcomes classification (NOC).* St. Louis: Mosby–Year Book.

Lang, N. M. & Murphy, M. (1995). International activities and perspectives on an international classification for nursing practice (ICNP). In N. M. Lang (Ed.), *Nursing data systems: The emerging framework.* (pp. 135–141). Washington, D.C.: American Nurses Association.

Leske, J. S. & Werley, H. H. (1992). Use of the Nursing Minimum Data Set. *Computers in Nursing, 10*(6), 259–263.

Lindberg, D. A. B. & Humphreys, B. L. (1995). The UMLS knowledge sources: Tool for building better user interfaces. In N. M. Lang (Ed.), *Nursing data systems: The emerging framework* (pp. 151–159). Washington, D.C.: American Nurses Association.

Lunney, M. (1997). *Posting on Nrsing-L.* Available: http://library.ummed.edu/lsv/wa.cgi?A1=ind9711&L=nrsing-l.

Martin, K.S., & Scheet, N. J. (1992). *The Omaha System: Applications for community health nursing.* Philadelphia: W. B. Saunders.

Martin, K. S., & Scheet, N. J. (1995). The Omaha System: Nursing diagnoses, interventions, and client outcomes. In N. M. Lang (Ed.), *Nursing data systems: The emerging framework.* (pp. 105–113). Washington, D.C.: American Nurses Association.

McCloskey, J. C. & Bulechek, G. M. (1996). *Nursing Intervention Classification (NIC)* (2nd ed). St. Louis: Mosby.

McCloskey, J. C. & Bulechek, G. M. (1994). Standardizing the language for nursing treatments: An overview of the issues. *Nursing Outlook, 42*(2), 56–63.

McCormick, K. A. (1995). An update on nursing's unified language system. In M J. Ball, K. J. Hannah, S. K. Newbold & J. V. Douglas (Eds.), *Nursing informatics: Where caring & technology meet* (2nd ed.; pp. 112–129). New York: Springer-Verlag.

McCormick, K. A. & Zielstorff, R. (1995). Building a unified nursing language system (UNLS). In N. M. Lang (Ed.), *Nursing data systems: The emerging framework.* (pp. 143–149). Washington, D.C.: American Nurses Association.

News from ICN. (1996). *CNF receives Kellogg grant toward development of an international nursing language.* Available: http://www.nursingworld.org/icn/release.htm.

Ozbolt, J. (1997, October). Multiple attributes for patient care data: Toward a multitiaxial combination vocabulary. In CD-ROM version of Proceedings of the AMIA Fall Symposium, Nashville, TN, October 25–28, 1997.

Renner, A. R. & Swart, J. C. (1997). Patient Care Data Set: Standard for a longitudinal health/medical record. *Computers in Nursing, 15*(2S), S7–S13.

Saba, V. K. (1995). Home health care classifications (HCCCs); Nursing diagnoses and nursing interventions. In N. M. Lang (Ed.), *Nursing data systems: The emerging framework.* (pp. 61–103). Washington, D.C.: American Nurses Association.

Shuttleworth, A. (1993). A common language for a shared purpose. *Professional Nurse, 8*(11), 692.

Simpson, R. L. (1997). Technology: Nursing the system, The Nursing Management Minimum Data Set. *Nursing Management, 26*(6), 20–21.

Telenurse. (1997). *Project summary telematics application.* Available: http://www.nethotel.dk/dihnr/telenurse/project/summary.htm.

Warren, J. J. & Hoskins, L. M. (1995). NANDA's nursing diagnosis taxonomy: A nursing database. In N. M. Lang (Ed.), *Nursing data systems: The emerging framework.* (pp. 49–59). Washington, D.C.: American Nurses Association.

Werley, H. H., Devine, E. C., & Zorn, C. R. (1988). *Nursing Minimum Data Set data collection manual.* Milwaukee, WI: University of Wisconsin-Milwaukee School of Nursing.

Werley, H. H., Ryan, P., & Zorn, C. R. (1995). The nursing minimum data set (NMDS): A framework for the organization of nursing language. In N. M. Lang (Ed.), *Nursing data systems: The emerging framework.* (pp. 19–30). Washington, D.C.: American Nurses Association.

CHAPTER 17

Computerized Patient Records

Objectives:

After studying this chapter you should be able to:

1 Define the CPR

2 Discuss the strengths and weaknesses of paper records

3 Examine the issues surrounding the CPR

4 Differentiate between the various computer-generated information systems

5 Identify ergonomic issues surrounding a computer system

Although health care professionals usually associate the acronym CPR with cardiopulmonary resuscitation, it also refers to a computerized patient record. The CPR is an electronic, lifelong record of health care for an individual. The system in which it resides will provide clinicians ready access to knowledge from many sources that is related to the patient's condition. The CPR system will also perform predetermined analyzes in real time to find things such as drug incompatibilities or other incipient problems, issuing alerts when necessary.

The CPR can be defined as "an electronically based, adaptable clinical tool for the primary input, storage, and recall of patient care—related information" (Tallon, 1996, p. 53). The Institute of Medicine (IOM), however, assigns a more definitive definition by stating that a CPR is ". . . an electronic patient record that resides in a system specifically designed to support users through the availability of 1) complete and accurate data, 2) practitioner reminders and alerts, 3) clinical decision support systems, 4) links to bodies of medical knowledge, and 5) other aids" (Dick & Steen, 1991, p. 2). The Computer-based Patient Record Institute (CPRI) adds that the patient record should contain information about an individual's lifetime health status and health care (Computer-based Patient Record Institute, 1998).

Thus, as envisioned, the CPR will have more than one focus. Not only will it provide a lifelong record of health care for an individual, but the system in which it resides will provide clinicians with ready access to knowledge from many sources that is related to the patient's condition. The CPR system will also perform predetermined analyses in real time to find things such as drug incompatibilities or other incipient problems, issuing alerts when it does.

▼ Background of the Computerized Patient Record

Work on the CPR grew out of discussions between staff at the National Institutes of Health (NIH) and the IOM, who were looking for a way to make patient records more useful for teaching and research (Dick & Steen, 1991). This discussion generated enough interest to introduce the issue at the June 1986 IOM program development workshop. In 1989, the IOM appointed the Committee on Improving the Patient Record to study the issue. The committee created several subcommittees who solicited information from more than 70 advisers, including nurses, patient groups, computer software and hardware vendors, and third-party payors.

The final result was the recommendation that public and private sectors join to establish a Computer-Based Record Patient Institute (CPRI) to promote the development of the CPR. The institute was established in 1992, with the goal to improve the quality of health care and access through the use of information technology. CPRI is a nonprofit organization composed of members of stakeholder groups, such as nursing, medical records, dentistry, patients, and third-party payors (Computer-based Patient Record Institute, 1998). Primary support for this group comes from organizations, although individuals can belong. The ANA is a member of the CPRI.

▼ Patient Records

The patient record is theoretically the repository of all information about a patient's health. It should not only serve as an active part of care but provide information on the origins, progress, and outcome of a disease (Levy & Lawrance, 1992). A patient record should also be a tool for auditing the quality of care. Additionally, it needs to serve health care planners, researchers, lawyers, and third-party payors. Today, all who visited more than one health care provider or institute have multiple patient records in many places. Thus, there is not one place to which health care professionals can go to retrieve pertinent health information, nor is it possible for policy planners to have a full picture of the health needs of a community, state, or nation.

▼ Strengths of Paper Records

Most institutions, including those with computerized systems, also use a paper record. When the IOM subcommittee studied the literature to determine strengths and weaknesses of the paper record, they found no substantive strengths, although they acknowledged that this factor may be due to widespread acceptance, which may have precluded defending their efficacy (Dick & Steen, 1991). Strengths of the paper record include familiarity, easy use, and easy customization. A paper record also can accommodate all necessary data and offers relatively good security against unauthorized access (McHugh, 1992).

Weaknesses of Paper Records

Many sources document the weakness of the paper record in today's information-intensive health care system. Owing to the organization of the record by department instead of by problem, it is difficult to reliably summarize information for discharge (Dick & Steen, 1991). Additionally, the records may be illegible or incomplete, data may be inaccurate, and information recorded is difficult and expensive to code for required reports due to lack of standardization of terms.

Paper records take a great deal of nursing time (McHugh, 1992). Estimates in the literature run from 25% to 50% of a nurse's time (Dick & Steen, 1991). Paper records often require the same data to be entered in more than one place. Clinicians may scribble notes on whatever paper is available, including paper towels, then transcribe the data later, a process that may lead to data being entered for the wrong patient or being lost. Unavailability of the record may also lead to errors or omissions in data entry, or time lost waiting to use the record.

Perhaps the biggest weakness of paper records is the difficulty of retrieving information. Not only is a requested record often not available, but finding information can be frustrating. For research purposes, access to information in paper records is very labor intensive. Before any analysis can be conducted, one must identify the records that contain the needed data, search the record to find the data, and manually enter it into a computer. All of these steps offer the potential for error, as well as increase the cost. They also prohibit timely reporting of needed data for making decisions.

Why is a CPR needed?

The necessity for health care data are increasing, demands that are difficult to meet with present medical records. Government and other third-party payors are requiring data from patient records. Meeting the quality assurance program for Joint Commission on Accreditation of Healthcare Organizations (JCAHO) also requires information from patient records. Internally, health care administrators require timely data from patient records to allocate resources. The various health care professionals need patient care data, some of it the same data, but formatted to meet the needs of their discipline. For example, the primary physician needs a view that will facilitate the management of the medical aspects of care, the pharmacist needs to see data about medications the patient is receiving, and nurses need a view of information that facilitates nursing care (Dick & Steen, 1991).

The explosion of knowledge has created a situation in which it is next to impossible to be continually aware of the latest research on a given condition, let alone have this knowledge in memory. Add to that the current health care environment, in which clinicians are being urged to care for more patients in less time, and a situation exists in which clinicians do not have time to search for treatments that can improve patient care. A system that provides this information as easily as recording patient information will improve this situation.

Today, many patients are seen by more than one health care provider. Relying on a patient to provide the necessary information to both clinicians or for the clinicians to communicate is not realistic. Universal access to a patient record that is structured in a way to make salient information easily available will vastly improve communication and patient care.

Today medical care is complex. In 50 years, we have moved from a time when physicians were familiar with most drugs to a situation in which new drugs appear weekly. In this climate, it is easy for a clinician to inadvertently prescribe a drug that is incompatible with one that she or he prescribed earlier (or another clinician prescribed). A system that is programmed to issue an alert is necessary for good patient care. Given the newness of some drugs, not all incompatibilities are known. A system that records results of clients and permits data in the aggregate to be used will uncover unknown incompatibilities long before traditional methods.

Not only are payors demanding more information, business organizations and labor unions, whose members ultimately pay for health care, are starting to ask questions of providers. Obtaining this information is not financially feasible without a CPR:

▼ Why is the rate of surgeries for a given condition greater in one city than another?
▼ Why does this variation seem to correlate with the number of specialists available?
▼ Why are new technologies introduced without evidence of efficacy?
▼ Why do costs for the same procedures vary even within the same community? (Shortliffe et al., 1992).

The reasons for adopting a CPR go beyond the convenience of health care professionals to access individual records in an acceptable format and the needs of the third-party payors for information to justify costs. Providing the best possible patient care requires access to the data generated in patient care situations and systems that can monitor for known problem areas and identify those that are unknown. Another positive feature of a CPR is the ability to offer immediate access to clinical information. It would be very labor intensive to provide these things without the CPR.

▼ Issues in Adopting the CPR

Despite the compelling reasons for adopting a CPR, there are many issues that need attention before it can become a reality. For example, standards for data format and transmission must be agreed upon, security concerns must be met, decisions need to be made about the ownership of data, and concerns about the sharing of market-sensitive information overcome. Additionally there are legal concerns.

STANDARDS FOR DATA TRANSMISSION

Computerization in health care institutions has generally been piecemeal. Different departments have various systems from an array of vendors. Difficulties arise when it becomes necessary to integrate the various information systems due to characteristics of each system that makes exchanging data difficult. For a CPR to be workable, it is necessary that the data stored in all these systems be exchanged. The exchange of data involves two different standards: data standards (length of fields, ASCII or binary data, how dates are represented, etc.) and the vocabularies used to identify the various phenomenon (McDonald & Hripcsak, 1992).

Data standards are fairly well developed due to HL7. Data exchange standards are also being defined for laboratory instruments, EKGs, and instruments such as infusion devices, ventilators, blood pressure measuring machines and cardiac monitoring devices.

Standardization of terms such as those being developed for the Unified Medical Language System (UMLS) and the Unified Nursing Language System (UNLS) are also necessary for the CPR. These are more difficult to develop, given the breadth of each healthcare practice area and the variety of practice arenas.

Much of a medical record today is free text, or natural language. It remains the richest form of expression, but presents an additional problem in standardizing language—that of finding specific information and determining how to code it so it is useful as aggregated data. Efforts are being made to develop text processing systems that will permit the extraction of needed information from free text. These, however, are not necessarily an efficient answer. Writing voluminous notes is time consuming; much of the information in these notes is routine and could be more quickly entered in a structured format. A well-designed CPR would require free text only for things that are truly unique.

SECURITY

One of the biggest issues confronting the development of the CPR is security. Without assurances that this concern has been met, the chance of success for the CPR is minimal. Security has three aspects: privacy, confidentiality, and protection against data loss. Privacy refers to the rights of individuals to decide when, where, and how information about themselves will be communicated to others. Confidentiality is the protection of information about individuals from unauthorized use. It is the professional responsibility of health care workers to protect both privacy and confidentiality of patient care data, whether in a paper record or a CPR. Protection against data loss involves ensuring that the data will always be available.

Privacy

The determination about what information about an individual will be shared is a valued commodity. There are instances in which people have been denied employment because of known medical conditions. This can make clients hesitant to share their health history with clinicians, especially when they know it will be entered into a record for anyone with access to read. Clients have a right to view their medical records and to determine what is revealed about themselves, both in print and on a computer. Protecting patient privacy is a primary professional responsibility.

Confidentiality

Confidentiality concerns with a CPR are different than those seen with paper records. Computerized records cannot be locked in a file cabinet, and by using a computer, it is easier to access several records. Plus, improperly protected data are vulnerable during transmission, especially transmission outside of the immediate institution. Misuse of patient care data can occur by both insiders and outsiders. Insiders may take advantage of their access to seek information for which they have no valid need and outsiders may gain access to patient information for personal or economic gain (Computer Science and Telecommunications Board & National Research Council, 1997). Preserving confidentiality involves balancing legitimate needs for data with threats of misuse.

There are practices that can minimize the danger of unauthorized access. Foremost is the authentication of users. Passwords and other identification devices, such as the use of a physical key along with a password, are one method. Biometric identification, such as fingerprints, retinal scans, or voice prints, may well be used in the future. Knowing where users have been in a system is another security measure. A well-designed system provides an *audit trail,* or a log that records what each user has done in the system. Knowledge of such a process can discourage misuse of data. One of the biggest dangers comes from individuals who forget to log off a system, which allows an unauthorized individual to use their access. Other problems stem from obtaining another's password. Encrypting data that is sent over public networks minimizes the danger of unauthorized access by outsiders.

Organizations need to develop security and confidentiality policies. These policies should state the types of information that are confidential, who has access to what information, who can release it to whom, and the penalties for violating the policies. Additionally, all employees need to be educated about the need for security and policies. A zero tolerance toward breaches of security will prevent most insider abuses. Unfortunately, information confidentiality must compete with other demands for scarce resources (Computer Science and Telecommunications Board & National Research Council, 1997). Too often, resources are not devoted to this issue until their has been a serious breach of security.

Protection Against Data Loss

Protection against data loss, or data security, deals with concerns related to hardware, software, and data integrity. These concerns involve such things as hardware failures, system program errors, and damage to data during acquisition, processing, storage, output, and distribution. Intensive testing can protect against program errors as well as damage to data during acquisition and processing. Protection against data loss can be achieved by the use of routine backups of data and provisions for off-site storage to protect against flood, fire, or other natural disasters. A disaster recovery plan that is tested periodically is another vital protection device.

Protection of data in long-term storage is another issue. A paper format for information has been shown to remain intact over centuries. Computerized data, however, has yet to pass that test. Anyone who has been working with computers for more than 10 years knows data that was carefully preserved on a 5¼ inch single-density diskette is practically unretrievable today due to the disappearance of disk drives that can read this diskette. The same thing has happened with larger computers. Technology continues to improve, and older technologies disappear.

Before committing data to a totally computerized format, it is necessary to ascertain that it will be possible to retrieve data that is 10, 25, or 50 years old. Not only is it necessary to ensure that it will be possible to read data from older mediums, but there should be thought given to the life span of data recorded on magnetic mediums, such as a disk or tape. Diskettes and files can become corrupt and unusable as many computer users can attest. There have even been some observations that data preserved on CD-ROMS begins to deteriorate after 5 years.

OWNERSHIP OF AND RESPONSIBILITY FOR ACCURACY OF DATA

Another issue in implementing a universal CPR is ownership of, and responsibility for, data accuracy. At present, physical patient records are the property of the organization or health care provider who created them, as is the responsibility for their accuracy (Dick & Steen, 1991). When data is added to a record from multiple sources, the ownership and responsibilities become blurred. Additional questions arise as to who will control access to the record and what data will be available to whom.

SHARING OF MARKET-SENSITIVE INFORMATION

Health care today is competitive. Institutions are necessarily reluctant to share information that could be used to advantage by their competitors. There is concern, therefore, about how data an institution or private practitioner records will be used.

LEGAL ISSUES

State legal requirements for medical records vary greatly. A large issue is electronic signatures. One format for entering electronic signatures is to assign an individual a separate password that she or he uses to authorize the addition of his or her name to an order or note. Several states have already passed laws legalizing electronic signatures. A National Conference of Commissioners on Uniform State Laws (NCCUSL) is working on drafting a uniform electronic transactions act for possible inclusion in state laws that covers a variety of legal issues (Brumfield, 1998). This is a worldwide concern, as evidenced by consideration given to digital and other forms of electronic signatures by the United Nations Commission on International Trade Law.

LEGACY SYSTEMS

Many health care institutions have computerized systems installed. Replacing these systems with technology that permits the exchange of data is a large expense. Forward thinking administrators, however, recognize that the need to be competitive will require additional expenditures in technology (Zinn, 1995).

COSTS

Many institutions report savings from using computerized records instead of paper (Adderley, Hyde, & Mauseth 1997). The jury, however, is still out on total costs, owing to a lack of consensus on how to measure benefits. There is agreement that the initial cost of a transition is high. It includes not only the hardware and software but

● ▼ ● ▲ ● ▼ ● ▲ ● ▼ ● ▲ ● ▼ ● ▲ ● ▼ ● ▲ ● ▼ ● ▲ ●

Display 17-1 ● **CONSIDERATIONS IN CALCULATING THE BENEFITS OF A COMPUTERIZED PATIENT RECORD**

1. Is there an improvement in patient care?
   a. Are antibiotics that are not effective against a specific microbe no longer being administered?
   b. Are drug incompatibilities uncovered?
   c. Is length of stay decreased and are outcomes improved by the availability of patient information and access to knowledge base or decision support system?
   d. Is there a reduction in lost data?
2. Are there time savings in:
   a. Recording information by all disciplines?
   b. Retrieving information (including a decrease in number of telephone calls, or gaining access to a chart)?
   c. Preparing data required for various internal and external reports?
   d. Follow-up time for incomplete records because records are more complete?
   e. Monitoring quality and outcomes?
3. Do the time savings result in increased patient satisfaction?
4. Is there a reduction in staff frustration that was due to inability to retrieve needed information? Does this reduce sick time or turnover?
5. Are charges reported more accurately?
6. Is there a reduction in incidents such as medication errors or patient falls due to better monitoring?
7. How much money is saved on paper purchases?

training of users. Unfortunately, like nursing care, agreed-on measures for interpreting the benefits of a CPR are lacking. How costs are calculated greatly affect the results. Some costs, such as paper savings, are easy to calculate. Others, such as time saved, can be calculated only if the items have been measured before the CPR was installed (Display 17-1).

▼ Benefits of a CPR

In noncomputerized systems, the IOM reported that 11% of test results are lost, causing the test to be repeated; 30% of ordered treatments are never documented; and in 40% of cases, a diagnosis is never recorded (Song, Ho, & Ho, 1997). Although the benefits of a CPR are more predicted than actual, the presence of a CPR could greatly reduce, if not eliminate, these percentages. It also seems likely that the availability of huge databases that permit the analysis of data on a local, state, national, and worldwide level will advance the knowledge of health care. Additionally, it is also the case that patients will benefit from having their health care data located in one place. Patient care should be improved when clinicians have access to the latest knowledge on a subject and when computers can catch possible omissions or conflicts in treatment (Display 17-2).

COMMUNITY HEALTH INFORMATION NETWORKS

A CPR will make possible Community Health Information Networks (CHINS). The purpose of CHINS is to make information available that will improve quality and cost factors in health care delivery systems. Ideally, they would facilitate the sharing of community-wide health care information in a standardized electronic format (Lake Superior, undated). The goal is to make this information available to health care providers such as hospitals, clinics, nursing homes, and other health interested organizations, such as public health, social services, employers, and educational institutions (Rural Health, undated). In addition to sharing information within the community, a focus of CHINs is to provide summary-oriented information about a

●▼●▲●▼●▲●▼●▲●▼●▲●▼●▲●▼●▲●

Display 17-2 • SOME BENEFITS OF A COMPUTERIZED PATIENT RECORD

1. To clinicians
   a. Availability of information when and where it is needed; this information includes patient data and bibliographical resources
   b. Decision support
   c. Organization of information specific to the discipline in a manner such that it is easily located
   d. Facilitation of the process of preparing reports for internal and external entities
   e. Ease of order entry
   f. Elimination of multiple entries of the same data
2. To patients
   a. Knowledge of who has access to their data
   b. Individualized treatment anywhere the CPR is available
   c. Ability to check the accuracy of their record
   d. One location for all health care data
   e. Evidence based health care
3. To researchers and policymakers
   a. Time savings in obtaining data
   b. Large databanks yielding more valid and precise research
   c. Ability to answer questions on a local, state, national, and possibly worldwide level

population for organizations such as public health groups. CHINS have not been readily accepted for many of the same reasons that are slowing the acceptance of the CPR, such as fear that providing this information will put institutions at a competitive disadvantage and concerns about confidentiality of records.

One system that is in may ways functioning as a CHIN is the Integrated Advanced Information Management System (IAIMIS), begun at the University of Washington in Seattle (Fuller, 1997). Originally devised to assist organizations in integrating the various computer systems that proliferated in the mid-1980s, the same methodology is used to assist regional institutions to integrate. IAIMISs face the same challenges CPRs face: political and social resistance, the need to build information linkages between institutions, and facilities that are under different ownership and who may even be competitors. The key in developing regional integrated health information systems is a planning process that successfully unites users and systems developers. IAMIS has found that the components of a successful regional information system are a robust technology that will support high-speed transmission of all types of data; high-quality, accurate, secure patient-focused information; decision-support tools; and adequate training and support.

▼ An Example of a Functioning Institutional CPR

A CPR that has been under development for more than 25 years is the Health Evaluation Through Logical Processing (HELP) hospital information system. The HELP system is both a centralized patient record and a knowledge base (Pryor, 1992). It consists of many different modules such as admitting, nursing, order entry, charge capture, respiratory therapy, pulmonary and blood gas analysis, and the laboratory. Users of each module can use the system to acquire patient data and for computerized decision making. In this system, the nurse serves as one of the main individuals who is responsible for data acquisition. Nursing is fully represented in the system.

An example of the use of the HELP system for decision making is the real-time review of antibiotic therapy. When microbiology culture and antibiotic susceptibility results are entered into the computer, the system checks the patient's files for medications (Goldszmidt, 1996). If the patient is not receiving an antibiotic to which the pathogen is susceptible, the system issues an antibiotic alert to the clinical pharmacist. In 1 year, 49% of the physicians contacted about these alerts were unaware of the situation. The system also monitors for adverse drug reactions by examining all drug orders, certain lab tests, and drug levels. If a problem is found, an alert is printed that is verified by either the pharmacist or a nurse. The first year this part of the system was operational, it facilitated the identification of 401 problems.

▼ Computer-Generated Information Systems

In the above-mentioned example of a CPR, a decision system was employed to review the use of antibiotic therapy for infections. The term decision system, along with the terms knowledge or expert systems and artificial intelligence are too often used interchangeably. Each has a separate meaning and use.

DECISION-SUPPORT SYSTEMS

A decision-support system furnishes the user with information to use in decision making. Care planning systems that provide standardized plans are not decision-support systems (Hannah, 1995). A decision-support system supplies help in formulating the problem, analyzing alternatives, and making a choice between alternatives. There are two overt types of decision-support systems: formatting tools and decision modeling.

Formatting Tools

Spreadsheets are an example of a formatting tool in that they are like a template into which information can be imputed. They allow a user to experiment with what if scenarios. They assist users in reducing and summarizing information.

Decision Models

The purpose of decision models is to assist the user in defining the problem. A model is a simplified, observable representation of a real entity that includes only those elements that are essential to the situation (Brennan, 1985). A map is an example; it depicts only relationships between the entities of interest. Depending on the need, a map can be very detailed, as in a map of a subdivision with the names of home owners, or very broad, as in a map of the world. A decision model assists in structuring or defining the problem, considering alternatives, weighting each one, and making a decision based on the results. When there are many criteria a decision must satisfy, the model of choice is a multiple criteria modeling system. These systems work similarly to the decision models, with the choice being made based on the numerical sums of the weighting.

EXPERT SYSTEMS

There are various names given to an expert system, such as an advisory system or a knowledge-based system. The purpose of an expert system is to evaluate data and make a recommendation that an expert would make, given the same situation. Expert systems have three overall parts: a data or knowledge base that contains the information needed for the domain of the system; a model base, or inference engine, which includes statistical and analytical methods for processing the data; and a user interface, or procedures for use in interacting with the system (Brennan, 1985). Two expert systems developed for nursing were COMMES and CYBERNURSE. However, both had difficulties. There are several problems inherent in developing an expert system for a domain as large as nursing. One difficulty is the existence of a multitude of conceptual and philosophical models that are not only different but in some cases incompatible (Ozbolt, 1995). Another difficulty is the development of nursing's knowledge base, which involves identifying and defining the phenomenon that comprise nursing, then determining how it is all related (Fig. 17-1).

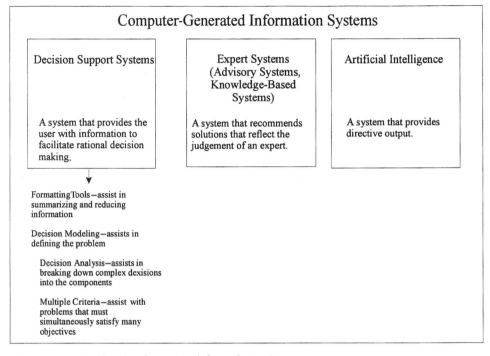

Figure 17-1 • Classification of computer information systems.

ARTIFICIAL INTELLIGENCE

True artificial intelligence is supposed to mimic the actions of an intelligent human in a given situation and be capable of substituting for a human. Artificial intelligence programs possess the ability to learn from users; thus, they develop a cumulative database. Although in the early 1980s, they were seen as the wave of the future, they have not lived up to expectations. They are very expensive to produce, and to date, they are helpful only in carefully defined situations.

▼ Ergonomics

Ergonomics is the consideration given to designing a product, or work environment, such that it is convenient to use and does not prove injurious to health. A well-designed computer system, whether part of a CPR or a small individual system, should be well designed ergonomically. Ergonomics is an important consideration for preventive health in terms of placement of terminals and keyboards, but it goes beyond the immediate physical environment and touches on the virtual environment of a system.

When planning any computer system, thought given to ergonomics in terms of how a user interacts with the software will affect its acceptance. A concept that can either hinder or help users is the overall organizing principle of a system (Staggers,

1995). Locus of control is another ergonomic factor. When the locus of control is with the user, there will be easy exits for the inevitable wrong selection. When the locus of control is with the computer, users who mistakenly select a wrong entry will be forced to go through a series of screens before being able to complete work (Zielstorff, Hudgings, & Grobe, 1993). When other mistakes are made, such as entering the wrong information on a patient, making the change should involve the same principle as using the undo icon in a word processor (Staggers, 1995). Errors in inputting information, such as entering the number 204 for a temperature, should be met with a clear message about the error and how to correct it. When possible, it is even better to assist the user to avoid the error in the first place.

A system needs to accommodate both novices and experts (Staggers, 1995). Also, too much information on a screen can be as disconcerting as too little. Progressive disclosure, in which more information on a topic is available with a mouse click, can serve the desires of both those who only seek immediate information and those with more extensive information needs. Data that is needed with other data should not require the user to memorize the information on a prior screen or to switch between screens. Acronyms or abbreviations can also be confusing. They may cause errors or confuse the novice.

As mentioned earlier, the physical ergonomics of a system should also be part of the planning. Looking at things from the users' point of view often reveals things that might not otherwise be considered. Nurses who have spent the better part of a day standing may appreciate being able to sit while using the computer. If the computer is also used by those standing, it should be at a height that does not require stooping. Stools can be provided for the nurse who has extensive uses to make of the computer. Touch screens and light pens may be ideal for quick entry, but for extended entries, they are very tiring to the arm. Providing dual means of entry may solve this situation. Resolution of a screen is also important. The higher the resolution, the easier the screen is on the eyes. Keyboards and mice should also be given consideration. Ideally, point-of-care terminals, that is bedside terminals, will be available for quick recording. Having too few terminals means that nurses will still need to record data and transcribe it to the computer, which is an error-prone procedure.

When planning a system, walk a day in the shoes of a user or several days in the shoes of several users before making firm decisions about computer placement or system interfaces. Computers are supposed to facilitate data recording, not impose additional burdens on health care personnel.

▼ Summary

Although the possibility of improving patient care with a CPR is great, acceptance depends on addressing many issues, the primary one, perhaps, being security of the data. Data security is a three-pronged issue involving protecting the patients' right to nondisclosure of information that they do not wish to share, shielding data from unauthorized uses, and preserving the data for a legal time limit.

Issues that are of concern in a regional or national CPR, such as ownership of and responsibility for the data, and sharing of market-sensitive information, are not problems at the institutional level. A CPR that includes a knowledge system and access to bibliographical data could be implemented at the institutional level, before the larger community or national issues are resolved.

Ergonomics in the design of a CPR system is as important in the overall acceptance of the system as physical considerations, such as design and placement of keyboards, mice, and terminals. Although it is ultimately the responsibility of vendors, health care professionals who are aware of good usability principles and are willing to work with a vendor to achieve them, can contribute greatly to the ease of using a system.

Despite the power of a CPR system, the output still requires human interpretation. Computer-generated knowledge, except in very circumscribed situations, is something that has not yet been attained. There are, however, decision-support systems and expert systems that can contribute information that will assist clinicians in their practice. Ultimately, however, the creation of knowledge and wisdom remain with humans. Even with the addition of expert systems, a CPR will not replace clinicians.

EXERCISES

1. In the present health care record situation, try to locate the dates of all your immunizations, childhood diseases, and surgeries.

2. How easy would it be for any individual wearing a white laboratory coat to read a record in the last patient unit in which you had clinical experience?

3. Explore the issue of professional responsibility in patient data privacy and confidentiality.

4. Prepare a case either against or for a national CPR.

5. What are some ways the CPR could be useful to health care professionals in
   a. Clinical practice?
   b. Administration?
   c. Education?
   d. Research?
   e. Entrepreneurial work?

6. Read the description of how a CPR could function for a client at the website http://www.acl.lanl.gov/sunrise/Medical/ota/08ch4.txt (Use the find option or scroll down to simplified administration for the start of the scenario.)

7. Experiment with the grammatical correction tool in a word processor. In which of the computer-generated information models would you classify it?

8. Evaluate a computer system for usability. What changes would you make to it? How does the system facilitate using it?

REFERENCES

Adderley, D., Hyde, C., & Mauseth, P. (1997). The computer age impacts nurses. *Computers in Nursing, 15*(1), 43–46.

Brennan, P. F. (1985). Decision support for nursing practice: The challenge and the promise. In K. Hannah, E. Guillemin, & D. Conklin (Eds.), *Nursing uses of computers and information science* (pp. 315–319). Amsterdam, Netherlands: Elsevier Science Publishers B.V.

Brumfield, P. (1998). Personal communication.

Computer Science and Telecommunications Board & National Research Council. (1997). *For the record: Protecting electronic health information.* Washington, D.C.: National Academy Press.

Computer-based Patient Record Institute. (1998). Available: http://www.cpri.org.

Dick, R., & Steen, E.V. (Eds.). (1991). *The computer-based patient record.* Washington, D.C.: National Academy Press.

Fuller, S. (1997). Regional Health Information Systems: Applying the IAMIS model. *Journal of the American Medical Informatics Association, 4*(2 Supplement), S47–S51.

Goldszmidt, E. (1996). *Applications of Medical Informatics in Antibiotic Therapy.* Available: http://mystic.biomed.mcgill.ca/~goldszmi/camel-2.html.

Hannah, K. J. (1995). Classification of decision-support systems. In M. J. Ball, K. J. Hannah, S. K. Newbold, & J. V. Douglas (Eds.), *Nursing informatics: Where caring & technology meet* (2nd ed.; pp. 260–266). New York: Springer-Verlag.

Lake Superior Region Community Health Information Network. (Undated). Available: http://www.d.umn.edu/superior/chin.html.

Levy, A. H. & Lawrance, D. P. (1992). Data acquisition and the computer-based patient record. In M. J. Ball & M. F. Cohen (Eds.), *Aspects of the computer-based patient record* (pp. 125–129). New York: Springer-Verlag.

McHugh, M. (1992). Nurses' needs for computer-based patient records. In M. J. Ball & M. F. Cohen (Eds.), *Aspects of the computer-based patient record* (pp. 16–29). New York: Springer-Verlag.

Medical informatics FAQ. (1995). Available: http://www.cis.ohio-state.edu/hypertext/faq/usenet/medical-informatics-faq/faq.html.

Ozbolt, J. (1995). Knowledge-based systems for supporting clinical nursing decisions. In M. J. Ball & M. F. Cohen (Eds.), *Aspects of the computer-based patient record* (pp. 274–285). New York: Springer-Verlag.

Pryor, A. T. (1992). Current state of computer-based patient record systems. In M. J. Ball & M. F. Cohen (Eds.), *Aspects of the computer-based patient record* (pp. 67–82). New York: Springer-Verlag.

Rural Health Futures. (Undated). *Community Health Information Networks.* Available: http://www.pageplus.com/~ruralfut/doc54.htm.

Shortliffe, E. H., Tang, P. C., Amatayakul, M. K., Cottington, E., Jencks, S. F., Martin, A. MacDonald, R., Morris, T. Q. & Nobel, J. J. (1992). Future vision and dissemination of computer-based patient records. In M. J. Ball & M. F. Cohen (Eds.), *Aspects of the computer-based patient record* (pp. 273–293). New York: Springer-Verlag.

Song, L., Ho, J., & Ho, S. (1997). The integrated patient information system. *Computers in Nursing, 15*(2 Supplement), S14–S22.

Staggers, N. (1995). Connecting points. Evaluating usability: Essential principles for evaluating the usability of clinical information systems. *Computers in Nursing, 13*(5), 207;211–213.

Tallon, R. W. (1996). Computer-based patient records: Hype versus reality. *Nursing Management, 27*(3), 53–57.

Zielstorff, R. D., Hudgings, C. I. & Grobe, S. J. (1993). *Next-generation nursing information systems: Essential characteristics for professional practice.* Washington, D.C.: American Nurses Association (NP 83 5M 5/93)

Zinn, T. K. (1995). Managing data sharing in the world of managed care. *Healthcare Information Management, 9*(4), 49–52.

Informatics

Computers permit nurses to access information, share knowledge, and manage data easily; therefore, they can assist in providing quality health care. The professional image and careers of nurses are also enhanced by computers. A developing field that combines nursing and computers is called nursing informatics, or the science of managing information.

Nursing Informatics

The American Nurses Association (ANA) defines the main characteristic of nursing informatics as managing information related to nursing (American Nurses Association, 1994). For example, nursing informatics specialists create databases to support nursing or help nursing managers develop systems to improve patient care. Nursing informatics specialists also use their knowledge to increase information acquisition, storage, analysis, retrieval, processing, and presentation of patient care data. Just like clinical nurses, informatics nurses must adhere to behavior standards that are expressed in a language that is understandable by the recipients of care. These are delineated in the ANA booklet *Standards of Practice for Nursing Informatics* (1995).

Nursing informatics is interdisciplinary in two ways (American Nurses Association, 1994). Knowledge from many disciplines, such as computer science, psychology, systems theory, organizational dynamics, and cognitive science make up its knowledge base. Second, nursing informatics specialists collaborate with other health care disciplines and services to provide the best possible patient care in the most efficient manner possible. Other health care disciplines have their own informatics specialists.

Careers in Nursing Informatics

There are many different careers available in nursing informatics. Most of the jobs are found in health care agencies, with vendors, in consulting, and in academe (Gassert, 1991).

Nursing informatics specialists interact with a variety of individuals at different organizational levels (Heller & Romano, 1988). Nursing informatics specialists often act as a user liaison. In this role, the nurse is the communications link between nurses and others involved in computer-related matters (Anderson, 1992; Hersher, 1995). Another role nursing informatics specialists might fill is that of nursing information systems specialist. In this job, the informaticist manages nursing applications and may head the nursing computer coordinating committee. Nursing informatics specialists might also act as a data systems manager for a speciality, such as oncology.

Nursing informatics specialists working for either a health care agency or a vendor may find themselves part of a team installing an information system or training new users. They might also be involved in product management or product definition. In this position, the nurse is responsible for seeing that the product is updated. This involves being aware of new developments in the field and current and future needs of clients.[1] Some nursing informatics specialists working for vendors are involved in marketing. Many nursing informatics specialists consult, either independently or for an organization. This role combines both that of a liaison and an expert. Nurses in academia who specialize in nursing informatics usually teach about the discipline or conduct research, or both (Display 18-1).

Educational Preparation

Before beginning a career in nursing informatics, it is helpful to have a thorough, in-depth understanding of clinical practice. Preparation can be acquired in a number of ways—by obtaining an academic degree, completing a certificate, taking courses, attending conferences, and through on-the-job learning. As more schools are offering graduate level courses in informatics, some of these are being offered online. Many speciality and professional societies provide seminars and workshops for informatics. Those certified in nursing informatics must meet a series of requirements (American Nurses Credentialing Center, 1995):

▼ Hold an active RN license in the US or its territories
▼ Hold a baccalaureate or higher degree in nursing
▼ Have practiced as a licensed RN for at least 2 years

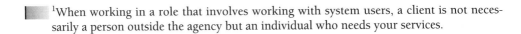

[1]When working in a role that involves working with system users, a client is not necessarily a person outside the agency but an individual who needs your services.

Display 18-1 • AN INFORMATICS NURSE SPECIALIST SPEAKS

My mother introduces me these days as "my daughter who used to be a nurse." But that's not true—I am and always will be a nurse. I'm just practicing in a *different* area. Advances in technology have improved our ability to care for patients. What nurses (or others, like my mother) don't often think about is that these technological advances also include computer systems. Nurses need to have the skills to be able to use a PC, a monitor, or other piece of equipment, just like they need the skills to be able to do a physical assessment. You cannot keep up with the information or reports needed in today's world unless you have some system (besides paper) to help you.

I got into the field of nursing informatics several years ago when I was manager of a hospital ambulatory services department. Being responsible for the business aspects of the department as well as the clinical, I was on the project team for implementation of the new computer systems. I found that my innate curiosity and need to always ask "Why" proved very helpful in this endeavor. I also discovered that computers are only a tool; it takes humans to analyze information needs and to plan how to best meet them—a discovery that led me to the field of nursing informatics.

I have never regretted the move! Just as in clinical nursing, you never know what to expect on a given day. Although you anticipate what you need to do each day, anything can happen to interrupt those plans and change your priorities. The next thing you know, it's 5:30 PM and you haven't been able to do one thing on your to-do list.

I start out each day by turning on my PC. Then I open my email system. I read my new messages and respond when necessary. This usually takes an hour or two. Sometimes an email I receive will require a telephone contact for follow-up, or users may contact me by telephone. Much of the time spent in my office I'm either answering a question, providing clarification, explaining how a function works, or troubleshooting. When I am troubleshooting, I often access the software system with which the caller is having difficulty. This allows me to try to do what the user has done or attempted to do, so I can assess whether the caller is using the right function or routine, and using it correctly. If the function is being used appropriately, I try to re-create what the user has done to see if I can elicit the same response or responses that she or he did. This method gives me a better picture of the difficulty and allows me either to solve the problem or to pinpoint a software problem. One day, I logged 6 hours and 45 minutes of telephone time; the majority of which was nonstop.

Sometimes I need to contact one of the vendors to get a problem resolved. Talking with vendors may also include discussing product enhancements, a new product or feature that they are developing and releasing to clients, or an upcoming class or meeting. Software testing is another function of the job. There may be new features or updates released that need to be tested. This process involves creating different scenarios in which you enter data and print reports to make sure the software does what it's supposed to do. This can take hours, days, or even weeks to complete.

Reports are the end result of information processing. When you buy software, you sometimes get *standard* reports (those that the majority of all users need) but you usually have to write *custom* reports. That is another role of the nurse informaticist: users give me requests for reports that they would like to have. To create them I may be able to modify an existing report, or I may need to create a new one. This involves determining which file or files the information resides in, how the output of the report should look, what fields the report needs to include, what to name it so that the users will know which report to run, and perhaps which menu to put it on. Writing reports can take anywhere from a few minutes to several days, depending on the complexity, as well as the amount of time you can devote. (Remember all those interruptions!) Testing a report is also part of modifying or creating one. As the creator, I need to test it to be certain that it produces what the user wants. Then I need to have the user test it to see if the data and design meet his or her needs.

Another role of the nurse informaticist is one of teacher. I develop the lesson plans and teaching materials to train the staff on the use of the computer systems. Training is done formally or informally, depending on the situation, and can take a few minutes to several days. In addition, I attend meetings, both in my department and with other departments. Many times, I am the

(continued)

▼●▲▼●▲▼●▲▼●▲▼●▲▼●▲●▼●▲▼●▲▼●▲▼●▲▼●▲▼●▲▼

Display 18-1 ● AN INFORMATICS NURSE SPECIALIST SPEAKS (Continued)

leader of the meeting, which also involves putting together the agenda and handouts, and doing minutes. There are also user group and informatics organizations to which I belong.

A key element in this role is communication. When you are working in nursing informatics, you are providing help and support to end users: staff, managers, directors, and vice-presidents, as well as the programmers/developers. (Very often, the programmer or developer is at your vendor's location and not in-

house.) Nursing informatics is extremely dynamic, and I love the challenge. It offers me the opportunity to work with many different people, do many different things, and to be creative. This role is never boring!

Judith Hornback, RN, BSN, MHSA
Informatics Nurse Specialist
Senior Consultant, RHI, Inc.
Highland, Indiana

▼ Have practiced at least 2000 hours in nursing informatics or practiced 1000 hours and completed at least 12 semester hours of academic credits in informatics in the last 5 years
▼ Have had 20 contact hours in nursing informatics education within the past 2 years
▼ Passed the nursing informatics examination, which includes the following topics:
  ▼ System analysis and design
  ▼ System implementation and support
  ▼ System testing and evaluation
  ▼ Human factors
  ▼ Computer technology
  ▼ Information/database management
  ▼ Professional practice trends and issues
  ▼ Theories

▼ Informatics Organizations

The major organizations in informatics are multidisciplinary. Healthcare Information and Management Systems Society (HIMSS) and International Medical Informatics Association (IMIA) are examples of two associations. These organizations provide journals and meetings, and are a source of up-to-date information in the field. They also establish a network of members so ideas can be shared.

HIMSS is a not-for-profit organization dedicated to promoting a better understanding of health care information and management systems. At present, HIMSS represents over 9000 health care professionals in four professional areas: clinical systems, information systems, management engineering, and telecommunications. Many nurses are involved in this organization, which meets annually. The organization publishes a quarterly journal and several guides to the field.

IMIA is a nonpolitical, international, scientific organization. IMIA's goals include promoting informatics in health care, biomedical research, and advancing international cooperation (International Medical Informatics Association General Information, 1997). IMIA sponsors many working groups on various topics. Nursing is one such group. The nursing working group sponsors a triennial international meeting that rotates between Europe, the Asian Pacific region, and North America.

The American Medical Informatics Association (AMIA) is the organization that represents the United States at IMIA. AMIA has working groups designed to give health care professionals the opportunity to convene and network with one another. One goal of the nursing informatics working group is to promote the advancement of nursing informatics within the larger multidisciplinary context of health informatics (AMIA, 1997). The nursing working group publishes a semiannual newsletter that is designed to keep the nursing community up to date with the changing health care informatics environment.

▼ Summary

Nursing informatics specialists use computers to identify, name, organize, group, collect, process, analyze, store, retrieve, or manage data and information. This factor does not negate the importance of other uses of computers by nurses. All nurses need a basic understanding of informatics, just as they need a basic understanding of other speciality areas in nursing. Nurses must think of the computer as a tool that is useful for identifying and solving problems.

Careers in nursing informatics are found in many different locations. One of the most important functions a nurse informaticist performs is as a liaison with other disciplines and people at all levels in an organization. There are many educational routes to becoming an informatics nurse specialist. However, no matter what route is used, the job is characterized by a need for continuous learning. Health care informatics organizations can provide some of this education.

EXERCISES

1. Define the main focus of nursing informatics
2. If you were to become a nursing informatics specialist, which career path would appeal to you? Give your reasons
3. List the health care informatics organizations

REFERENCES

American Nurses Association. (1994). *The scope of practice for nursing informatics.* Washington, D.C.: American Nurses Publishing, NP-90 7.5M 5/94.

American Nurses Association. (1995). *Standards of practice for nursing informatics.* Washington, D.C.: American Nurses Publishing, NP-100 7.5M 3/95.

American Nurses Credentialing Center. (1995). *Informatics certification catalog.* Washington, D.C.: American Nurses Credentialing Center.

AMIA Nursing Informatics Working Group. (1997.) Available: http://www.gl.umbc.edu/~abbott/nurseinfo.html.

Anderson, B. L. (1992). Nursing informatics: Career opportunities inside and out. *Computers in Nursing, 10*(4), 165–170.

Educational paths in clinical informatics. (1996). In *Guide to Effective Health Care Clinical Systems* (pp. 67–76). Chicago: Healthcare Information and Management Systems Society.

Gassert, C. A. (1991). Preparing for a career in nursing informatics. In P. B. Marr, R. L. Axford, & S. K. Newbold (Eds.), *Lecture Notes in Medical Informatics*, 163–166.

Heller, B. R., & Romano, C. A. (1988). Nursing informatics: The pathway to knowledge. *Nursing & Health Care, 9*(9) 483–484.

Hersher, B. S. (1995) Careers for nurses in healthcare information systems. In Ball, M. J., Hannah, K. J., Newbold, S. K., & Douglas, J. V. (Eds.), *Nursing informatics: Where caring and technology meet* (2nd ed.; pp. 77–83). New York: Springer-Verlag.

International Medical Informatics Association General Information. (1997). Available: http://www.imia.org/.

Special Keys on a Computer Keyboard

NOTE: The term *insertion point* refers to the place on the screen where the character that you type will be placed. Originally this was called the *cursor*.

Key	What it does
Any key	When you see this in instructions, it means to tap any of the character or numeric keys on the keyboard. There is not a key that is labeled *Any*.
Enter (or return key)	The exact procedure the computer follows when you tap this key is context dependent. That is, what happens depends on what you are doing. The function that is executed at the time, however, is always related to the concept of accepting data that has been entered. In a word processor, tapping Enter tells the word processor to accept everything since the last time this key was tapped as a paragraph and to insert the code for end of paragraph. When entering data into a spreadsheet or database, tapping Enter tells the computer that you are through entering the data for that cell (spreadsheet) or field (database). In many cases, you can use it as an alternative to mouse-clicking on OK. For example, if you have entered a term for which you wish the computer to search, tapping the Enter key gives the computer the go-ahead to start the search, producing the same result as moving the mouse pointer to the OK box and clicking once.
Alt (called an option key on a Macintosh)	Acts along with other keys. Instructions will be written **Alt-D.** This means that you should press and hold down the Alt key, tap the letter d, and release the Alt key. That is, it is used like a shift key—you hold it down while tapping the key given in the instruction.
Ctrl (an open Apple on a Macintosh)	This is the Control key. From a user standpoint, it is used exactly like the Alt key. In the old days, when it was tapped with the letter C, it was often used to interrupt a program and return to what is called DOS. Instructions will be written **Ctrl-xx key.** One holds down the Control key, taps whatever key is in place of the xx key, and releases the Control key.
Shift	Although this key is similar to that of a typewriter, there are some differences. When the Caps Lock is off, holding the Shift key down and tapping a letter produces an uppercase letter. When the caps lock is on, this same procedure creates a lowercase letter. With non-letter keys, when the Shift key is depressed and one of them is tapped, the symbol over the non-letter key is inverted on the screen, regardless of the position of the caps lock.
F1–F12 on a desktop PC F1–F15 on a Macintosh PF1–PF24 on a mainframe	These are called function keys. Tapping them causes different things to happen, depending on the program you are using. For example, in one word processor, tapping F3 tells the computer to save a document, while tapping F9 brings up a dialog box that allows you to change the typeface (font) that you are using. They can also be used with the Shift, Alt, and Ctrl keys to allow more than one function per key. If you see an instruction written **Shift-F9,** you should hold down the shift key and tap the F9 key.
Arrow keys	Arrow keys move the insertion point (the place on the screen where what you type is placed) in the direction of the arrow. They allow you to move the insertion point without changing any other characters on the screen.
Esc	Called the Escape key, this key is used to exit (escape) from some programs (not all) and from some conditions. For example, most word processors provide an option that lets you clear the screen of all tool bars and menus. Tapping the Esc key will put these tools back on the screen. This key is always used alone, that is, it is never held down while another key is tapped.

Fn	Seen on laptops and other smaller computers, the lettering is generally of a different color than that on the other keys. How it functions is dependent on the brand of computer. On some laptops, Fn-F5 (that is, hold down the Fn key and tap the F5 key) will toggle the various display modes between the screen; an external image (could be another monitor or a computer image projector); and images in both places.
Caps Lock	Creates a condition in which upper case letters are typed when a letter is tapped. Only affects letter keys; has no effect on whether the symbol on the top or bottom of other keys is entered.
Backspace	Tapping this key results in the character to the left of the insertion point being deleted.
Del (delete)	Tapping this key will remove the character at the location of the insertion point. In databases and spreadsheets, it may erase the information in a given field or cell (rectangles in both programs that contain data).
Ins (insert)	The exact function of this key varies with the program. In a word processor, tapping it will toggle between a condition in which the characters that you enter are inserted in the text, or are typed over the existing text. In a database or spreadsheet, tapping this key will insert a blank record or row above where the insertion point is.
PgUp (Page Up)	Using this key alters the view on the screen. The exact number of lines that are moved depends on how many lines of the document or file on which you are working are in view. If you are currently seeing 18 lines, tapping the PgUp key will move the view up one screen to the 18 lines above the ones you are currently viewing.
PgDn (Page Down)	Operates in the same manner as the Page Up key, but for the screen lines below those currently being viewed.
Prt Sc (Print Screen)	What Print Screen does varies with the operating system being used. If you are running programs under DOS, tapping it will send the text on a screen to a printer. If you are using Windows, tapping the Print Screen key places the contents of the screen onto the clipboard, from where it can be inserted in another program by tapping Shift-Insert. On a Macintosh, the keystroke combination Apple Key + Shift + 3 places a snapshot of the screen on the clipboard.
Num Lock (numbers lock)	The Num Lock toggles the condition of the numeric key pad. When it is off (many keyboards have lights that are on when the num lock is on and off when it is off), tapping any of the keys on the numeric key pad will produce the function printed on the lower part of the key. When the num lock is on, tapping the keys on the numeric key pad inserts the numbers or indicated mathematical symbols in the document on which you are working. The numeric key pad is set up to mimic the "10 key" or adding maching that accountants use. If you enter a lot of numbers, learning to touch type this key pad will save many hours.
Home	In most programs, tapping Home places the insertion point at the beginning of a line or cell. When used in conjunction with other keys, its function is program dependent. In any Windows-compliant program, holding down the Ctrl (control) key and tapping Home moves the insertion point to the top of the document file.
End	In most programs, tapping the End key moves the insertion point at the end of the line. In any Windows-compliant program, holding down the Ctrl (control) key and tapping End moves the insertion point to the end of the document file.
Tab (the key labeled with two arrows—one pointing left, the other pointing right)	In word processors, tapping this key moves the insertion point to the next tab stop, like it does on a typewriter. When using a spreadsheet, a database, or a table in a word processor, tapping it moves the insertion point to the next box (called a cell). When filling in a form on a computer, tapping it often moves the insertion point to the next spot on the form where you are to enter data.

Index

Note: Page numbers followed by "f" indicate figures; page numbers followed by "t" indicate tabular material.

A

Admission, discharge, transfer (ADT) data
  in hospital information system, 239
Adobe Acrobat Reader, 221
Advanced Research Projects Agency NETwork
      (ARPANET), 190
AIDSLINE, 151–152
AIDSNET, 227
ALU. *See* Arithmetic logic unit (ALU)
American Medical Informatics Association (AMIA),
      293
American Nurses Association (ANA)
  membership in Computer-based Patient Record
      Institute, 274
American Standard Code for Information Exchange
      (ASCII), 15
AMIA. *See* American Medical Informatics Association
      (AMIA)
Analog format. *See also* Digital format
  for telephone transmission, 191
Analog signal, 26, 26f
Ancillary systems
  in hospital information system, 240
Applets, Java programs from Internet, 222
Application software, 37–43
  computer-to-computer, 38–40
  copyright and, 44
  database managers, 38
  desktop publishers, 37
  educational, 176–178
  news reader, 204
  presentation, 38
  programming, 40–43
    languages for, 39–40
  spiders, 218
  spreadsheets, 37, 79–81
  statistical packages, 89–90
  for test construction, 181
  for testing, 180–181
  user groups for learning, 43
  word processors, 37
Archie and Wide-Area Information Server, 211
Arithmetic logic unit (ALU), 14

ARPANET (Advanced Research Projects Agency
      NETwork), 190
Artificial intelligence, 284
ASCII (American Standard Code for Information Ex-
      change) format, 73
  for data export and import, 123
  for mail list message replies, 208
Assembly language, 39–40, 40f
Asynchronous communication
  on non-world wide web communications, 209, 209t
Attributes
  for visuals, 111t
  in word processing programs, 49–50
AVLINE, 151

B

Bandwidth
  for transmission speed, 192, 193f
Bar charts, 93, 94f, 94–95
Bar codes, 22–23
Basic Input Output System (BIOS), 17
Bibliographical database(s), 128, 129. *See also* Literature
      search citation *versus* full-text, 150–151
  full-text, 153
  indexing of, 155, 156f
  Internet, 153
  National Library of Medicine, 151–152
  for nursing, 151–153
  personal
    benefits of managers for, 166–167
    versus card file system, 165
    software for development of, 166
    Z39–50 compliant, 166
  versus print indexes, 149
  relationship of MEDLARS to each other and print
      products, 151,152f
  specialized, 153
  structure of, 153–155
  subject headings in, 154
    organization of, 154–155
BIOETHICSLINE, 152, 157
BIOS. *See* Basic Input Output System (BIOS)
Bits, 15

297